Gastrointestinal Pathology: Common Questions and Diagnostic Dilemmas

Editor

RHONDA K. YANTISS

SURGICAL PATHOLOGY CLINICS

www.surgpath.theclinics.com

Consulting Editor
JASON L. HORNICK

December 2017 • Volume 10 • Number 4

ELSEVIER

1600 John F. Kennedy Boulevard • Suite 1800 • Philadelphia, Pennsylvania, 19103-2899

http://www.theclinics.com

SURGICAL PATHOLOGY CLINICS Volume 10, Number 4
December 2017 ISSN 1875-9181, ISBN-13: 978-0-323-55302-5

Editor: Stacy Eastman
Developmental Editor: Donald Mumford

Surgical Pathology Clinics (ISSN 1875-9181) is published quarterly by Elsevier Inc., 360 Park Avenue South, New York, NY 10010. Months of issue are March, June, September, and December. Business and Editorial Office: Elsevier Inc., 1600 John F. Kennedy Blvd., Ste. 1800, Philadelphia, PA 19103-2899. Accounting and Circulation Offices: Elsevier Inc., 3251 Riverport Lane, Maryland Heights, MO 63043. Periodicals postage paid at New York, NY and at additional mailing offices. Subscription prices are $206.00 per year (US individuals), $274.00 per year (US institutions), $100.00 per year (US students/residents), $258.00 per year (Canadian individuals), $312.00 per year (Canadian Institutions), $258.00 per year (foreign individuals), $312.00 per year (foreign institutions), and $120.00 per year (international & Canadian students/residents). Foreign air speed delivery is included in all *Clinics'* subscription prices. All prices are subject to change without notice. **POSTMASTER:** Send address changes to *Surgical Pathology Clinics*, Elsevier, 3251 Riverport Lane, Maryland Heights, MO 63043. **Customer Service: 1-800-654-2452 (US). From outside the United States, call 1-314-447-8871. Fax: 1-314-447-8029. E-mail: JournalsCustomerServiceusa@elsevier.com (for print support) and JournalsOnlineSupport-usa@elsevier.com (for online support).**

Reprints. For copies of 100 or more, of articles in this publication, please contact the Commercial Reprints Department, Elsevier Inc., 360 Park Avenue South, New York, NY 10010-1710. Tel. 212-633-3874; Fax: 212-633-3820; E-mail: reprints@elsevier.com.

Surgical Pathology Clinics of North America is covered in *MEDLINE/PubMed (Index Medicus).*

Contributors

CONSULTING EDITOR

JASON L. HORNICK, MD, PhD
Director of Surgical Pathology and
Immunohistochemistry, Brigham and Women's
Hospital, Professor of Pathology, Harvard
Medical School, Boston, Massachusetts, USA

EDITOR

RHONDA K. YANTISS, MD
Professor, Department of Pathology and
Laboratory Medicine, Weill Cornell Medicine,
New York, New York, USA

AUTHORS

HENRY D. APPELMAN, MD
M.R. Abell Professor of Surgical Pathology,
Department of Pathology, University of
Michigan, Ann Arbor, Michigan, USA

FÁTIMA CARNEIRO, MD, PhD
Professor, Department of Pathology,
Centro Hospitalar de São João, Department
of Pathology, Faculty of Medicine of the
University of Porto (FMUP), Institute of
Molecular Pathology and Immunology of
the University of Porto (Ipatimup), Institute
for Research Investigation Innovation in
Health (i3S), Universidade do Porto, Porto,
Portugal

WEI CHEN, MD, PhD
Assistant Professor, Department of Pathology,
The Ohio State University Wexner Medical
Center, Columbus, Ohio, USA

EUN-YOUNG KAREN CHOI, MD
Assistant Professor, Department of Pathology,
University of Michigan, Ann Arbor, Michigan,
USA

WON-TAK CHOI, MD, PhD
Assistant Professor, Department of Pathology,
University of California San Francisco,
San Francisco, California, USA

WENDY L. FRANKEL, MD
Professor and Chair, Department of Pathology,
The Ohio State University Wexner Medical
Center, Columbus, Ohio, USA

JOHN HART, MD
Professor, Department of Pathology,
The University of Chicago, Chicago, Illinois,
USA

JOSE JESSURUN, MD
Professor, Department of Pathology and
Laboratory Medicine, Weill Cornell Medicine
New York, New York, USA

HEEWON A. KWAK, MD
Gastrointestinal and Liver Pathology Fellow,
Department of Pathology, The University of
Chicago, Chicago, Illinois, USA

LAURA W. LAMPS, MD
Professor, Department of Pathology, University of Michigan, Ann Arbor, Michigan, USA

GREGORY Y. LAUWERS, MD
Senior Member, Gastrointestinal Pathology Service, Department of Pathology, Moffitt Cancer Center, Tampa, Florida, USA

MAURICE B. LOUGHREY, MD, MRCP, FRCPath
Department of Histopathology, Royal Victoria Hospital, Belfast, Northern Ireland, United Kingdom

MICHAEL MARKOW, MD
Gastrointestinal Pathology Fellow, Department of Pathology, The Ohio State University Wexner Medical Center, Columbus, Ohio, USA

ELIZABETH A. MONTGOMERY, MD
Professor of Pathology, Oncology, and Orthopedic Surgery, Department of Pathology, Johns Hopkins Medicine, Baltimore, Maryland, USA

SCOTT R. OWENS, MD
Associate Professor of Pathology, University of Michigan, Ann Arbor, Michigan, USA

NICOLE C. PANARELLI, MD
Associate Professor, Department of Pathology, Albert Einstein College of Medicine, Bronx, New York, USA

NEIL A. SHEPHERD, DM, FRCPath
Professor of Gastrointestinal Pathology, Gloucestershire Cellular Pathology Laboratory, Cheltenham General Hospital, Cheltenham, Gloucestershire, United Kingdom

THOMAS C. SMYRK, MD
Professor, Department of Pathology, Mayo Clinic, Rochester, Minnesota, USA

EFSEVIA VAKIANI, MD, PhD
Assistant Attending Member, Department of Pathology, Memorial Sloan Kettering Cancer Center, New York, New York, USA

RACHEL S. VAN DER POST, MD
Department of Pathology, Radboud University Medical Centre, Nijmegen, The Netherlands

LYSANDRA VOLTAGGIO, MD
Assistant Professor, Department of Pathology, Johns Hopkins Medicine, Baltimore, Maryland, USA

MARIA WESTERHOFF, MD
Associate Professor, Department of Pathology, University of Michigan, Ann Arbor, Michigan, USA

RHONDA K. YANTISS, MD
Professor, Department of Pathology and Laboratory Medicine, Weill Cornell Medicine, New York, New York, USA

Contents

Preface   xi

Rhonda K. Yantiss

Other Forms of Esophagitis: It Is Not Gastroesophageal Reflux Disease, So Now
What Do I Do?   765

Nicole C. Panarelli

Esophagitis results from diverse causes, including gastroesophageal reflux, immune-mediated or allergic reactions, therapeutic complications, and infections. The appropriate clinical management differs in each of these situations and is often guided by pathologic interpretation of endoscopic mucosal biopsy specimens. This article summarizes the diagnostic features of unusual forms of esophagitis, including eosinophilic esophagitis, lymphocytic esophagitis, esophagitis dissecans superficialis, drug-induced esophageal injury, and bullous disorders. Differential diagnoses and distinguishing features are emphasized.

Diagnosis and Management of Barrett-Related Neoplasia in the Modern Era   781

Lysandra Voltaggio and Elizabeth A. Montgomery

In the past, pathologists were hesitant to diagnose high-grade dysplasia in patients with Barrett esophagus because this diagnosis prompted esophagectomy, whereas current international consensus is that endoscopic treatment is the management for high-grade dysplasia and intramucosal carcinoma. Furthermore, many centers advocate endoscopic ablation for low-grade dysplasia. As such, establishing a diagnosis of dysplasia has become the key step; differentiation between the grades of dysplasia is less critical. This article offers some criteria for differentiating dysplasia from reactive changes, discusses pitfalls in interpreting endoscopic mucosal resection specimens, and outlines management strategies.

Patterns of Gastric Injury: Beyond *Helicobacter pylori*   801

Won-Tak Choi and Gregory Y. Lauwers

Gastric biopsies are routinely obtained from patients with symptoms related to the gastrointestinal tract and, as a result, a variety of histologic changes are observed in patients with or without endoscopic evidence of mucosal injury. Although *Helicobacter pylori*–related gastritis is still common, several other patterns of mucosal injury are increasingly encountered. These patterns of injury are classified based on the nature and distribution of inflammation, location of epithelial cell injury, presence of crystal or pigment deposition, and/or other unique features. This article discusses each of these patterns and provides a differential diagnosis for each.

Practical Approach to the Flattened Duodenal Biopsy   823

Thomas C. Smyrk

Celiac disease features duodenal intraepithelial lymphocytosis with or without villous atrophy. Lymphocytosis without villous atrophy has been proved to represent celiac disease in 10% to 20% of cases. The differential diagnosis is broad: *Helicobacter pylori* gastritis, nonsteroidal antiinflammatory drug injury, and bacterial overgrowth are considerations. Lymphocytosis with villous atrophy is very likely to be celiac disease, but there are mimics to consider, including collagenous sprue, tropical sprue, drug injury, and common variable immunodeficiency. Histologic clues to a diagnosis other than celiac disease include paucity of plasma cells, excess of neutrophils, granulomas, and relative paucity of intraepithelial lymphocytes.

Chronic Colitis in Biopsy Samples: Is It Inflammatory Bowel Disease or Something Else?   841

Eun-Young Karen Choi and Henry D. Appelman

Chronic colitis, regardless of type, is defined histologically by chronic inflammation, mainly plasmacytosis, in the lamina propria. Specific diagnosis of chronic colitides in biopsies can be challenging for practicing pathologists. This article focuses on discussing specific histologic features in biopsies of the inflammatory bowel diseases (IBDs), including ulcerative colitis, Crohn colitis, and colitis of indeterminate type. It also offers suggestions as to how to differentiate the IBDs from other chronic colitides, such as lymphocytic colitis, collagenous colitis, diverticular disease–associated colitis, diversion colitis, and chronic colitides, that are due to drugs. Normal histology in colon biopsies is also briefly discussed.

The Differential Diagnosis of Acute Colitis: Clues to a Specific Diagnosis   863

Jose Jessurun

This article describes a systematic approach to the interpretation of colonic biopsy specimens of patients with acute colitis. Five main histologic patterns are discussed: acute colitis, focal active colitis, pseudomembranous colitis, hemorrhagic colitis, and ischemic colitis. For each pattern, the most common etiologic associations and their differential diagnoses are presented. Strategies based on histologic analysis and clinical considerations to differentiate acute from chronic colitides are discussed.

The Many Faces of Medication-Related Injury in the Gastrointestinal Tract   887

Heewon A. Kwak and John Hart

Every year many new medications are approved for clinical use, several of which can cause clinically significant gastrointestinal tract toxicity. This article emphasizes the histologic features and differential diagnosis of drug-induced injury to the gastrointestinal mucosa. Ultimately, clinical correlation and cessation of a drug with resolution of symptoms are needed to definitively confirm a drug as a causative factor in mucosal injury. Recognizing histologic features in gastrointestinal biopsies, however, can allow surgical pathologists to play a key role in establishing a diagnosis of drug-induced gastrointestinal toxicity.

Mucosal Biopsy After Bone Marrow Transplantation   909

Maria Westerhoff and Laura W. Lamps

Gastrointestinal mucosal biopsies in the hematopoietic stem cell transplantation setting are challenging because histologic features of graft-versus-host disease (GVHD), which is treated by increasing immunosuppression, overlap with those of other conditions, such as infection, which can get worse with GVHD treatment. More than one condition can occur at the same time. It is important to understand the histologic features of GVHD, drug toxicity, infection, and clinical factors surrounding patients, including timing of biopsy in relation to transplantation, medi-cation history, and laboratory data. Rendering a correct diagnosis and generating a pathology report with standard language that can direct clinical management ensure proper management.

Emerging Concepts in Gastric Neoplasia: Heritable Gastric Cancers and Polyposis Disorders   931

Rachel S. van der Post and Fátima Carneiro

Hereditary gastric cancer is a relatively rare disease with specific clinical and histo-pathologic characteristics. Hereditary gastric cancer of the diffuse type is predom-inantly caused by germline mutations in *CDH1*. The inherited cause of familial intestinal gastric cancer is unknown. Gastric adenocarcinoma and proximal polypo-sis of the stomach is a hereditary cancer syndrome caused by germline mutations in promoter 1B of *APC*. Other well-defined cancer syndromes, such as Lynch, Li-Fraumeni, and hereditary breast or ovarian cancer syndromes, are associated with an increased risk of gastric cancer. This article reviews important histopatho-logic features and emerging concepts regarding gastric carcinogenesis in these syndromes.

Problematic Colorectal Polyps: Is It Cancer and What Do I Need to Do About It?   947

Maurice B. Loughrey and Neil A. Shepherd

Two issues commonly arise for pathologists reporting adenomatous polyps of the colorectum. Particularly problematic within large sigmoid colonic adenomas is the distinction between benign misplacement of epithelium into the submucosa and invasive malignancy. This distinction requires careful morphologic evaluation of key discriminatory features, assisted only rarely by the application of selected adjunctive immunohistochemistry. Following a diagnosis of adenocarcinoma within a polypectomy or other local excision specimen, systematic assessment is required of features that may indicate the risk of residual local and/or nodal neoplastic dis-ease and inform management decision making regarding the need for further endo-scopic or surgical intervention.

Persistent Problems in Colorectal Cancer Reporting   961

Rhonda K. Yantiss

Tumor stage, as determined by the Tumor, Node, Metastasis (TNM) staging system, is the single most influential factor determining treatment decisions and outcome among patients with colorectal cancer. Several stage-related elements in pathology reports consistently pose diagnostic challenges: recognition of serosal penetration by tumor (ie, pT3 vs pT4a), evaluation of regional lymph nodes, distinction between tumor deposits and effaced lymph nodes, and assessment of tumor stage in the neoadjuvant setting. This article discusses each of these issues in detail and pro-vides practical tips regarding colorectal cancer staging.

Immunohistochemical Pitfalls: Common Mistakes in the Evaluation of Lynch Syndrome   977

Michael Markow, Wei Chen, and Wendy L. Frankel

At least 15% of colorectal cancers diagnosed in the United States are deficient in mismatch repair mechanisms. Most of these are sporadic, but approximately 3%

of colorectal cancers result from germline alterations in mismatch repair genes and represent Lynch syndrome. It is critical to identify patients with Lynch syndrome to institute appropriate screening and surveillance for patients and their families. Exclusion of Lynch syndrome in sporadic cases is equally important because it reduces anxiety for patients and prevents excessive spending on unnecessary surveillance. Immunohistochemistry is one of the most widely used screening tools for identifying patients with Lynch syndrome.

Molecular Testing of Colorectal Cancer in the Modern Era: What Are We Doing and Why?   1009

Efsevia Vakiani

A plethora of tests are routinely ordered and interpreted by pathologists to assist the management of patients with colorectal cancer. Many of these tests are immunohistochemistry assays using antibodies against prognostically relevant proteins, some of which predict therapeutic response. This article focuses on tissue DNA–based tests. It presents novel methodologies for assessing well-established biomarkers, updates the expanding spectrum of genetic alterations that are associated with resistance to inhibition of epidermal growth factor receptor signaling, and briefly discusses emerging actionable alterations that may translate into new therapeutic options for patients with colorectal cancer. The utility of next-generation sequencing is emphasized.

Lymphoproliferative Diseases of the Gut: A Survival Guide for the General Pathologist   1021

Scott R. Owens

The gastrointestinal tract is the most common extranodal site of involvement by lymphoma, with B-cell tumors outnumbering T-cell tumors by a wide margin. Diffuse large B-cell lymphoma is the most common lymphoid neoplasm involving the gastrointestinal tract, but a variety of other B- and T-cell neoplasms occur in the gastrointestinal organs, often with characteristic associations or manifestations. Although the diagnosis of gastrointestinal lymphomas can sometimes seem daunting to general pathologists, a knowledge of the most commonly encountered entities, in combination with a reasoned and pragmatic approach to the diagnostic workup, makes it possible to approach most cases with confidence.

SURGICAL PATHOLOGY CLINICS

FORTHCOMING ISSUES

March 2018
Breast Pathology
Laura C. Collins, *Editor*

June 2018
Liver Pathology
John Hart, *Editor*

September 2018
Cytopathology
Vickie Jo, *Editor*

RECENT ISSUES

September 2017
Bone Tumor Pathology
Judith V.M.G. Bovée, *Editor*

June 2017
Dermatopathology
Thomas Brenn, *Editor*

March 2017
Head and Neck Pathology
Raja R. Seethala, *Editor*

RELATED INTEREST

Clinics in Laboratory Medicine, June 2015 (Volume 35, Issue 2)
Diagnostic Testing for Enteric Pathogens
Alexander J. McAdam, *Editor*

THE CLINICS ARE AVAILABLE ONLINE!
Access your subscription at:
www.theclinics.com

Preface

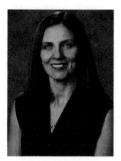

Rhonda K. Yantiss, MD
Editor

Gastrointestinal pathology emerged as a subspecialty in the early 1980s, roughly coincident with development of endoscopy and mucosal biopsy for diagnosis and management of patients with gastrointestinal disorders. Since that time, changes in tissue acquisition techniques and ancillary testing have drastically altered the field, such that current practice bears little resemblance to that of our mentors. The past two decades have seen an explosion in the number and types of biopsy samples pathologists encounter in daily practice. Virtually every part of the tubular gut is now amenable to visualization and sampling. As a result, pathologists are expected to generate comprehensive and accurate differential diagnoses for a variety of inflammatory and neoplastic disorders that occur throughout the gastrointestinal tract. Although we have always played an important role in the care of patients with persistent gastrointestinal symptoms, we are increasingly involved in the management of immunosuppressed patients, particularly those with hematopoietic malignancies receiving stem cell transplants. Most of these individuals require medical therapies notorious for their negative effects on the gastrointestinal tract. Unfortunately, immune-mediated injury, infections, and medication effects are common in this population and evoke similar patterns of mucosal damage in biopsy material. Pathologists must be able to hone in on key features in order to narrow the differential diagnosis and facilitate patient management.

Advanced endoscopic techniques have led to changing expectations of pathologists, as nonsurgical approaches to superficial neoplasms are now the rule, rather than the exception. Although most patients with dysplasias and early invasive carcinomas were referred to surgeons in the past, most are now completely treated by gastroenterologists, who require pathologists to provide information regarding tumor stage and adequacy of excision based on limited excisional material. For these and many other reasons, surgical pathologists are challenged to stay abreast of new developments in the diagnosis and management of neoplastic gastrointestinal diseases and to distinguish malignancies from their mimics in small samples.

Finally, colorectal and gastric carcinomas are global health problems, together ranking second only to lung cancer as a leading cause of cancer-related death in developed countries. The roles of pathologists in their diagnosis and management continue to be defined. Not only do pathologists report accurate staging information to oncologists in order to plan postoperative chemotherapeutic strategies but also they provide clinical colleagues with guidance for usage of ancillary tests and interpretation of test results. In fact, pathologists are often the first physicians to suspect, or diagnose, heritable gastrointestinal cancers in many centers.

This issue of *Surgical Pathology Clinics* is intended to address all of these needs in a succinct and pragmatic fashion. It contains 14 articles that describe practical approaches to diagnosis of inflammatory gastrointestinal disorders, including

Surgical Pathology 10 (2017) xi–xii
http://dx.doi.org/10.1016/j.path.2017.07.015
1875-9181/17/© 2017 Published by Elsevier Inc.

sections that discuss biopsies in the bone marrow transplant setting and newly described medication-related injuries. The reader is provided with helpful criteria to facilitate recognition and reporting of neoplasia in endoscopically obtained material. Emerging concepts important to the diagnosis of heritable gastric and colorectal carcinomas are discussed in detail, as are ancillary tests relevant to the treatment of patients with these cancers. I sincerely thank all of the authors for their exceptional efforts; all of the articles are beautifully illustrated and include helpful tables and key points that provide easy references to the reader.

Rhonda K. Yantiss, MD
Department of Pathology and
Laboratory Medicine
Weill Cornell Medicine
525 East 68th Street
New York, NY 10065, USA

E-mail address:
Rhy2001@med.cornell.edu

Other Forms of Esophagitis
It Is Not Gastroesophageal Reflux Disease, So Now What Do I Do?

Nicole C. Panarelli, MD

KEYWORDS

• Eosinophilic • Lymphocytic • Esophagitis dissecans superficialis • Sloughing • Pill

Key points

- Several biopsy samples from multiple levels in esophagus and remaining gastrointestinal tract facilitate distinction between entities that cause esophageal eosinophilia.

- Distribution and nature of inflammatory infiltrate are useful in formulating a differential diagnosis when esophageal lymphocytosis is encountered.

- Endoscopic and pathologic correlation is critical when evaluating for esophagitis dissecans superficialis (sloughing esophagitis).

- Characteristic histologic features are clues to cause when infectious esophagitis is suspected.

ABSTRACT

Esophagitis results from diverse causes, including gastroesophageal reflux, immune-mediated or allergic reactions, therapeutic complications, and infections. The appropriate clinical management differs in each of these situations and is often guided by pathologic interpretation of endoscopic mucosal biopsy specimens. This review summarizes the diagnostic features of unusual forms of esophagitis, including eosinophilic esophagitis, lymphocytic esophagitis, esophagitis dissecans superficialis, drug-induced esophageal injury, and bullous disorders. Differential diagnoses and distinguishing features are emphasized.

related to the esophagus. As a result, less common forms of esophagitis are now recognized by clinicians and pathologists. Accurate classification of esophageal injury is important to management, although many disorders show overlapping histologic features with gastroesophageal reflux disease (GERD) and remain a source of diagnostic confusion among surgical pathologists. The purpose of this review is to provide readers with helpful practice points that aid distinction between GERD and its potential mimics as well as other types of esophageal injury.

OVERVIEW

Upper endoscopy with mucosal biopsy is increasingly used to evaluate patients with symptoms

EOSINOPHILIC ESOPHAGITIS

CLINICAL AND ENDOSCOPIC FEATURES

Eosinophilic esophagitis is a chronic immune-mediated disorder that shows a predilection for children and adults under 50 years of age. Patients typically present with dysphagia to solids and recurrent food impaction, although nausea

Disclosure: Dr N.C. Panarelli receives royalties from Elsevier, Inc for book chapter authorship.
Department of Pathology, Albert Einstein College of Medicine, 1300 Morris Park Avenue, Bronx, NY 10467, USA
E-mail address: npanarel@montefiore.org

Surgical Pathology 10 (2017) 765–779
http://dx.doi.org/10.1016/j.path.2017.07.001

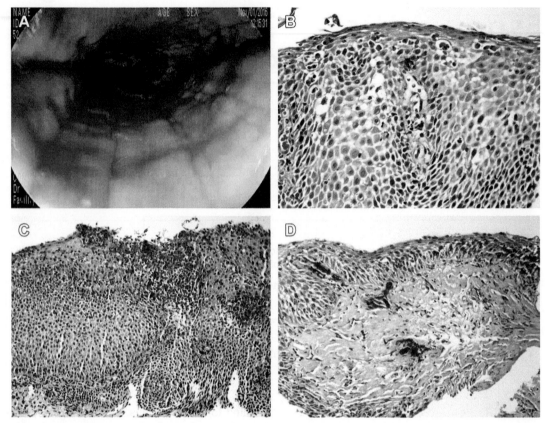

Fig. 1. Linear furrows are present in the esophagus of a patient with eosinophilic esophagitis (*A*). Biopsy specimens show luminally oriented eosinophils in clusters and intercellular edema (*B*). Eosinophils coat the mucosal surface in a severe case (*C*). Subepithelial fibrosis is a consequence of long-standing disease (*D*) (H&E, original magnifications, [*B*] ×200 [*C,D*] ×100).

and vomiting are more common in pediatric patients.[1,2] Affected individuals often have a history of atopic disorders, including asthma, dermatitis, and food allergies. Endoscopic findings include esophageal rings, linear furrows, white plaques, strictures, and a crepe-paper–like appearance, although the esophagus is essentially normal in at least 20% of patients (**Fig.** 1A).[3]

MICROSCOPIC FEATURES AND DIAGNOSIS

Eosinophilic esophagitis can affect any level of the esophagus and is a disease with a patchy distribution, necessitating multiple tissue samples to establish a diagnosis.[4,5] Endoscopists are encouraged to obtain 2 to 4 tissue samples from the proximal and distal esophagus when eosinophilic esophagitis is suspected, to increase the likelihood of including diagnostic tissue.[6] Mucosal biopsies show eosinophil-rich inflammatory infiltrates, sometimes exceeding 250 eosinophils per 400× field.[7] Eosinophils are more concentrated in the superficial squamous epithelium. Degranulated eosinophils, clusters of greater than or equal to 4 eosinophils (eosinophil microabscesses), and striking intercellular edema are typical (see **Fig.** 1B, C). Lamina propria fibrosis is common and may contribute to dysphagia and stricture development in patients with eosinophilic esophagitis (see **Fig.** 1D).

Key Pathologic Features

- Luminally oriented eosinophil-rich inflammatory infiltrates present in multiple levels of the esophagus

- Eosinophil microabscesses, degranulatd eosinophils, surface scale crust of eosinophils and granules

- Intercellular edema

- Subepithelial fibrosis

DIFFERENTIAL DIAGNOSIS

The features of eosinophilic esophagitis simulate those of GERD, although these entities can usually be distinguished based on clinical and histologic grounds (Table 1). Dellon and colleagues[8] compared clinical, endoscopic, and histologic features of 151 patients with eosinophilic esophagitis and 226 with GERD. They reported significantly higher mean eosinophil counts in patients with eosinophilic esophagitis than GERD (76 vs 16, P<.001) as well as more frequent degranulated eosinophils and eosinophil microabscesses in the former group. Parfitt and colleagues[9] also found eosinophils more numerous in biopsies from patients with eosinophilic esophagitis (mean: 39 per 400× field) compared with GERD (mean: 1 per 400× field; P<.001) and found eosinophil microabscesses to be much less common in patients with GERD. Lamina propria fibrosis is also more common in patients with eosinophilic esophagitis than GERD.[10] Li-Kim-Moy and colleagues[11] reviewed biopsy specimens from 51 patients and found lamina propria fibrosis in 89% of those with eosinophilic esophagitis compared with 38% of those with GERD.

Unfortunately, GERD may produce changes indistinguishable from eosinophilic esophagitis, particularly in severe cases or when sampling is limited to the distal esophagus; final classification may depend on clinical response to therapy.[7] Rodrigo and colleagues[12] evaluated histologic features in biopsy specimens from 6 patients with eosinophilic esophagitis and 28 with severe GERD. They found substantial overlap in maximum eosinophil counts between eosinophilic esophagitis (range: 51–204) and GERD (range: 20–168); eosinophil microabscesses were identified in both groups as were eosinophils at multiple levels in the esophagus. Some patients with clinical, endoscopic, and histologic features of eosinophilic esophagitis completely respond to proton pump inhibitor (PPI) therapy.[13,14] Wen and colleagues[15] evaluated biopsies from such patients with "PPI-responsive esophageal eosinophilia" using a panel of 94 mRNA transcripts associated with eosinophilic esophagitis, including those encoding proteins for barrier function, promotion of eosinophil and mast cell chemotaxis, and tissue remodeling. They found transcriptomes of PPI-responsive esophageal eosinophilia overlapped substantially with those of eosinophilic esophagitis. These data suggest that PPI-responsive esophageal eosinophilia may represent an extreme reflux-related injury that develops in patients at risk for eosinophilic esophagitis or a continuum of allergic disease related to eosinophilic esophagitis.

Finally, esophageal biopsy specimens do not distinguish eosinophilic esophagitis from eosinophilic gastroenteritis, which may affect any segment of the gastrointestinal tract. The mucosal form of eosinophilic gastroenteritis, in particular, shows a predilection for men and children and association with food allergies and hypersensitivity similar to eosinophilic esophagitis. Biopsies from the gastric antrum and duodenum show aggregates of eosinophils around glands and/or eosinophils infiltrating the epithelium and muscularis mucosae (see Table 1).[16] Therefore, biopsies from these sites should also be evaluated in patients with suspected eosinophilic esophagitis to exclude the possibility of more generalized disease.

PROGNOSIS

Eosinophilic esophagitis responds to a combination of dietary elimination and/or topical corticosteroid therapy, whereas eosinophilic gastroenteritis generally requires systemic corticosteroid treatment. Strictures are managed with endoscopic dilatation. The disorder does not seem to be associated with neoplasia.

Table 1
Differential diagnosis of eosinophilic esophagitis

Disorder	Features That Aid Distinction from Eosinophilic Esophagitis
GERD	• Eosinophils usually limited to distal esophagus • Eosinophils evenly distributed in the squamous mucosa or predominantly in deeper mucosa • Microabscesses and scale crust uncommon
Eosinophilic gastroenteritis	• Indistinguishable from eosinophilic esophagitis when evaluation limited to esophageal biopsy samples • Eosinophilia in samples of gastric antrum and small intestine; colorectal involvement uncommon
PPI-responsive esophageal eosinophilia	• Indistinguishable from eosinophilic esophagitis based on endoscopy and histology; treatment response determines final classification of disease

Pitfalls

! Eosinophils may be numerous in severe GERD, particularly in samples from the distal esophagus.

! Eosinophilic esophagitis is indistinguishable from eosinophilic gastroenteritis in samples from the esophagus; exclusion of eosinophilic gastroenteritis requires biopsy of other sites in the gastrointestinal tract.

LYMPHOCYTIC ESOPHAGITIS

CLINICAL AND ENDOSCOPIC FEATURES

Lymphocytic esophagitis is an increasingly recognized histologic abnormality of unclear clinical significance. The largest study to date described an incidence of only 0.1% in greater than 100,000 patients undergoing esophageal biopsy.[17] Another study reported that 80% of cases were diagnosed in the most recent 3 years of an 11-year period, coincident with a trend toward submission of more esophageal biopsy specimens from several levels in the esophagus and increased awareness of the entity among pathologists.[18]

The clinical and endoscopic features of patients with lymphocytic esophagitis are heterogeneous. Dysphagia is a common presenting symptom, acknowledged by 43% to 76% of patients, although approximately one-third of patients with histologic lymphocytic esophagitis are clinically asymptomatic.[17–20] Purdy and colleagues[19] found that only 26% of patients with lymphocytic esophagitis had GERD-type symptoms. Similarly, Haque and Genta[17] noted that only 19% of 119 patients with lymphocytic esophagitis presented with GERD symptoms compared with 37% of 40,654 controls. Endoscopic examination is normal in approximately one-third of patients and a similar proportion show features that overlap with eosinophilic esophagitis, namely longitudinal furrows, rings, or webs.[17–20] Cohen and colleagues[18] evaluated 81 patients with lymphocytic esophagitis and found that 20% had esophageal rings, whereas plaques and furrows were less common (2% and 1%, respectively).

MICROSCOPIC FEATURES AND DIAGNOSIS

Lymphocytic esophagitis is characterized by increased numbers of intraepithelial lymphocytes, intercellular edema, and rare, if any, granulocytes (Fig. 2). Lymphocytes are predominantly CD8+ T cells concentrated around esophageal papillae.

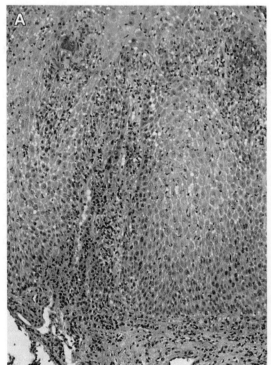
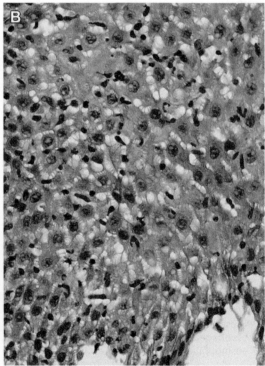

Fig. 2. Intraepithelial lymphocytes are concentrated around esophageal papillae in lymphocytic esophagitis (*A*). The lymphocytes have irregular contours and are associated with intercellular edema (*B*) (H&E, original magnifications, [*A*] ×200, [*B*] ×400).

Rubio and colleagues[20] found significantly more peripapillary lymphocytes per high power field than interpapillary lymphocytes (mean: 55 vs 20, respectively) in lymphocytic esophagitis, whereas esophagitis due to other causes showed mixed inflammation with denser lymphocytic infiltrates in interpapillary fields (mean: 13 vs 7 per high power field, respectively). This pattern of distribution has been subsequently observed by other investigators.[17,19]

Key Pathologic Features

- Increased lymphocytes in a peripapillary distribution
- Absence or near-absence of granulocytes
- Intercellular edema

ASSOCIATIONS AND PROPOSED CAUSES

Lymphocytic esophagitis is a pattern of injury that may be seen in association with some medications, immune-mediated disorders, and dysmotility. Lymphocytic esophagitis is clearly associated with Crohn disease among pediatric patients but much less so in adults. Sutton and colleagues[21] evaluated esophageal biopsies from 545 pediatric patients and found that 19% of patients with lymphocytic esophagitis also had Crohn disease but only 8% of patients without lymphocytic esophagitis had Crohn disease. Ebach and colleagues[22] found that lymphocytic esophagitis was more common among pediatric patients with Crohn disease (28%) compared with ulcerative colitis (7%). On the other hand, Basseri and colleagues[23] studied esophageal biopsy samples from 47 adult patients with inflammatory bowel disease and found only 1 (2%) who met criteria for lymphocytic esophagitis. Lymphocytic esophagitis is commonly seen in patients with esophageal dysmotility, in particular achalasia. Xue and colleagues[24] detected motility disorders by manometry or barium esophagram in 16 of 45 (36%) patients with lymphocytic esophagitis, 88% of whom had CD4+ T-cell–predominant inflammatory infiltrates in their biopsies. In a subsequent study, the same investigators reported lymphocytic esophagitis in 22 of 69 (32%) patients with dysmotility but only 6% of GERD patients.[25] Finally, Kissiedu and colleagues[26] studied 102 patients with Barrett esophagus and dysplasia who underwent ablative therapy. They reported a higher rate of lymphocytic esophagitis in postablation biopsies compared with preintervention samples.

DIFFERENTIAL DIAGNOSIS

The features of lymphocytic esophagitis overlap with those of several other types of esophagitis (**Table 2**). Lichen planus is a chronic immune-mediated disease of the skin and mucous membranes; it occurs in middle-aged adults and affects both genders equally. Esophageal lichen planus is extremely uncommon and occurs almost exclusively in patients with concomitant oral disease. Affected patients may develop strictures and, rarely, squamous cell carcinoma.[27] Endoscopically, the upper two-thirds of the esophagus show lacy white papules, erosions, desquamation, and stenosis.[28] Histologic features include lymphocyte-rich inflammation, including subepithelial bandlike infiltrates, degenerated basal epithelial cells, scattered necrotic keratinocytes, and parakeratosis. Direct immunofluorescence studies reveal globular IgM deposits at the junction of the squamous epithelium and lamina propria as well as complement staining in apoptotic keratinocytes. These features overlap considerably with those of lymphocytic esophagitis and the 2 cannot be distinguished in the absence of immunofluorescence studies and extraesophageal disease manifestations. The term, *lichenoid esophagitis*, has proposed to describe cases that have histologic features of lichen planus but lack confirmatory immunofluorescence studies.[29]

Biopsy samples from patients with GERD and eosinophilic esophagitis may also contain increased intraepithelial lymphocytes and, in the former situation, lymphocytes often outnumber

Table 2 Differential diagnosis of lymphocytic esophagitis	
Disorder	**Features That Aid Distinction from Lymphocytic Esophagitis**
Esophageal lichen planus/lichenoid esophagitis	- Indistinguishable in biopsy samples - May account for some cases of lymphocytic esophagitis - Some investigators list dyskeratotic cells (Civatte bodies) as a distinguishing feature.
GERD	- Lymphocytes may be numerous but are usually mixed with eosinophils. - Lacks peripapillary distribution of lymphocytes

mucosal eosinophils. Basseri and colleagues[30] reported mean lymphocyte counts of 23 per 400× field in GERD (n = 40) and 20 per 400× field in eosinophilic esophagitis (n = 40). An analysis of 78 adults with GERD-like symptoms and normal endoscopic examinations found that 41% had increased intraepithelial lymphocytes compared with only 14% of asymptomatic controls.[31] Dunbar and colleagues[32] discontinued PPI therapy in 12 patients with severe GERD and performed mucosal biopsies 2 weeks after cessation of acid suppression. Recurrent esophagitis was marked by increased intraepithelial lymphocytes, basal cell hyperplasia, and papillary elongation but only rare neutrophils and eosinophils, suggesting that lymphocytes play a role in the early evolution of GERD.

PROGNOSIS

Data regarding the natural history of lymphocytic esophagitis are scarce, but prognosis depends on the presence and nature of any underlying disorders. Some patients with dysphagia and/or GERD-type symptoms respond to PPI therapy, whereas the clinical picture may be dominated by associated immune-mediated disorders, such as inflammatory bowel disease or dysmotility in other cases. Patients who participated in a telephone follow-up survey reported good quality of life and satisfaction with their health status.[18]

Pitfalls

! The esophageal mucosa normally contains lymphocytes (squiggle cells); these should not be interpreted as pathologic in the absence of other features of mucosal injury.

! Lymphocytes are common in GERD; a diagnosis of lymphocytic esophagitis should not be made based on findings limited to the gastroesophageal junction.

SLOUGHING ESOPHAGITIS (ESOPHAGITIS DISSECANS SUPERFICIALIS)

CLINICAL AND ENDOSCOPIC FEATURES

Sloughing esophagitis is a poorly understood disorder that is most often incidentally detected during upper endoscopy performed for unrelated reasons. It may be related to chronic debilitation and certain medications. Purdy and colleagues[33] compared 31 patients with sloughing esophagitis to 34 controls. They found a majority of study patients to be older women (55%); the most common presenting symptom was dysphagia (32%), although more than half (55%) of patients were asymptomatic. Patients with sloughing esophagitis were significantly more likely than controls to have chronic illnesses, such as cardiac or renal failure (P = .01) and to be taking 5 or more prescription medications (77% vs 32%). In particular, central nervous system depressants (narcotics or benzodiazepines) or medications that cause dry mouth or interfere with swallowing (opioids and selective serotonin reuptake inhibitors, and antiepileptics) were more frequently used by the study group (65% vs 32%). Hart and colleagues[34] retrospectively identified 41 cases of sloughing esophagitis. They also found most affected patients to be women (mean age: 65 years) who complained of dysphagia (47%), abdominal pain (49%), and/or heartburn (42%). A high proportion of patients were taking psychoactive drugs, including selective serotonin reuptake inhibitors (51%), opiates (22%), or benzodiazepines (20%). Endoscopic features are more pronounced in the distal two-thirds of the esophagus and include longitudinal white casts of desquamated epithelium alternating with intact, healthy mucosa (Fig. 3A).[35]

MICROSCOPIC FEATURES AND DIAGNOSIS

Biopsy specimens reveal two-toned strips of squamous epithelium with an intraepithelial cleft: sloughed epithelial layers above the split are

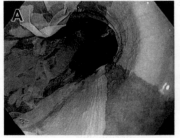
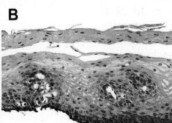
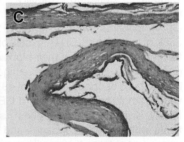

Fig. 3. Linear casts of squamous epithelium peel from the surface in sloughing esophagitis (*A*). Biopsy specimens show an intraepithelial cleft with parakeratosis (*B*) and necrosis (*C*) of the sloughed layers (H&E, original magnification [*B*,*C*] ×200).

Table 3
Differential diagnosis of esophagitis dissecans superficialis

Disorder	Distinguishing Features
Epidermoid metaplasia	• Granular cell layer subjacent to compact hyperorthokeratosis • Lack of intraepithelial split and necrosis
Parakeratosis	• Compact surface layers of hypereosinophilic squamous cells with pyknotic nuclei • Lack of intraepithelial split and necrosis
Candidal esophagitis	• Desquamated epithelial cells associated with neutrophils and lymphocytes • Yeast and pseudohyphae

hypereosinophilic and display parakeratosis and/or confluent necrosis, whereas the deeper layers are normal or show basal zone expansion (see Fig. 3B, C). Inflammation is not characteristic, but neutrophils and eosinophils may be present in some cases. Bacterial or fungal colonies are often observed in the intraepithelial cleft or at the surface of necrotic parakeratotic debris.[34] Other disorders can simulate sloughing esophagitis endoscopically and histologically; thus, pathologic and endoscopic correlation is critical to the diagnosis (Table 3).

Key Pathologic Features

• Tubular white casts of sloughed squamous mucosa

• Intraepithelial split: squamous mucosa under the split is normal or shows basal zone expansion; layers above the split show parakeratosis and/or coagulative necrosis

• Usually little or no inflammation

DIFFERENTIAL DIAGNOSIS

Epidermoid metaplasia usually involves the mid to lower esophagus and occurs in middle-aged women who present with dysphagia. Epidermoid metaplasia is characterized basal zone expansion and a granular cell layer subjacent to

superficial hyperorthokeratosis, the latter of which imparts a 2-toned appearance to the mucosa (Fig. 4A). Singhi and colleagues[36] reported an association between epidermoid metaplasia and tobacco (61%) or alcohol (39%) use in 18 patients and found that 3 cases (17%) were associated with high-grade squamous dysplasia or squamous cell carcinoma. Cottreau and colleagues[37] compared the incidence of epidermoid metaplasia in 58 cases of squamous dysplasia or carcinoma to 1048 controls and found it in 2 study patients (3%) and 2 controls (0.2%) ($P<.05$). Benign parakeratosis is a common finding in patients with chronic esophageal injury for any reason. It is characterized by compact layers of squamous epithelial cells with pyknotic nuclei and hypereosinophilic cytoplasm at the luminal surface (see Fig. 4B).[38] Necrosis and intraepithelial splitting are not features of epidermoid metaplasia or parakeratosis, helping to distinguish these findings from sloughing esophagitis.

PROGNOSIS

Esophagitis dissecans superficialis is a benign self-limited condition. All reported patients who have undergone follow-up endoscopic examination experienced resolution of sloughing and none has developed related complications.[34]

Pitfalls

! Diagnosis requires endoscopic and pathologic correlation.

! Endoscope-induced trauma may cause artifactual intraepithelial splitting but does not produce casts of sloughed mucosa.

! Graft-versus-host disease and medications can cause squamous denudation but do not show histologic features of esophagitis dissecans superficialis.

MEDICATION-INDUCED ESOPHAGEAL INJURY

CLINICAL AND ENDOSCOPIC FEATURES

A growing list of medications causes injury to the esophagus, usually by direct contact with the mucosa. Drug-related esophageal injury, also referred to as pill esophagitis, tends to occur at points of extrinsic compression, including the junction of the proximal and middle third of the

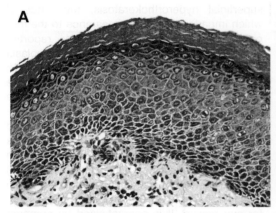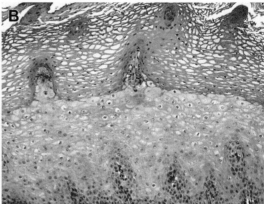

Fig. 4. A granular cell layer subjacent to orthokeratosis is the hallmark of epidermoid metaplasia (*A*). Parakeratosis displays layers of keratinized epithelial cells with pyknotic nuclei (*B*) (H&E, original magnification, [*A,B*] ×200).

esophagus, where is passes over the aortic arch, the gastroesophageal junction, and the segment overlying the left atrium in patients with left atrial enlargement. It is more common among elderly patients and those who take multiple medications. Endoscopic features include discrete ulcers or localized areas of erythema and mucosal friability. Strictures and circumferential wall thickening may simulate malignancy in some cases. Medications that are commonly reported to cause pill esophagitis include bisphosphonates, potassium chloride, nonsteroidal anti-inflammatory drugs, antibiotics, and antihypertensives.[39]

MICROSCOPIC FEATURES AND DIAGNOSIS

Histologic features of drug-related injury are nonspecific and include neutrophilic inflammation, erosions, and granulation tissue, although some clues can point to a specific etiology. Ulcers may contain fragments of refractile cellulose that is used as a filler in many medications; this substance is not specific for any agent but does point toward a medication-related injury.[40] Bisphosphonates are osteoclast inhibitors that are well known to be corrosive to the esophageal mucosa. Bisphosphonate-induced esophageal injury is severe and characterized by extensive mucosal necrosis that may result in desquamation of squamous epithelium that simulates the endoscopic appearance of esophagitis dissecans superficialis.[40,41]

Tetracycline antibiotics, in particular doxycycline, are used to treat acne and characteristically cause severe esophageal injury. They produce a highly acidic environment when dissolved in small volumes, as may be the case when pills become lodged in the esophagus. Absorption of the drug causes marked intercellular edema in the deep to mid layers of the squamous mucosa and

neutrophilic inflammation. Eventually vacuolar degeneration of the basal cell layers causes them to separate from the superficial layers, creating an intramucosal cleft. The superficial layers undergo coagulative necrosis and slough into the lumen.[42] Tetracyclines should be suspected when esophageal biopsies show severe injury predominantly affecting the deeper layers of the squamous mucosa, especially in a young adult patient.

Kayexalate is a cation exchange resin used to treat hyperkalemia; the most common formulation consists of Kayexalate in sorbitol. The sodium polystyrene crystals cause direct mucosal injury in the esophagus.[43] Endoscopic findings include mural thickening, ulcers, and white plaques that simulate *Candida* infection. Kayexalate crystals can be found adherent to intact mucosa and granulation tissue or within inflammatory debris. They are deeply basophilic and display an internal mosaic pattern that has been likened to fish scales or stacked bricks (**Fig. 5**).

Ferrous sulfate is used to treat iron deficiency anemia and is frequently implicated as a cause of injury to the upper gastrointestinal tract. Iron deposition and associated mucosal damage are more common in the stomach and duodenum, but injury is well documented in the esophagus. Endoscopic examination reveals ulcers containing brown pigment that corresponds to iron encrustation in the squamous epithelium and ulcer debris in biopsy samples (**Fig. 6**). Some cases show iron deposits within blood vessel walls or as components of intravascular thrombi.[44]

PROGNOSIS

Pill esophagitis usually resolves on discontinuation of the offending agent combined with PPI therapy,

Fig. 5. Kayexalate crystals are basophilic and have an internal mosaic pattern (H&E, original magnification, ×600).

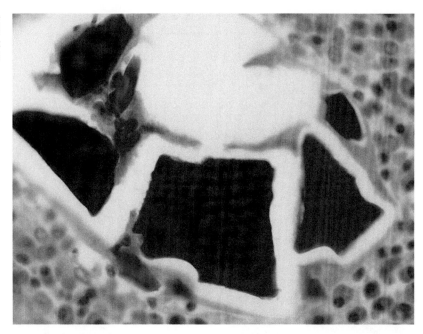

but untreated cases may prove fatal due to esophageal perforation.[45]

INFECTIOUS ESOPHAGITIS

HERPES ESOPHAGITIS

Clinical and Endoscopic Features

Gastrointestinal involvement by herpes simplex virus (HSV) is most common in the esophagus and affects immunocompromised and immunocompetent hosts.[46,47] Esophageal disease is usually caused by HSV-1, but HSV-2 infection also occurs.[47] Varicella-zoster virus (VZV) rarely causes esophagitis in immunocompromised individuals. Herpesviruses have a predilection to cause injury in the mid and distal esophagus, producing multiple, discrete ulcers (**Fig. 7**A). The ulcers are shallow with slightly raised edges and may be confluent; intact vesicles are uncommon.

Microscopic Features and Diagnosis

Diagnostic inclusions are present in injured squamous epithelial cells at the edges of ulcers or in sloughed squamous epithelial cells. Infected cells generally contain hard eosinophilic or orangophilic cytoplasm and are often associated with a macrophage-rich inflammatory infiltrate. They contain single or multiple enlarged nuclei bearing viral inclusions surrounded by a peripheral rim of marginated chromatin; viral inclusions may have an eosinophilic, glassy appearance (Cowdry type A inclusions) or appear basophilic with a powdery or homogeneous quality (Cowdry type B inclusions). Nuclear molding is characteristic (see **Fig. 7**B). VZV infection produces changes indistinguishable from HSV infection, but patients often have a rash (**Table 4**). Immunohistochemical stains directed against the VZV glycoprotein 1 represent a sensitive and specific means of distinguishing it from HSV infection.[48]

Prognosis

HSV esophagitis is generally self-limited in immunocompetent patients, but immunocompromised hosts require acyclovir therapy. Prognosis is related to etiology of underlying immunodeficiency.

CYTOMEGALOVIRUS ESOPHAGITIS

Clinical and Endoscopic Features

Reactivation of cytomegalovirus infection is a common cause of esophageal injury in immunocompromised individuals, in particular those receiving immunosuppressive drugs or chemotherapy and patients with HIV infection or AIDS.[49] It rarely produces clinical symptoms in immunocompetent patients. Cytomegalovirus tends to affect the mid to distal esophagus, where it produces large, discrete ulcers that may be confluent or circumferential. Strictures and acute necrotizing esophagitis are less common presentations.[50,51]

Microscopic Features and Diagnosis

Unlike HSV, which affects squamous epithelial cells, cytomegalovirus shows tropism for

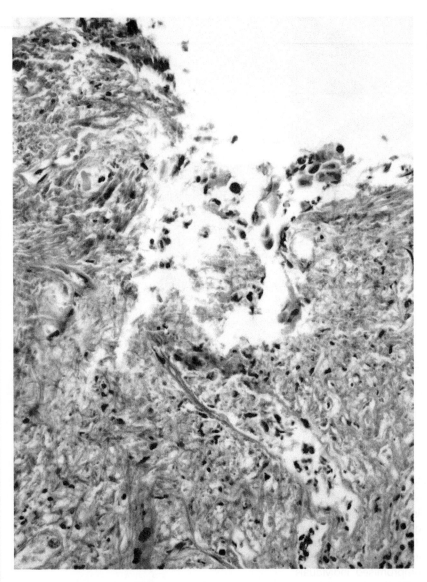

Fig. 6. Golden-brown crystalline material in an esophageal ulcer reflects injury from iron pill ingestion (H&E, original magnification, ×200).

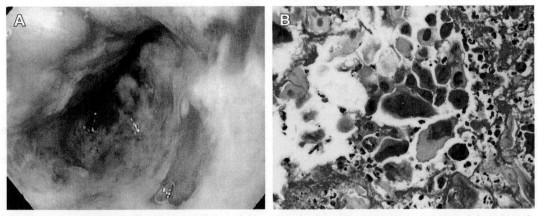

Fig. 7. Multiple, discrete ulcers are present in the distal esophagus of a patient with HSV esophagitis (*A*). Multinucleated squamous cells display nuclear molding and margination of chromatin associated with intranuclear inclusions (*B*) (H&E, original magnification, ×400).

Table 4
Differential diagnosis of viral esophagitis

Disorder	Distinguishing Features
Other viral infections	• Site and appearance of viral inclusions • Patients with VZV infection often have a rash. • Immunostains aid identification of specific pathogen.
Other causes of erosive esophagitis (eg, pill esophagitis, toxin ingestion)	• Clinical history of immunosuppression favors infectious etiology. • Sudden onset of retrosternal pain favors medication or toxin ingestion. • Lack of viral cytopathic changes

endothelial and stromal cells as well as glandular epithelium. For this reason, esophageal infections are most readily detected when the ulcer bed is sampled. Viral inclusions may be intranuclear or intracytoplasmic. Nuclear inclusions are amphophilic and have a peripheral clearing, imparting an owl's eye appearance that resembles the nuclear inclusions of HSV infection. Cytoplasmic inclusions appear as multiple, small, brightly eosinophilic granules (**Fig. 8**).

Prognosis

Cytomegalovirus is a deadly opportunistic infection in immunocompromised hosts; thus, antiviral prophylaxis is commonly used in patients with AIDS and transplant recipients. Active infection is usually treated with intravenous ganciclovir. Although many patients respond well to antiviral therapy, the prognosis is variable depending on the nature of underlying immunosuppression.

Key Pathologic Features
VIRAL ESOPHAGITIS

• Ulcers, erosions, neutrophil-rich infiltrates, and granulation tissue should prompt search for inclusions.

• HSV: red or amphophilic intranuclear inclusions with peripheral rim of chromatin

• Cytomegalovirus: intranuclear and cytoplasmic inclusions

Pitfalls
VIRAL ESOPHAGITIS

! Multinucleated squamous epithelial cells are seen in multiple types of esophageal injury but lack inclusions of HSV.

! Activated stromal cells in esophagitis may simulate cytomegalovirus inclusions.

CANDIDAL ESOPHAGITIS

CLINICAL AND ENDOSCOPIC FEATURES

Candidiasis is the most common infection of the esophagus. The gastrointestinal tract is a common entry portal for *Candida* spp, which may disseminate and cause life-threatening systemic disease.[52] *C albicans* is the most common species, but *C tropicalis* and *C glabrata* are also isolated from the esophagus.[53] Endoscopic features are characteristic and include patchy or confluent yellow-white plaques that are easily removed from the underlying mucosa. The esophageal lining is usually intact but may be edematous or friable; gross ulcers are uncommon.

MICROSCOPIC FEATURES AND DIAGNOSIS

Biopsy specimens show expansion of the squamous mucosa with parakeratosis and desquamated luminal keratin debris. The inflammatory infiltrate consists of neutrophils and lymphocytes distributed throughout the mucosa as well as superficial neutrophilic microabscesses. Severe cases may be characterized by tissue invasion and ulcers. Yeasts are ovoid and measure 3 μm to 5 μm, and pseudohyphae are elongated with incomplete septa. The latter are often arranged perpendicularly to squamous cells in a shish kabob–like configuration (**Fig. 9**A). Histochemical stains, such as periodic acid–Schiff with diastase (PAS-D) and Grocott methenamine silver (GMS), highlight the organisms (see **Fig. 9**B).

PROGNOSIS

Candida esophagitis usually responds to treatment with fluconazole and similar medications, but immunocompromised hosts may require amphotericin to clear the infection.

ESOPHAGEAL INVOLVEMENT IN CUTANEOUS BULLOUS DISORDERS

The esophagus may be involved by disorders affecting intercellular and epithelial basement

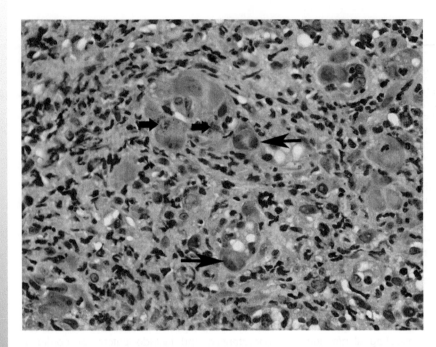

Fig. 8. Cytomegalovirus intranuclear inclusions have a peripheral clearing (*arrows*); whereas intracytoplasmic inclusions are granular (*block arrows*) (H&E, original magnification, ×400).

membrane adhesion of squamous cells, resulting in dysphagia, bleeding, and strictures. Pemphigus vulgaris is a rare blistering disorder of the skin and mucous membranes caused by autoantibodies to intercellular binding proteins, desmoglein 3 and desmoglein 1. Trattner and colleagues[54] detected esophageal involvement in 5 of 12 (42%) patients with pemphigus vulgaris, although only 2 reported esophageal symptoms, raising the possibility that the incidence of esophageal involvement is underestimated. Esophageal findings include flaccid bullae, superficial erosions, and ulcers. Biopsy samples show separation between basal keratinocytes and more superficial epithelial cells with a mild inflammatory infiltrate. Squamous cells above the split have a rounded appearance, whereas basal epithelial cells cling to the basement membrane, resembling tombstones. Direct immunofluorescence shows intercellular IgG and C3 deposits.

Epidermolysis bullosa is genetic disorder that causes blisters to form at sites of mild trauma. Esophageal blisters form at sites of external compression, presumably reflecting a response to friction from food boluses. Webs and strictures may develop at sites of healed blisters.[55] Subepithelial blisters are characteristic but may not be evident in biopsy samples. Direct

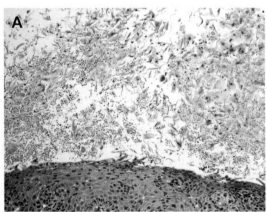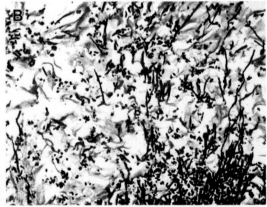

Fig. 9. Candida esophagitis is characterized by neutrophils and lymphocytes in the superficial squamous epithelium and sloughed keratin debris (*A*). Yeast and pseudohyphae are highlighted by a periodic acid–Schiff with diastase stain (*B*) (H&E, original magnification, [*A*] ×100, [*B*] ×200).

immunofluorescence shows linear IgG deposits on the roof of blisters in both junctional and dystrophic forms, whereas immunoglobulins deposit on the blister floor in epidermolysis bullosa simplex.[56]

Bullous pemphigoid affects older adults and is caused by autoantibodies to hemidesmosomes that attach squamous epithelial cells to the basement membrane. Subepithelial bullae are typically associated with eosinophil infiltrates. Direct immunofluorescence demonstrates linear IgG and C3 deposition on the roof of blisters and/or along the basement membrane. The disease affects the esophagus in less than 5% of cases.[56]

SUMMARY

Inflammatory disorders of the esophagus display a broad range of histologic abnormalities. Although many features of these diseases overlap, pathologists are often able to distinguish among them with careful attention to subtle details. Every effort should be made to correlate histologic findings with the endoscopic features to facilitate timely interventions and optimize patient care.

REFERENCES

1. Dellon ES. Epidemiology of eosinophilic esophagitis. Gastroenterol Clin North Am 2014;43(2):201–18.
2. Liacouras CA, Spergel JM, Ruchelli E, et al. Eosinophilic esophagitis: a 10-year experience in 381 children. Clin Gastroenterol Hepatol 2005;3(12): 1198–206.
3. Hirano I, Moy N, Heckman MG, et al. Endoscopic assessment of the oesophageal features of eosinophilic oesophagitis: validation of a novel classification and grading system. Gut 2013;62(4): 489–95.
4. Nielsen JA, Lager DJ, Lewin M, et al. The optimal number of biopsy fragments to establish a morphologic diagnosis of eosinophilic esophagitis. Am J Gastroenterol 2014;109(4):515–20.
5. Salek J, Clayton F, Vinson L, et al. Endoscopic appearance and location dictate diagnostic yield of biopsies in eosinophilic oesophagitis. Aliment Pharmacol Ther 2015;41(12):1288–95.
6. Dellon ES, Gonsalves N, Hirano I, et al. ACG clinical guideline: evidenced based approach to the diagnosis and management of esophageal eosinophilia and eosinophilic esophagitis (EoE). Am J Gastroenterol 2013;108(5):679–92, [quiz: 693].
7. Shah A, Kagalwalla AF, Gonsalves N, et al. Histopathologic variability in children with eosinophilic esophagitis. Am J Gastroenterol 2009;104(3): 716–21.
8. Dellon ES, Gibbs WB, Fritchie KJ, et al. Clinical, endoscopic, and histologic findings distinguish eosinophilic esophagitis from gastroesophageal reflux disease. Clin Gastroenterol Hepatol 2009; 7(12):1305–13, [quiz: 1261].
9. Parfitt JR, Gregor JC, Suskin NG, et al. Eosinophilic esophagitis in adults: distinguishing features from gastroesophageal reflux disease: a study of 41 patients. Mod Pathol 2006;19(1):90–6.
10. Chehade M, Sampson HA, Morotti RA, et al. Esophageal subepithelial fibrosis in children with eosinophilic esophagitis. J Pediatr Gastroenterol Nutr 2007;45(3):319–28.
11. Li-Kim-Moy JP, Tobias V, Day AS, et al. Esophageal subepithelial fibrosis and hyalinization are features of eosinophilic esophagitis. J Pediatr Gastroenterol Nutr 2011;52(2):147–53.
12. Rodrigo S, Abboud G, Oh D, et al. High intraepithelial eosinophil counts in esophageal squamous epithelium are not specific for eosinophilic esophagitis in adults. Am J Gastroenterol 2008;103(2): 435–42.
13. Dellon ES, Speck O, Woodward K, et al. Clinical and endoscopic characteristics do not reliably differentiate PPI-responsive esophageal eosinophilia and eosinophilic esophagitis in patients undergoing upper endoscopy: a prospective cohort study. Am J Gastroenterol 2013;108(12): 1854–60.
14. Moawad FJ, Schoepfer AM, Safroneeva E, et al. Eosinophilic oesophagitis and proton pump inhibitor-responsive oesophageal eosinophilia have similar clinical, endoscopic and histological findings. Aliment Pharmacol Ther 2014;39(6): 603–8.
15. Wen T, Dellon ES, Moawad FJ, et al. Transcriptome analysis of proton pump inhibitor-responsive esophageal eosinophilia reveals proton pump inhibitor-reversible allergic inflammation. J Allergy Clin Immunol 2015;135(1):187–97.
16. Yantiss RK. Eosinophils in the GI tract: how many is too many and what do they mean? Mod Pathol 2015; 28(Suppl 1):S7–21.
17. Haque S, Genta RM. Lymphocytic oesophagitis: clinicopathological aspects of an emerging condition. Gut 2012;61(8):1108–14.
18. Cohen S, Saxena A, Waljee AK, et al. Lymphocytic esophagitis: a diagnosis of increasing frequency. J Clin Gastroenterol 2012;46(10): 828–32.
19. Purdy JK, Appelman HD, Golembeski CP, et al. Lymphocytic esophagitis: a chronic or recurring pattern of esophagitis resembling allergic contact dermatitis. Am J Clin Pathol 2008;130(4):508–13.
20. Rubio CA, Sjodahl K, Lagergren J. Lymphocytic esophagitis: a histologic subset of chronic esophagitis. Am J Clin Pathol 2006;125(3):432–7.

21. Sutton LM, Heintz DD, Patel AS, et al. Lymphocytic esophagitis in children. Inflamm Bowel Dis 2014; 20(8):1324–8.

22. Ebach DR, Vanderheyden AD, Ellison JM, et al. Lymphocytic esophagitis: a possible manifestation of pediatric upper gastrointestinal Crohn's disease. Inflamm Bowel Dis 2011;17(1):45–9.

23. Basseri B, Vasiliauskas EA, Chan O, et al. Evaluation of peripapillary lymphocytosis and lymphocytic esophagitis in adult inflammatory bowel disease. Gastroenterol Hepatol 2013;9(8):505–11.

24. Xue Y, Suriawinata A, Liu X, et al. Lymphocytic esophagitis with CD4 T-cell-predominant Intraepithelial lymphocytes and primary esophageal motility abnormalities: a potential novel clinicopathologic entity. Am J Surg Pathol 2015;39(11): 1558–67.

25. Putra J, Muller KE, Hussain ZH, et al. Lymphocytic esophagitis in nonachalasia primary esophageal motility disorders: improved criteria, prevalence, strength of association, and natural history. Am J Surg Pathol 2016;40(12):1679–85.

26. Kissiedu J, Thota PN, Gohel T, et al. Post-ablation lymphocytic esophagitis in Barrett esophagus with high grade dysplasia or intramucosal carcinoma. Mod Pathol 2016;29(6):599–606.

27. Schwartz MP, Sigurdsson V, Vreuls W, et al. Two siblings with lichen planus and squamous cell carcinoma of the oesophagus. Eur J Gastroenterol Hepatol 2006;18(10):1111–5.

28. Chryssostalis A, Gaudric M, Terris B, et al. Esophageal lichen planus: a series of eight cases including a patient with esophageal verrucous carcinoma. A case series. Endoscopy 2008; 40(9):764–8.

29. Salaria SN, Abu Alfa AK, Cruise MW, et al. Lichenoid esophagitis: clinicopathologic overlap with established esophageal lichen planus. Am J Surg Pathol 2013;37(12):1889–94.

30. Basseri B, Levy M, Wang HL, et al. Redefining the role of lymphocytes in gastroesophageal reflux disease and eosinophilic esophagitis. Dis Esophagus 2010;23(5):368–76.

31. Ronkainen J, Aro P, Storskrubb T, et al. High prevalence of gastroesophageal reflux symptoms and esophagitis with or without symptoms in the general adult Swedish population: a Kalixanda study report. Scand J Gastroenterol 2005;40(3): 275–85.

32. Dunbar KB, Agoston AT, Odze RD, et al. Association of acute gastroesophageal reflux disease with esophageal histologic changes. JAMA 2016; 315(19):2104–12.

33. Purdy JK, Appelman HD, McKenna BJ. Sloughing esophagitis is associated with chronic debilitation and medications that injure the esophageal mucosa. Mod Pathol 2012;25(5):767–75.

34. Hart PA, Romano RC, Moreira RK, et al. Esophagitis dissecans superficialis: clinical, endoscopic, and histologic features. Dig Dis Sci 2015;60(7): 2049–57.

35. Longman RS, Remotti H, Green PH. Esophagitis dissecans superficialis. Gastrointest Endosc 2011; 74(2):403–4.

36. Singhi AD, Arnold CA, Crowder CD, et al. Esophageal leukoplakia or epidermoid metaplasia: a clinicopathological study of 18 patients. Mod Pathol 2014;27(1):38–43.

37. Cottreau J, Gruchy S, Kamionek M, et al. Prevalence of oesophageal epidermoid metaplasia in 1048 consecutive patients and 58 patients with squamous neoplasms. Histopathology 2016;68(7):988–95.

38. Waintraub DJ, Serouya S, Wang LS. An incidental finding of esophageal parakeratosis. Clin Gastroenterol Hepatol 2016;14(2):A23.

39. De Petris G, Caldero SG, Chen L, et al. Histopathological changes in the gastrointestinal tract due to medications: an update for the surgical pathologist (part II of II). Int J Surg Pathol 2014; 22(3):202–11.

40. Abraham SC, Cruz-Correa M, Lee LA, et al. Alendronate-associated esophageal injury: pathologic and endoscopic features. Mod Pathol 1999;12(12): 1152–7.

41. Hokama A, Ihama Y, Nakamoto M, et al. Esophagitis dissecans superficialis associated with bisphosphonates. Endoscopy 2007;39(Suppl 1):E91.

42. Banisaeed N, Truding RM, Chang CH. Tetracycline-induced spongiotic esophagitis: a new endoscopic and histopathologic finding. Gastrointest Endosc 2003;58(2):292–4.

43. Abraham SC, Bhagavan BS, Lee LA, et al. Upper gastrointestinal tract injury in patients receiving kayexalate (sodium polystyrene sulfonate) in sorbitol: clinical, endoscopic, and histopathologic findings. Am J Surg Pathol 2001;25(5):637–44.

44. Abraham SC, Yardley JH, Wu TT. Erosive injury to the upper gastrointestinal tract in patients receiving iron medication: an underrecognized entity. Am J Surg Pathol 1999;23(10):1241–7.

45. Kim SH, Jeong JB, Kim JW, et al. Clinical and endoscopic characteristics of drug-induced esophagitis. World J Gastroenterol 2014;20(31): 10994–9.

46. Lavery EA, Coyle WJ. Herpes simplex virus and the alimentary tract. Curr Gastroenterol Rep 2008;10(4): 417–23.

47. Wishingrad M. Sexually transmitted esophagitis: primary herpes simplex virus type 2 infection in a healthy man. Gastrointest Endosc 1999;50(6): 845–6.

48. Eyzaguirre E, Haque AK. Application of immunohistochemistry to infections. Arch Pathol Lab Med 2008;132(3):424–31.

49. Huppmann AR, Orenstein JM. Opportunistic disorders of the gastrointestinal tract in the age of highly active antiretroviral therapy. Hum Pathol 2010; 41(12):1777–87.

50. Olmos M, Sanchez Basso A, Battaglia M, et al. Esophageal strictures complicating cytomegalovirus ulcers in patients with AIDS. Endoscopy 2001;33(9):822.

51. Barjas E, Pires S, Lopes J, et al. Cytomegalovirus acute necrotizing esophagitis. Endoscopy 2001; 33(8):735.

52. van de Veerdonk FL, Kullberg BJ, Netea MG. Pathogenesis of invasive candidiasis. Curr Opin Crit Care 2010;16(5):453–9.

53. Antinori S, Milazzo L, Sollima S, et al. Candidemia and invasive candidiasis in adults: a narrative review. Eur J Intern Med 2016;34:21–8.

54. Trattner A, Lurie R, Leiser A, et al. Esophageal involvement in pemphigus vulgaris: a clinical, histologic, and immunopathologic study. J Am Acad Dermatol 1991;24(2 Pt 1):223–6.

55. Hillemeier C, Touloukian R, McCallum R, et al. Esophageal web: a previously unrecognized complication of epidermolysis bullosa. Pediatrics 1981;67(5):678–82.

56. Smoller BR, Woodley DT. Differences in direct immunofluorescence staining patterns in epidermolysis bullosa acquisita and bullous pemphigoid. J Am Acad Dermatol 1992;27(5 Pt 1):674–8.

Diagnosis and Management of Barrett-Related Neoplasia in the Modern Era

Lysandra Voltaggio, MD, Elizabeth A. Montgomery, MD*

KEYWORDS

- Barrett neoplasia • Barrett dysplasia • Endoscopic mucosal resection
- Endoscopic submucosal dissection • Radiofrequency ablation

Key points

- The definition of Barrett esophagus is undergoing evolution, such that 1 of the 2 main United States gastroenterology societies has introduced the concept of a length requirement of 1 cm of columnar esophagus for a diagnosis of Barrett esophagus.

- Treatment of high-grade dysplasia is no longer esophagectomy except in unusual circumstances.

- There are a few pitfalls in interpreting specimens that are derived from endoscopic procedures that are intended to treat high-grade dysplasia and early carcinomas in Barrett esophagus.

ABSTRACT

Whereas in the past, pathologists were hesitant to diagnose high-grade dysplasia in patients with Barrett esophagus, because this diagnosis prompted esophagectomy, current international consensus is that endoscopic treatment is the management for high-grade dysplasia and intramucosal carcinoma. Furthermore, many centers advocate endoscopic ablation for low-grade dysplasia. As such, establishing a diagnosis of dysplasia has become the key step; separation between the grades of dysplasia is less critical. This article offers some criteria for separating dysplasia from reactive changes, discusses pitfalls in interpreting endoscopic mucosal resection specimens, and outlines management strategies.

OVERVIEW

Esophageal adenocarcinoma is an increasing burden to the medical system in the United States.

The incidence increased from 0.3 per 100,000 to 2.7 per 100,000 between 1973 and 2011.[1] It is estimated that in 2016 there were 17,000 new cases and approximately 16,000 deaths related to esophageal carcinoma in the United States.[2] Gastroesophageal reflux disease (GERD) is a major risk factor for esophageal adenocarcinoma.[3] As such, evaluation of patients with GERD symptoms for Barrett esophagus and dysplasia is an indication for many endoscopic procedures.

The risk factors for Barrett esophagus include chronic (>5 years) GERD, age over 50 years, male gender, smoking, central obesity, and white ethnicity. Alcohol use is not a significant factor and wine drinking may be protective.[4]

Barrett esophagus has been defined differently by various societies in the United States and abroad. The American Gastroenterological Association (AGA) requires the presence of goblet cells (intestinal metaplasia) and a tongue of columnar mucosa but specifies no required length.[5] In contrast, the American College of Gastroenterologists (ACG) proposes the following definition for

There are no disclosures.
Department of Pathology, Johns Hopkins Medical Institutions, 401 North Broadway, Baltimore, MD 21231, USA
* Corresponding author.
E-mail address: emontgom@jhmi.edu

Surgical Pathology 10 (2017) 781–800
http://dx.doi.org/10.1016/j.path.2017.07.002

Barrett esophagus: "Barrett esophagus should be diagnosed when there is extension of salmon-colored mucosa into the tubular esophagus extending ≥1 cm proximal to the gastroesophageal junction with biopsy confirmation of intestinal metaplasia" and further suggests that endoscopic biopsy be avoided in the presence of a normal Z line or a Z line with less than 1 cm of variability.[4] British criteria do not require the presence of goblet cells for a diagnosis of Barrett esophagus and include a segment length requirement of greater than or equal to 1 cm.[6]

The recommendation by the ACG to introduce a disease-length criterion causes difficulty for pathologists because endoscopic data are often unavailable. If a pathologist has documentation that the segment is less than 1 cm, the term, *specialized intestinal metaplasia of the esophagogastric junction*, can be used.[4]

When the authors receive samples labeled "esophagus" that contain goblet cells and are unaware of the segment length, the following comments are incorporated into the reports:

> *Note: The above diagnosis of Barrett esophagus is made due to presence of goblet cells (intestinal metaplasia) with the assumption that the biopsies were obtained from columnar mucosa in the distal esophagus located at least 1 cm proximal to the top of the gastric folds as per 2016 ACG guidelines.[4]*

If a sample is labeled "gastroesophageal junction" and goblet cells are present, the following comment is used:

> *Note: This biopsy shows gastric-type mucosa with scattered goblet cells. The diagnosis in this case depends on the location of this biopsy. If this biopsy was taken from the tubular esophagus at least 1 cm above the gastric folds, it shows Barrett mucosa of the distinctive type. If this biopsy was taken from the gastric cardia, it shows intestinal metaplasia of the gastric cardia.[4]*

Barrett esophagus (with goblet cells) was present in approximately 1% to 2% of the general population in a Scandinavian study[7] and in up to 15% of people with GERD. Life expectancy is not shortened as a result of Barrett esophagus.[8] Danish colleagues reported the annual incidence of cancer progression in Barrett esophagus to be only 0.12%, implying that 1000 patients must be screened to prevent 1 cancer, indicating that surveillance is of no value.[9] The AGA later commissioned a study in the United States and noted that in the first 5 years of follow-up, a mean 0.19% annual rate of progression could be expected, whereas a 9.1% to 9.5% cumulative cancer incidence was predicted after 20 years of disease. These data suggest that intensive surveillance is indicated for patients with longstanding Barrett esophagus, but longer surveillance intervals are adequate in the early years after diagnosis.[10] Identification of high-risk patients for screening and surveillance is suboptimal; thus, many patients present with symptoms of advanced, incurable disease.[1]

CLASSIFICATION OF DYSPLASIA IN BARRETT ESOPHAGUS

Consensus criteria for evaluation of Barrett esophagus can be used to distinguish between biopsies that are negative for dysplasia and those that are positive for dysplasia, although some variations in morphology exist.[11,12]

There are 4 key features to note in samples from Barrett esophagus:

1. Surface maturation compared with underlying glands
2. Architecture of the glands
3. Cytologic features
4. Inflammation, erosions/ulcers

Surface maturation is assessed at low magnification. In nondysplastic Barrett esophagus, the nuclei in the basal regions of glands are larger and more hyperchromatic than those at the surface. The surface nuclei are arranged in a monolayer with polarized basal nuclei. The glands of Barrett esophagus are mildly atypical, especially compared with adjacent oxyntic or cardiac glands.

Glandular architecture describes the relationships between glands and the lamina propria and also encompasses the shapes of the glands. Architectural abnormalities include both increased numbers of glands and changes in their shapes. In nondysplastic mucosa, the glands are round with little budding in abundant lamina propria. Crowding of normal-appearing glands is considered a mild architectural abnormality and a reparative change. Crowding of abnormal glands is a feature of dysplasia or early carcinoma. Cribriform glands, cystic dilation, and necrotic luminal debris are severe architectural abnormalities.

Cytologic features are the heart of diagnosis. Some degree of nuclear alteration is inherent in nondysplastic Barrett metaplasia, especially in the basal zone and in columnar epithelium adjoining squamous mucosa. Cytologic atypia in Barrett esophagus can indicate (1) dysplasia; (2)

reactive changes, particularly when associated with inflammation; and (3) inherent changes in the deeper glands of Barrett esophagus.

Once dysplasia is diagnosed, assigning a low-grade and high-grade category reflects a matter of degree along a morphologic continuum.[13] An important component of assessment of cytologic features is the relationship of one nucleus to another—nuclear polarity. In normal polarity, the long axis of the nucleus remains perpendicular to the basement membrane, and the nuclei are aligned parallel to one another. Loss of nuclear polarity indicates loss of this perpendicular orientation and a random arrangement of the nuclei in relation to the basement membrane and each other.

BARRETT ESOPHAGUS: NEGATIVE FOR DYSPLASIA

In nondysplastic Barrett esophagus (Fig. 1), the surface appears more mature than the underlying glands. That is, the nuclear-to-cytoplasmic ratio of surface cells is lower than that of the deeper glands. The architecture is normal with abundant lamina propria. The cytologic features are normal, noting that mitoses may be present in deeper glands. Individual nuclei have smooth nuclear membranes and nucleoli, if present, are small with smooth contours. Nuclear polarity is maintained.

A helpful clue to nondysplastic reactive changes is the presence of 4 lines/tiers. Starting at the surface, the first tier is formed by the gastric foveolar type mucin droplet, the second by the base of the foveolar mucin vacuole, the third by the cytoplasm below the mucin vacuole, and the fourth by the row of nuclei. This pattern is found in both gastric cardiac mucosa and non-dysplastic Barrett mucosa (Figs. 2–6). Using this criterion helps reduce the number of lesions regarded as indefinite for dysplasia (discussed later).

BARRETT ESOPHAGUS: INDEFINITE FOR DYSPLASIA

The indefinite for dysplasia category includes cases that show cytologic changes suggestive of dysplasia in the deep mucosa in combination with surface maturation or those in which inflammation obscures the findings (Fig. 7).

BARRETT ESOPHAGUS: LOW-GRADE DYSPLASIA

In low-grade dysplasia (Figs. 8–9), the surface appears similar to the underlying glands at low magnification or displays only slight maturation. The architecture may be mildly to markedly distorted with glandular crowding, although lamina propria should be identifiable between glands. The cytologic changes extend at least focally to the surface. Abrupt transitions between nondysplastic and atypial epithelium are a clue that the changes are neoplastic. Superficially

Fig. 1. Barrett esophagus, negative for dysplasia. Lamina propria is abundant and the nuclei mature toward the surface [Original magnification ×40].

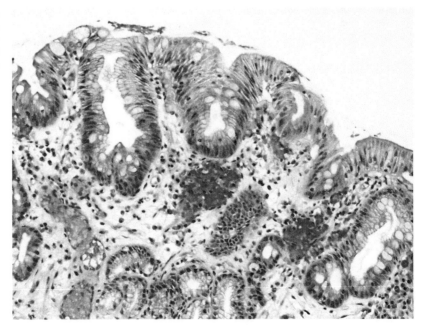

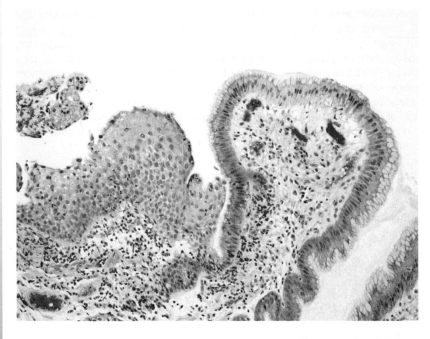

Fig. 2. Gastric cardiac mucosa adjoining reactive squamous mucosa. Despite acute inflammation, 4 levels are apparent in the columnar epithelium [Original magnification ×20].

located nuclei are irregular, hyperchromatic, and mildly enlarged. Dysplastic epithelial cells show some degree of stratification and mucin loss, and the 4 lines/4 tiers typical of reactive epithelia are lost.

Some examples of low-grade dysplasia resemble colorectal tubular adenomas and may be polypoid or nonpolypoid (**Fig. 10**). The term, *tubular adenoma*, should not be used. Terminology similar to *polypoid low-grade columnar epithelial dysplasia* is more appropriate.

BARRETT ESOPHAGUS: HIGH-GRADE DYSPLASIA

As in low-grade dysplasia, surface maturation is lacking in high-grade dysplasia (**Figs. 11** and **12**). The architecture may show crowding of cytologically abnormal glands or be markedly distorted with prominent glandular crowding and little intervening lamina propria, but many cases show normal amounts of lamina propria. Most examples lack prominent nucleoli, which tend to be present

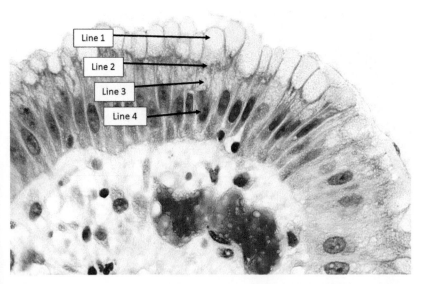

Line 1
Line 2
Line 3
Line 4

Fig. 3. Cardiac mucosa (epithelium and superficial lamina propria). The 4 levels (*lines*) are annotated and consist of the cap of foveolar mucin, the base of the cap, the cytoplasm of the columnar cells, and the row of nuclei [Original magnification ×100].

Fig. 4. Barrett mucosa with inflammation and reactive changes. The nuclei are enlarged in the bases of the pits and become smaller toward the surface. Note that the 4 levels are apparent in the surface epithelium [Original magnification ×20].

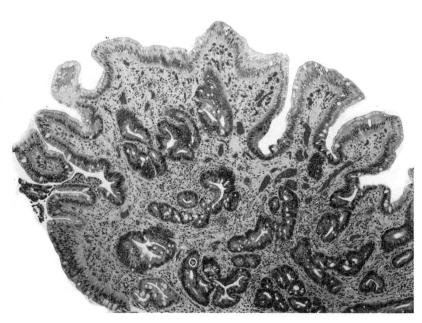

in either reactive changes or invasive carcinoma, both of which are often associated with ulcers. Cells with markedly enlarged hyperchromatic nuclei often extend to the surface and loss of nuclear polarity is typical.

INTRAMUCOSAL CARCINOMA

The distinction between high-grade dysplasia and the earliest carcinomas (invasion through the basement membrane into the lamina propria or muscularis mucosae; T1a) is difficult. Certain features should raise concern for carcinoma, including (1) cribriform architecture, (2) dilated tubules containing necrotic debris, (3) ulceration of the lesion, (4) neutrophils within dysplastic glands, and (5) pagetoid growth of neoplastic cells in the overlying squamous epithelium. The last finding is always associated with invasive carcinomas that penetrate the muscularis mucosae at a minimum, whereas the others may be seen in deeply invasive tumors or intramucosal carcinoma or even some cases of high-grade dysplasia (**Fig. 13**).[14]

Fig. 5. Barrett mucosa with inflammation and reactive changes. Higher magnification of the lesion seen in **Fig. 4** [Original magnification ×40].

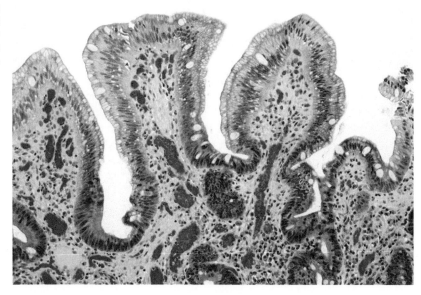

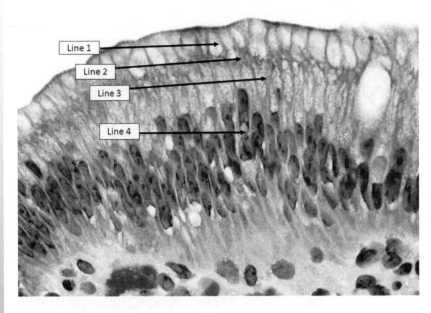

Line 1
Line 2
Line 3
Line 4

Fig. 6. Barrett mucosa with inflammation and reactive changes with annotation of the levels/lines [Original magnification ×100].

Carcinomas in the mucosa generally show effacement of lamina propria architecture and a syncytial growth pattern, extensive back-to-back microglands, cells with prominent nucleoli, and an intermingling of single cells and small clusters within the lamina propria (**Figs. 14–16**). Desmoplasia ranges from absent to incomplete at this stage. According to some observers, the earliest sign of mucosal invasion is the presence of glands with round, hyperchromatic nuclei that grow sideways rather than perpendicular to the surface.

Interobserver variability can be a factor when diagnosing intramucosal carcinoma in small biopsies. Fortunately, this distinction is less important than it was in the past because both high-grade dysplasia and intramucosal carcinoma are managed endoscopically.[4,5]

VARIANT DYSPLASIA PATTERNS

Some biopsy samples from patients with Barrett esophagus show cytologic atypia in the basal

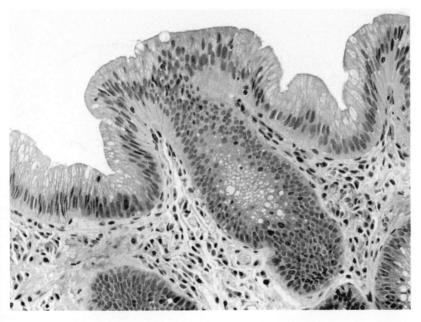

Fig. 7. Indefinite for dysplasia. These epithelial changes may be reactive but the levels of the epithelium at the surface are obscured in a well-oriented focus and the nuclei are enlarged [Original magnification ×40].

Fig. 8. Low-grade dysplasia. The surface appears involved [Original magnification ×20].

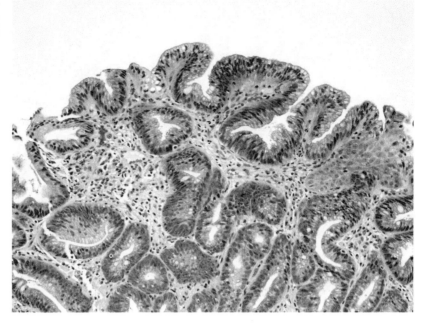

pits with surface maturation; the term, *basal crypt dysplasia*, has been used to describe this finding[15] (**Figs. 17** and **18**). Cytologic atypia may be low grade or high grade, although most cases show high-grade dysplasia because low-grade atypia confined to the deep mucosa is often classified as indefinite for dysplasia. No clear guidelines exist regarding follow-up for basal crypt dysplasia, although most patients are followed per guidelines for low-grade dysplasia. Although p53 immunostaining is not suggested for all cases, basal crypt dysplasia often shows strong nuclear labeling.[16]

Other examples of dysplasia show differentiation along gastric foveolar or pyloric/cardiac-type lines (**Figs. 19–23**) or extend laterally on the surface of non-neoplastic cardiac or cardiac-oxyntic glands (**Fig. 24**). The terms, *nonadenomatous dysplasia*[17] and *gastric dysplasia*,[18] have been

Fig. 9. Low-grade dysplasia. The surface lines/levels are lost [Original magnification ×100].

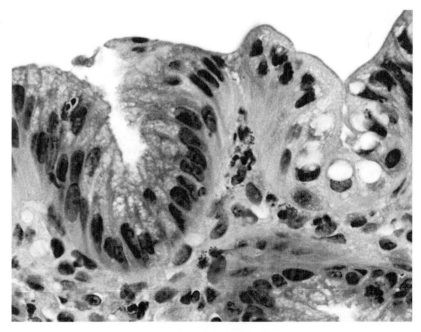

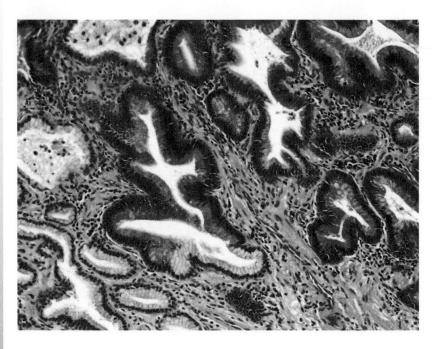

Fig. 10. Low-grade dysplasia. This example shows cytologic features resembling those of a tubular adenoma of the colon — intestinal differentiation. Note the abrupt transition between the dysplastic and foveolar epithelium [Original magnification ×40].

applied to lesions lacking the classic stratification of intestinal-type dysplasia. Nonadenomatous dysplasia typically displays numerous, tiny glands that may seem bland at low magnification but display nuclear alterations at high magnification. Criteria for grading such lesions are not well established because the cells contain round nuclei arranged in a monolayer, rather than crowded, pseudostratified nuclei.[12] Proposed criteria for low-grade dysplasia include the presence of closely packed tubules, whereas criteria for high-grade dysplasia simply involve loss of polarity. Gastric forms of dysplasia account for approximately 15% of dysplasia cases and seem to have similar progression rates compared with conventional intestinal-type dysplasia.

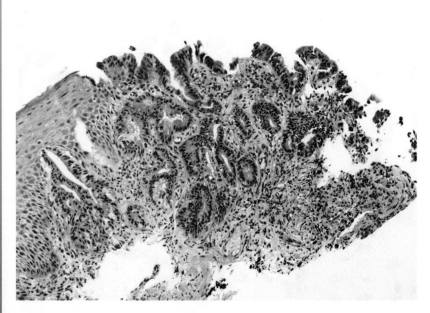

Fig. 11. High-grade dysplasia. The amount of lamina propria is similar to that in nondysplastic Barrett mucosa. A very irregular gland at the left is buried beneath the squamous epithelium, but most of the lesion is on the surface. At the upper right, the nuclei are hyperchromatic and have lost their alignment with one another and with the basement membrane [Original magnification ×20].

Fig. 12. High-grade dysplasia. Note the loss of nuclear polarity [Original magnification ×100].

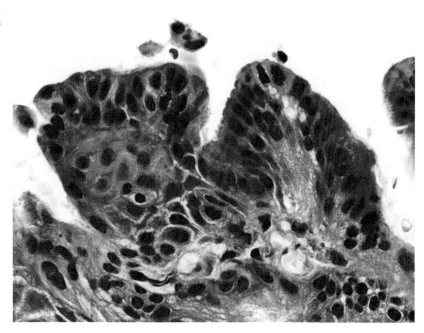

ROLE OF IMMUNOLABELING

Immunolabeling to confirm a dysplasia diagnosis can be of use but there are limitations, as summarized by other investigators.[16] The best studied adjuncts include Mib1/ki-67, p53, and alpha-methylacyl-CoA racemase (AMACR). AMACR has proved disappointing because it is apt to label nondysplastic lesions and fail to highlight dysplastic ones. Ki-67 labels regenerating mucosa as readily as it does dysplasia. Mutations in *TP53* lead to aberrant nuclear accumulation of p53 protein, which can be detected on immunolabeling. In 1 study of p53 immunolabeling, aberrant expression was detected in approximately 10% of cases regarded as nondysplastic, 40% of cases

Fig. 13. Pagetoid spread of single cells of deeply invasive adenocarcinoma into the overlying squamous epithelium [Original magnification ×100].

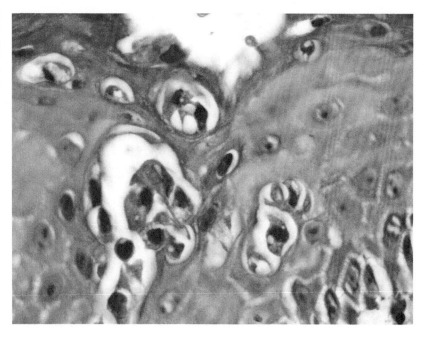

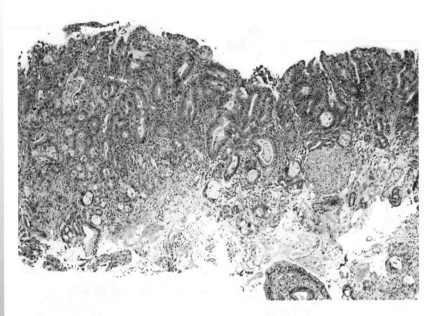

Fig. 14. Biopsy appearance of intramucosal adenocarcinoma. There is no desmoplasia but the mucosa is overrun with glands [Original magnification ×20].

classified as low-grade dysplasia, 85% of cases classified as high-grade dysplasia, and all adeno-carcinomas.[19] This marker can confirm a diagnosis of high-grade dysplasia; some investigators believe its presence can predict an increased probability of progression from low-grade dysplasia to adenocarcinoma. Reflex staining of all Barrett esophagus for p53, however, yields a subset of clearly nondysplastic cases that show aberrant expression. Some examples of high-grade dysplasia show complete lack of nuclear staining; this null pattern reflects biallelic loss of the *TP53* gene (**Fig. 25**).

TREATMENT AND POST-TREATMENT CHANGES

Esophagectomy was the treatment of patients with high-grade dysplasia in the past, although endoscopic treatment is now the standard of care for high-grade dysplasia and early carcinoma

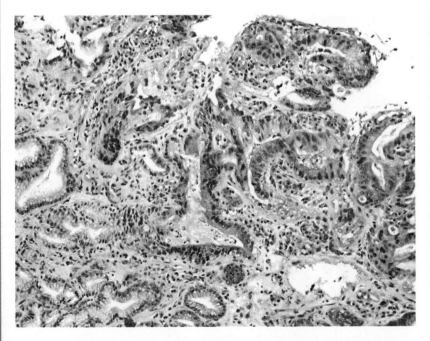

Fig. 15. Biopsy appearance of intramucosal adenocarcinoma. A gland at the center is aligned parallel to the surface, an abnormal arrangement. In the deeper left portion of the sample, however, there are a few maloriented benign cardiac glands, so using gland alignment as a criterion for invasion is suspect in the authors' view. In this case, however, there are small glands that have budding and luminal necrosis at the right of the image [Original magnification ×20].

Fig. 16. Biopsy appearance of intramucosal adenocarcinoma. Note the nucleoli [Original magnification ×100].

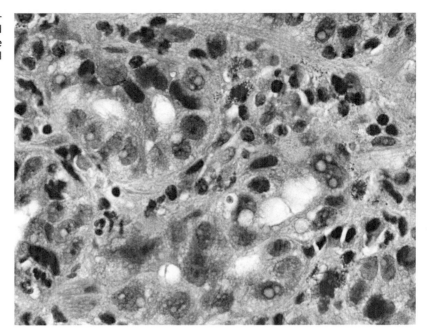

(ie, tumor confined to mucosa).[4,5,20] Current management practices include aggressive sampling to exclude more deeply invasive carcinoma, followed by endoscopic resection of visible lesions and radiofrequency ablation (RFA).

In addition to endoscopic mucosal resection (EMR), other endoscopic treatments include multipolar electrocoagulation, argon plasma coagulation, photodynamic therapy, RFA, and cryotherapy. RFA is the preferred technique because it has fewer complications than other methods.[21,22] Photodynamic therapy has largely been replaced by other techniques, especially cryopotherapy.[23–25] Endoscopic submucosal dissection offers a greater likelihood of achieving negative margins but is not necessary for most

Fig. 17. Dysplasia with apparent surface maturation. There are markedly atypical nuclei in the glands at the lower right and unremarkable Barrett epithelium in the top center. On closer inspection, however, the surface at the left is abnormal [Original magnification ×40].

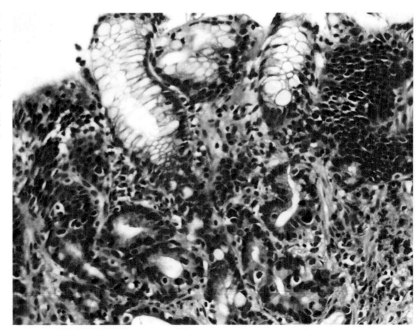

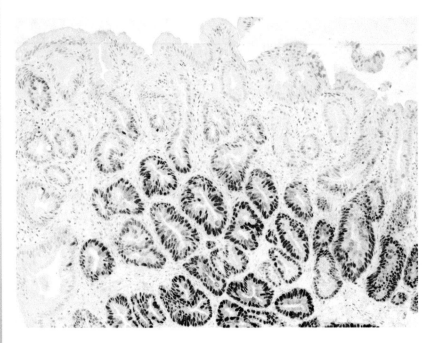

Fig. 18. Dysplasia with apparent surface maturation. This is a p53 immunostain. The deep nuclei are strongly labeled whereas the surface nuclei are not [Original magnification ×20].

esophageal lesions.[26] Although a worry may be that all these techniques fail to ablate dysplastic mucosa underneath squamous mucosa, this is rarely a clinical problem.[25] Most patients enjoy favorable initial responses after luminal therapy; recurrences of Barrett mucosa during subsequent surveillance are not uncommon, but recurrent neoplasia is much less problematic.[27,28] Not surprisingly, patients with extensive intramucosal carcinoma are the most likely to have recurrences.[27]

EVALUATION OF ENDOSCOPIC MUCOSAL RESECTION SPECIMENS

EMRs and submucosal dissections allow removal of mucosa and submucosa, usually by a

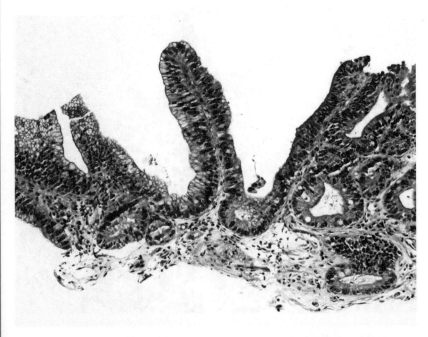

Fig. 19. Dysplasia with prominent gastric foveolar differentiation. There are a few goblet cells to the right but the villiform structure in the center shows low-grade dysplasia with gastric foveolar differentiation. On the right, there is loss of nuclear polarity and closely packed glands, which are features of a high-grade dysplasia component [Original magnification ×20].

Fig. 20. Dysplasia with prominent gastric foveolar differentiation [Original magnification ×100].

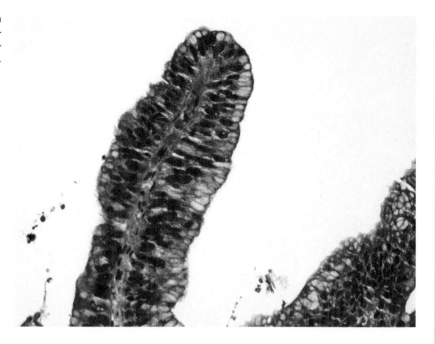

suck-and-cut method. After injection of the submucosa with fluid, the endoscopist applies a cap to the lesion, followed by suction through the endoscope that creates an artificial polyp that can be resected. These methods allow for good characterization of neoplasia but have a few pitfalls:

1. Because the plastic cap is applied to the mucosal surface, the epithelium may be damaged such that dysplasia must be evaluated in the absence of an intact surface.

2. Duplicated muscularis mucosae is found in many cases of Barrett esophagus, attributable to many cycles of reflux injury (**Figs. 26–29**). The original muscularis mucosae is accompanied by a second delicate smooth muscle layer closer to the luminal surface; this feature has been identified in more than 90% of resection

Fig. 21. Dysplasia with prominent gastric foveolar differentiation, periodic acid–Schiff/Alcian blue stain [Original magnification ×100].

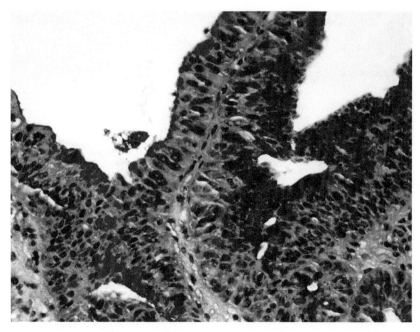

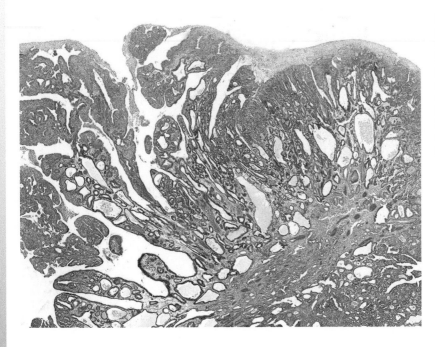

Fig. 22. High-grade dysplasia with gastric cardiac differentiation (pyloric gland adenoma-like lesion). The cells are not as hyperchromatic as those seen in classic intestinal-type dysplasia. Note the closely packed tubules [Original magnification ×2].

samples[29] and approximately 70% of endoscopic resection specimens.[30] Care must be taken to avoid interpreting the duplicated muscularis mucosae as the deepest extent of the mucosa, particularly because the lamina propria subjacent to the duplicated layer simulates the submucosa. Distinction between invasive carcinoma restricted to the lamina propria (T1a) and submucosal invasion (T1b) is important because T1a lesions can be treated endoscopically whereas tumors in the submucosa often require esophagectomy.

3. Diathermy causes the muscularis mucosae to contract, pulling the lateral edges of the sample together such that the sample becomes convex (see **Figs. 26** and **28**) resulting in the false

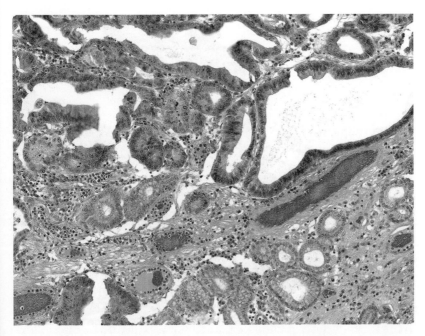

Fig. 23. High-grade dysplasia with gastric cardiac differentiation (pyloric gland adenoma-like lesion). There are nondysplastic cardiac glands at the lower right. The cytoplasm of the neoplastic cells in the upper half of the image has a ground glass appearance. The nuclei are not hyperchromatic but they have lost their polarity [Original magnification ×20].

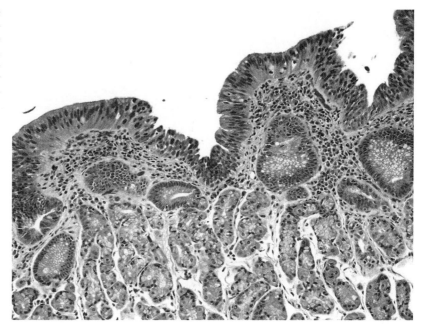

Fig. 24. Intestinal-type high-grade dysplasia extending along the surface of gastric oxyntic mucosa. The nuclei are hyperchromatic and have lost their polarity [Original magnification ×20].

impression that lateral margins are instead deep margins.

Depth of tumor invasion into the submucosa and margin status should be assessed in all endoscopic resection specimens. Although the mucosa can be subdivided into layers (Table 1), depth of invasion in the mucosa is of little clinical importance because all intramucosal carcinomas are similarly managed. It is the authors' practice to provide both a description, such as "invading the lamina propria" and the m level, with an explanatory note regarding the depth of invasion. Reporting the precise depth of invasion

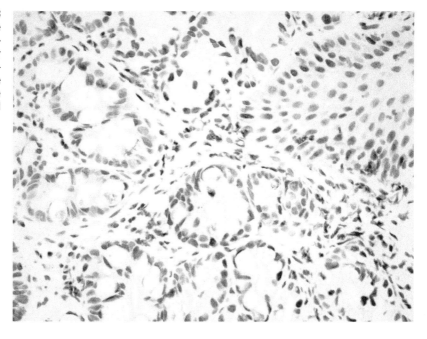

Fig. 25. Null pattern p53 immunolabeling. There are a few basal squamous cells at the upper right with immunolabeling (normal) but the dysplastic glands are nonreactive [Original magnification ×100].

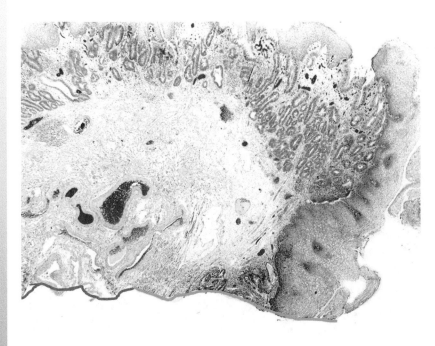

Fig. 26. EMR. A dysplastic lesion partly buried under squamous epithelium is at the upper right. The sample has curled so the lateral and deep margins all appear as a deep edge. The green line indicates the lateral margin, consisting of epithelium at the right, lamina propria containing buried nondysplastic Barrett mucosa with diathermy changes, and disorganized muscularis mucosae. There are slender muscle bundles close to the squamous epithelium at the right (duplicated muscularis mucosae) and a thicker one curling around the center of the sample (original muscularis mucosae). The deep portion of the curled muscularis mucosae (lateral margin) is marked by the left part of the green line. The blue line shows the deep submucosal margin [Original magnification ×2].

facilitates dialogue when patients are referred between institutions. Depth of invasion into the submucosa can be classified as sm1, sm2, or sm3 by dividing the submucosa into thirds, although most endoscopic resection specimens do not contain muscularis propria, so the deepest aspect of the submucosa is not evident.[31] The authors find it more valuable to measure the depth of invasion into the submucosa, because this information facilitates treatment decisions regarding potential esophagectomy.[32]

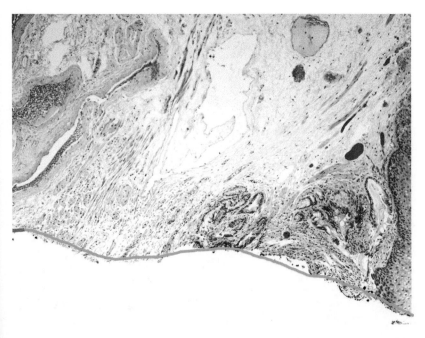

Fig. 27. EMR. This is a high magnification of the lesion shows in **Fig. 26.** The lateral margin is indicated with the green line, and a small portion of the deep margin is at the lower left. Note delicate wisps of duplicated muscularis mucosae at the upper right and the submucosal vessels at the left [Original magnification ×20].

Fig. 28. EMR. There is a buried dysplastic lesion at the top. Green lines indicate curled lateral margins and a blue deep line indicates the deep submucosal margin. An attempt has been made at drawing the delineation between the mucosa and the submucosa with a dashed pale blue line. The muscularis mucosae at the right part of the sample, however, is so disorganized that the accuracy of the depiction is somewhat in doubt [Original magnification ×2].

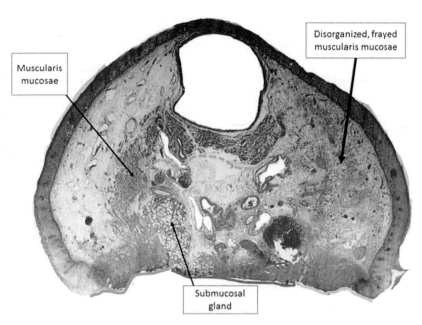

The ideal endoscopic resection sample is pinned to a corkboard and floated upside down in formalin with assurance that the pins do not pierce the lesion. In reality, most samples are dropped into formalin, in which case the tissue curls. The deep (submucosal) and lateral (mucosal) margins are painted with ink. The sample is then serially sectioned and entirely submitted. This does not allow precise evaluation of every lateral margin but ensures evaluation of the deep margin, which is the most important.

Pathologists should expect frequent positive lateral margins because the nature of the procedure requires removal of several adjoining zones in a piecemeal fashion to treat the field of dysplasia.

FOLLOW-UP OF BARRETT ESOPHAGUS PATIENTS

Guidelines for screening and surveillance intervals for patients with Barrett esophagus were

Fig. 29. EMR. This is a higher magnification of the lesion shown in Fig. 28. The green line indicates the lateral margin and the blue line highlights the deep submucosal margin [Original magnification ×10].

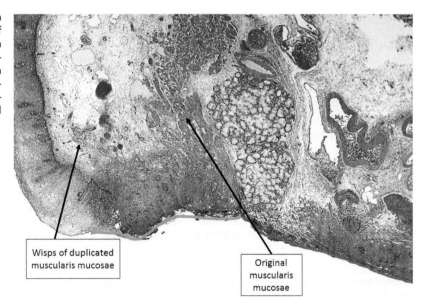

Table 1
Reported subclassification schemes for assessing extent of intramucosal carcinoma (T1a)

Description of Invasion	Dutch Method[31]	German Method[33]	United States Method[34]
None (Tis, high-grade dysplasia)	m1	High-grade dysplasia	High-grade dysplasia
Tumor cells invade beyond basement membrane into lamina propria	m2	m1	Lamina propria
Tumor cells invade (inner) duplicated muscularis mucosae	m2	m2	Inner muscularis mucosae
Tumor cells in the space between the duplicated muscularis mucosae and original muscularis mucosae	m2	m3	Between the layers of muscularis mucosae
Tumor cells into (outer) original muscularis mucosae	m3	m4	Outer muscularis mucosae

developed by the ACG (Table 2).[4] The ACG does not suggest screening everyone but endorses screening of men over 50 years of age with long-standing GERD, especially those with central obesity (>102 cm [>40 in] waist circumference) who smoke cigarettes. If initial endoscopy fails to identify Barrett esophagus, repeat examination is indicated only if a patient has severe esophagitis that requires assessment for response to therapy. Patients with Barrett esophagus should undergo surveillance with high-definition methodology at 3 years to 5 years. Biopsies interpreted as indefinite for dysplasia are followed by repeat screening at 3 months to 6 months after acid-suppressive therapy. Any detected dysplasia is confirmed by peer review and managed by ablation.

PROGNOSTICATION

Patients with dysplasia are at increased risk for cancer, especially if diagnosis is confirmed by more than 1 pathologist or the dysplasia is high grade. The risk of cancer progression is 0.2% to 0.5% per year among patients without dysplasia, compared with 0.7% per year for those with low-grade dysplasia. Patients with high-grade dysplasia have an annual progression rate of approximately 6% to 7%.[4] Immunohistochemical panels are not sufficiently useful to be routinely used for prognostication. In situ hybridization, aneuploidy, and other assays have been offered to predict which patients are most likely to progress to cancer, but the added value of these tests is not known at this writing.[16]

Table 2
American College of Gastroenterology recommendations regarding surveillance for Barrett esophagus and related dysplasia

Dysplasia Grade	Specific Further Documentation	Follow-up Interval
Negative for dysplasia	None	3–5 y
Indefinite for dysplasia	Repeat at 3–6 mo after optimization of acid suppression If again indefinite, follow-up	12 mo
Low-grade dysplasia	Expert confirmation Ablation	Every 6 mo during the first year, then annually
High-grade dysplasia or intramucosal carcinoma	Expert confirmation EMR recommended if biopsies are taken from an area of mucosal irregularity RFA performed on perilesional area	Every 3 mo for first year, every 6 mo for second year, then annually

Adapted from Shaheen NJ, Falk GW, Iyer PG, et al, American College of Gastroenterology. ACG clinical guideline: diagnosis and management of Barrett's esophagus. Am J Gastroenterol 2016;111(1):30–50. [quiz: 51].

SUMMARY

Barrett esophagus is currently defined as the presence of intestinal metaplasia (goblet cells) in samples obtained from a visible mucosal abnormality in the distal esophagus. Barrett esophagus is a precursor to esophageal adenocarcinoma, and the greatest risk factor among affected patients is the presence of dysplasia. Pathologic diagnosis and grading of dysplasia are the most reliable method for assessing risk for neoplastic progression. Unfortunately, the diagnosis and classification of dysplasia can be challenging, especially when superimposed inflammatory changes are present. Both low-grade dysplasia and high-grade dysplasia are endoscopically managed in the modern era, and superficially invasive carcinomas are increasingly resected using minimally invasive techniques. Thus, surgical pathologists are increasingly expected to provide information regarding extent of disease as well as prognostic data based on review of limited material.

REFERENCES

1. Vaughan TL, Fitzgerald RC. Precision prevention of oesophageal adenocarcinoma. Nat Rev Gastroenterol Hepatol 2015;12(4):243–8.
2. Siegel RL, Miller KD, Jemal A. Cancer statistics, 2016. CA Cancer J Clin 2016;66(1):7–30.
3. Lagergren J, Bergstrom R, Lindgren A, et al. Symptomatic gastroesophageal reflux as a risk factor for esophageal adenocarcinoma [see comments]. N Engl J Med 1999;340(11):825–31.
4. Shaheen NJ, Falk GW, Iyer PG, et al, American College of Gastroenterology. ACG Clinical guideline: diagnosis and management of Barrett's esophagus. Am J Gastroenterol 2016;111(1):30–50, [quiz: 51].
5. American Gastroenterological Association, Spechler SJ, Sharma P, Souza RF, et al. American gastroenterological association medical position statement on the management of Barrett's esophagus. Gastroenterology 2011;140(3):1084–91.
6. Fitzgerald RC, di Pietro M, Ragunath K, et al. British society of gastroenterology guidelines on the diagnosis and management of Barrett's oesophagus. Gut 2014;63(1):7–42.
7. Ronkainen J, Aro P, Storskrubb T, et al. Prevalence of Barrett's esophagus in the general population: an endoscopic study. Gastroenterology 2005;129(6):1825–31.
8. Sikkema M, de Jonge PJ, Steyerberg EW, et al. Risk of esophageal adenocarcinoma and mortality in patients with Barrett's esophagus: a systematic review and meta-analysis. Clin Gastroenterol Hepatol 2010;8(3):235–44, [quiz: e32].
9. Hvid-Jensen F, Pedersen L, Drewes AM, et al. Incidence of adenocarcinoma among patients with Barrett's esophagus. N Engl J Med 2011;365(15):1375–83.
10. Kroep S, Lansdorp-Vogelaar I, Rubenstein JH, et al. An accurate cancer incidence in Barrett's esophagus: a best estimate using published data and modeling. Gastroenterology 2015;149(3):577–85.e4, [quiz: e14–5].
11. Montgomery E, Bronner MP, Goldblum JR, et al. Reproducibility of the diagnosis of dysplasia in Barrett esophagus: a reaffirmation. Hum Pathol 2001;32(4):368–78.
12. Vieth M, Montgomery EA, Riddell RH. Observations of different patterns of dysplasia in barretts esophagus - a first step to harmonize grading. Cesk Patol 2016;52(3):154–63.
13. Reid BJ, Haggitt RC, Rubin CE, et al. Observer variation in the diagnosis of dysplasia in Barrett's esophagus. Hum Pathol 1988;19(2):166–78.
14. Abraham SC, Wang H, Wang KK, et al. Paget cells in the esophagus: assessment of their histopathologic features and near-universal association with underlying esophageal adenocarcinoma. Am J Surg Pathol 2008;32(7):1068–74.
15. Lomo LC, Blount PL, Sanchez CA, et al. Crypt dysplasia with surface maturation: a clinical, pathologic, and molecular study of a Barrett's esophagus cohort. Am J Surg Pathol 2006;30(4):423–35.
16. Panarelli NC, Yantiss RK. Do ancillary studies aid detection and classification of Barrett esophagus? Am J Surg Pathol 2016;40(8):e83–93.
17. Rucker-Schmidt RL, Sanchez CA, Blount PL, et al. Nonadenomatous dysplasia in barrett esophagus: a clinical, pathologic, and DNA content flow cytometric study. Am J Surg Pathol 2009;33(6):886–93.
18. Mahajan D, Bennett AE, Liu X, et al. Grading of gastric foveolar-type dysplasia in Barrett's esophagus. Mod Pathol 2010;23(1):1–11.
19. Kastelein F, Biermann K, Steyerberg EW, et al. Aberrant p53 protein expression is associated with an increased risk of neoplastic progression in patients with Barrett's oesophagus. Gut 2013;62(12):1676–83.
20. Pech O, May A, Manner H, et al. Long-term efficacy and safety of endoscopic resection for patients with mucosal adenocarcinoma of the esophagus. Gastroenterology 2014;146(3):652–60.e1.
21. Shaheen NJ, Sharma P, Overholt BF, et al. Radiofrequency ablation in Barrett's esophagus with dysplasia. N Engl J Med 2009;360(22):2277–88.
22. Spechler SJ, Fitzgerald RC, Prasad GA, et al. History, molecular mechanisms, and endoscopic treatment of Barrett's esophagus. Gastroenterology 2010;138(3):854–69.
23. Marchesi F, Tendas A, Giannarelli D, et al. Cryotherapy reduces oral mucositis and febrile episodes

in myeloma patients treated with high-dose melphalan and autologous stem cell transplant: a prospective, randomized study. Bone Marrow
Transplant 2016;52(1):154–6.

24. Canto MI, Shin EJ, Khashab MA, et al. Safety and efficacy of carbon dioxide cryotherapy for treatment of
neoplastic Barrett's esophagus. Endoscopy 2015;
47(7):591.

25. Bronner MP, Overholt BF, Taylor SL, et al. Squamous
overgrowth is not a safety concern for photodynamic
therapy for Barrett's esophagus with high-grade
dysplasia. Gastroenterology 2009;136(1):56–64,
[quiz: 351–2].

26. Terheggen G, Horn EM, Vieth M, et al. A randomised
trial of endoscopic submucosal dissection versus
endoscopic mucosal resection for early Barrett's
neoplasia. Gut 2016;66(5):783–93.

27. Agoston AT, Strauss AC, Dulai PS, et al. Predictors of
treatment failure after radiofrequency ablation for intramucosal adenocarcinoma in Barrett esophagus:
a multi-institutional retrospective cohort study. Am
J Surg Pathol 2016;40(4):554–62.

28. Krishnamoorthi R, Singh S, Ragunathan K, et al. Risk
of recurrence of Barrett's esophagus after successful endoscopic therapy. Gastrointest Endosc 2016;
83(6):1090–106.e3.

29. Abraham SC, Krasinskas AM, Correa AM, et al.
Duplication of the muscularis mucosae in Barrett
esophagus: an underrecognized feature and its
implication for staging of adenocarcinoma. Am J
Surg Pathol 2007;31(11):1719–25.

30. Lewis JT, Wang KK, Abraham SC. Muscularis
mucosae duplication and the musculo-fibrous
anomaly in endoscopic mucosal resections for
barrett esophagus: implications for staging of
adenocarcinoma. Am J Surg Pathol 2008;32(4):
566–71.

31. Westerterp M, Koppert LB, Buskens CJ, et al.
Outcome of surgical treatment for early adenocarcinoma of the esophagus or gastro-esophageal junction. Virchows Arch 2005;446(5):497–504.

32. Greene CL, Worrell SG, Attwood SE, et al. Emerging
concepts for the endoscopic management of superficial esophageal adenocarcinoma. J Gastrointest
Surg 2016;20(4):851–60.

33. Vieth M, Stolte M. Pathology of early upper GI cancers. Best Pract Res Clin Gastroenterol 2005;19(6):
857–69.

34. Kaneshiro DK, Post JC, Rybicki L, et al. Clinical significance of the duplicated muscularis mucosae in
Barrett esophagus-related superficial adenocarcinoma. Am J Surg Pathol 2011;35(5):697–700.

Patterns of Gastric Injury
Beyond *Helicobacter Pylori*

Won-Tak Choi, MD, PhD[a], Gregory Y. Lauwers, MD[b],*

KEYWORDS

- Autoimmune • Collagenous • Eosinophilic • Granulomatous • Lymphocytic • Stomach

---

Key points

- Non–*Helicobacter pylori* gastritis can be broadly categorized into 4 distinct patterns based on the distribution and nature of inflammation, and other unique features.
- Chronic inflammation in the lamina propria raises consideration for autoimmune gastritis, collagenous gastritis, and lymphocytic gastritis.
- Granulomatous inflammation is associated with Crohn's disease, sarcoidosis, and some forms of infectious gastritis.
- Limited lamina propria inflammation can be seen in the setting of viral infection, caustic gastritis, ulcero-hemorrhagic gastritis, reactive gastropathy, graft-versus-host disease, drug-induced gastritis, and chemoradiation-induced injury.
- Crystal or pigment deposition is present in iron-pilled gastritis, gastric mucosal calcinosis, lanthanum carbonate, and Kayexalate in sorbitol.

ABSTRACT

Gastric biopsies are routinely obtained from patients with symptoms related to the gastrointestinal tract and, as a result, a variety of histologic changes are observed in patients with or without endoscopic evidence of mucosal injury. Although *Helicobacter pylori*–related gastritis is still common, several other patterns of mucosal injury are increasingly encountered. These patterns of injury are classified based on the nature and distribution of inflammation, location of epithelial cell injury, presence of crystal or pigment deposition, and/or other unique features. This article discusses each of these patterns and provides a differential diagnosis for each.

OVERVIEW

Several patterns of gastric injury have been recognized since the identification of *Helicobacter pylori* as a cause of chronic gastritis. Several classification schemes for gastritis have been described, most of which are based on the presence of active (neutrophilic) or chronic (lymphoplasmacytic) inflammation. Herein, we describe a classification system that includes 4 broad groups of non–*H. pylori*–related gastric injury: gastritis with prominent inflammatory infiltrates in the lamina propria, gastritis with granulomatous inflammation, gastritis with focal lamina propria inflammation, and mucosal injury with crystal or pigment deposition.

Disclosure Statement: The authors have nothing to disclose.
[a] Department of Pathology, University of California at San Francisco, 505 Parnassus Avenue, M554, Box 0102, San Francisco, CA 94143, USA; [b] Gastrointestinal Pathology Service, Department of Pathology, Moffitt Cancer Center, 12902 Magnolia Drive, Tampa, FL 33612, USA
* Corresponding author.
E-mail address: Gregory.Lauwers@Moffitt.org

GASTRITIS WITH PROMINENT INFLAMMATORY INFILTRATES IN THE LAMINA PROPRIA

GASTRITIS WITH LYMPHOPLASMACYTIC INFLAMMATION

Autoimmune Gastritis

Autoimmune gastritis presumably develops from a complex interaction between circulating auto-antibodies directed against intrinsic factor and H+/K+ ATPase proton pumps of parietal cells (Fig. 1). Progressive destruction of parietal cells leads to lack of intrinsic factor, vitamin B12 deficiency, and hypochlorhydria, as well as iron deficiency due to decreased duodenal uptake. The resultant atrophic mucosa is thin with loss of folds, although patchy preservation of oxyntic mucosa produces a polypoid appearance in early stages of disease.[1] Other abnormalities include low serum pepsinogen I and high serum gastrin concentrations, the latter resulting from hyperplasia of antral gastrin-producing G-cells.

Early histologic features are subtle; patchy lymphoplasmacytic inflammation is centered on oxyntic glands and may be associated with surface foveolar hyperplasia.[2] Fully developed autoimmune gastritis displays dense, diffuse lymphoplasmacytic inflammation with rare eosinophils and neutrophils, predominantly affecting the deep mucosa where it is associated with gland infiltration and damage (Fig. 2A). The pit region of the mucosa is relatively spared.[2] Over time, oxyntic glands are replaced by metaplastic epithelium with pseudopyloric, intestinal, and/or pancreatic differentiation (Fig. 2B).[2,3] Completely atrophic oxyntic mucosa is composed of metaplastic glands mimicking antral mucosa; a negative gastrin immunostain ensures that a biopsy is from the fundus or body.

Decreased acidity of gastric juices leads to proliferation of G-cells in the antrum that secrete gastrin, resulting in hypergastrinemia. Gastrin is a trophic hormone that stimulates endocrine cells, including enterochromaffin-like (ECL) cells of oxyntic mucosa to proliferate.[2] "Linear ECL-cell hyperplasia" is defined by at least 2 linear groups of 5 consecutive cells lining a gland. "Micronodular hyperplasia" consists of clusters of 5 or more cells bounded by basement membrane and not exceeding 150 μm (ie, approximately the diameter of a gastric gland). Five or more clusters of micronodules are classified as "adenomatoid ECL-cell hyperplasia," whereas "ECL-cell dysplasia" applies to fused micronodules that show loss of basement membrane or span greater than 150 μm in diameter. Linear, micronodular, and adenomatoid ECL-cell hyperplasia have essentially no neoplastic potential,[4] whereas some patients with ECL-cell dysplasia develop well-differentiated gastric tumors (type 1 carcinoid tumors). Of note, even these lesions are associated with a very low risk of progressive disease, especially when compared with type 3 (sporadic) endocrine tumors of the stomach. Autoimmune gastritis with atrophy is also associated with an increased risk of adenocarcinoma.[3]

Syphilitic Gastritis

Gastric syphilis should be considered in high-risk patients who complain of nausea, vomiting, abdominal pain, gastrointestinal bleeding, and/or early satiety. Variable endoscopic findings include diffuse mucosal edema, erythema, multiple erosions and ulcerations, and thickened rugal folds that simulate an infiltrative process.[5] Rare patients develop gastric perforation. Symptoms may wane after a few days of antibiotherapy and, thus, the diagnosis is uncommonly made on biopsies with its true incidence unknown.[5]

Characteristic features include a dense lymphoplasmacytic infiltrate with gland destruction and

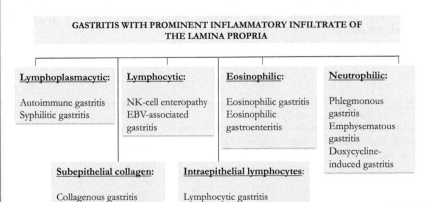

Fig. 1. Differential diagnosis of gastritis with prominent inflammation in the lamina propria.

GASTRITIS WITH PROMINENT INFLAMMATORY INFILTRATE OF THE LAMINA PROPRIA

Lymphoplasmacytic:	Lymphocytic:	Eosinophilic:	Neutrophilic:
Autoimmune gastritis Syphilitic gastritis	NK-cell enteropathy EBV-associated gastritis	Eosinophilic gastritis Eosinophilic gastroenteritis	Phlegmonous gastritis Emphysematous gastritis Doxycycline-induced gastritis

Subepithelial collagen:	Intraepithelial lymphocytes:
Collagenous gastritis	Lymphocytic gastritis

Fig. 2. (*A*) Autoimmune gastritis characterized by a dense lymphoplasmacytic infiltrate (H&E, original magnification, ×10). (*B*) The fundic-type gastric mucosa became atrophic with pseudopyloric and intestinal metaplasia (H&E, original magnification, ×4).

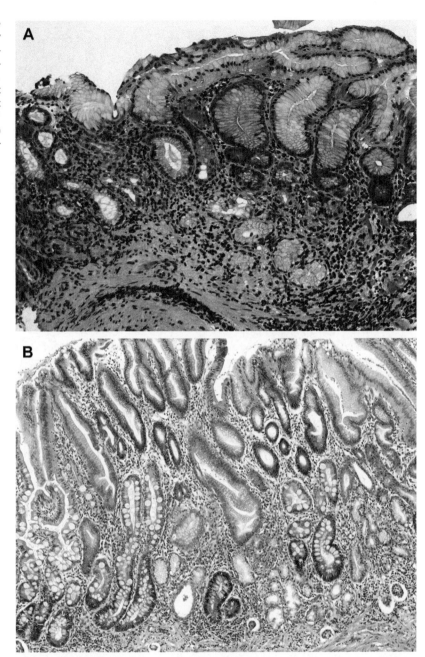

relative sparing of the superficial mucosa. Proliferative endarteritis and ill-formed granulomata are particularly suggestive in the appropriate clinical setting (Fig. 3A).[5,6] Although silver stains (Steiner) have been historically used to detect the organism, recently developed immunohistochemical stains are more sensitive. Other detection methods include immunofluorescent stains for *Treponema pallidum* (Fig. 3B) and/or detection of treponemal DNA sequences by polymerase chain reaction (PCR).[7] Co-infection with *H pylori* is not uncommon; gastric

syphilis should be ruled out in patients with peptic ulcers resistant to an anti-ulcer therapy.[5]

GASTRITIS WITH PROMINENT INFLAMMATION AND SUBEPITHELIAL COLLAGEN DEPOSITION

Collagenous Gastritis

Patients with collagenous gastritis may complain of dyspepsia, anemia, and/or chronic diarrhea.[8,9] Adult and pediatric forms of disease

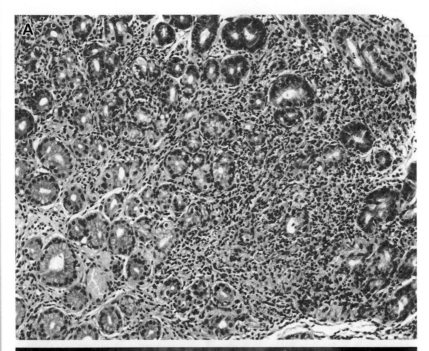

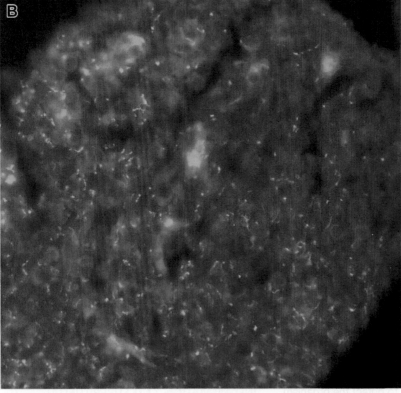

Fig. 3. (*A*) Syphilitic gastritis shows a dense lymphoplasmacytic infiltrate (H&E, original magnification, ×4). (*B*) Immunofluorescent stain specific for *Treponema pallidum* is confirmatory.

have been described. The adult form may be associated with diffuse involvement of the gastrointestinal tract and chronic watery diarrhea, whereas children and young adults have limited disease in the stomach and present with abdominal pain, bleeding, and anemia.[9] More recent data suggest substantial overlap across both age groups.[8] Endoscopic findings include nodular or "cobblestone" mucosa, erythema, erosions, and ulcers. Normal gastric mucosa is also seen in many patients.[9]

Collagenous gastritis is characterized by a thickened, often discontinuous, subepithelial collagen band spanning at least 10 μm and usually averaging 30 to 70 μm in thickness (**Fig. 4**).[10] The subepithelial collagen displays an irregular interface with the underlying lamina propria, entrapment of capillaries and inflammatory cells, and surface epithelial attenuation with detachment. Collagenous gastritis is also characterized by a diffuse lymphoplasmacytic infiltrate of the lamina propria with scattered eosinophils and rare neutrophils. Some cases may show eosinophil-rich inflammation (>30 eosinophils/high-power field [HPF]) or diffuse intraepithelial lymphocytosis.[10] Inflammation eventually causes mucosal atrophy

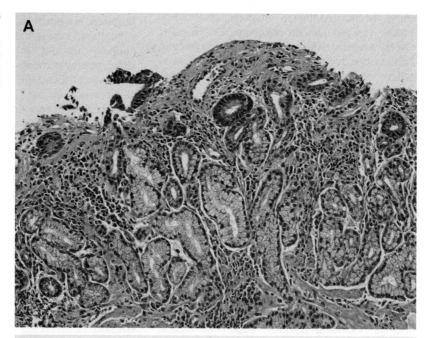
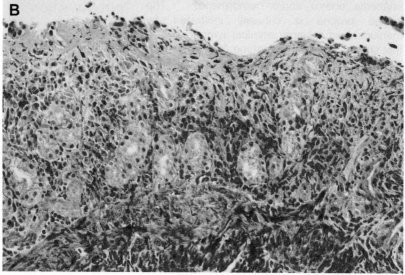

Fig. 4. (*A*) Collagenous gastritis with a thickened, subepithelial collagen band, readily highlighted by a Trichrome stain (*B*) (H&E, [*A*, *B*] original magnification, ×4).

that produces a depressed endoscopic mucosal pattern.[11] Some patients have shown improvement after steroid or sulfasalazine therapy, although collagen deposits generally do not decrease as a result of treatment.[12]

GASTRITIS WITH PREDOMINANTLY LYMPHOCYTIC INFLAMMATION

Epstein-Barr Virus–Associated Gastritis

Epstein-Barr virus (EBV)-associated gastritis can develop in immunocompetent individuals as a manifestation of infectious mononucleosis.[13] Symptoms include nausea, abdominal pain, and diarrhea.[13] Diffuse granular mucosa, wall thickening, edema, erythema, erosions, ulcerations, and/or necrosis can be observed.[13,14] Biopsies display a dense, diffuse, polymorphic lymphocytic infiltrate that typically lacks a prominent plasma cell or neutrophil infiltrate, *Helicobacter* organisms, intestinal metaplasia, or endocrine cell hyperplasia.[13] Lymphoepithelial lesions may be present. The diagnosis can be confirmed by *in situ* hybridization, which highlights EBV-encoded RNA (EBER)-positive lymphocytes in the lamina propria.[13] Scattered EBV-positive cells can be detected in other forms of chronic gastritis, including up to 2% of *H pylori* gastritis and 1.2% of autoimmune gastritis cases.

Lymphomatoid Gastropathy (Natural Killer Cell Enteropathy)

Lymphomatoid gastropathy is a rare, benign natural killer (NK) cell proliferation that can mimic malignant lymphoma.[15–17] Patients may present with vague symptoms and variable endoscopic findings, including plaques, superficial ulcers, erythema, edema, and/or hemorrhage.[15–17] The lamina propria is diffusely infiltrated by medium-sized to large atypical lymphoid cells that show an NK-cell phenotype (ie, cytoplasmic CD3+, CD4−, CD5−, CD8−, CD56+, T-cell−restricted intracellular antigen-1+, granzyme B+), but lack overtly malignant cytologic features (Fig. 5).[15,16] Because NK cells are rare in other types of gastrointestinal disease, this infiltrate can be misdiagnosed as malignant lymphoma, particularly extranodal NK/T-cell lymphoma, nasal type, or intestinal enteropathy-associated T-cell lymphoma.[17] Unlike malignant lymphoma, lymphomatoid gastropathy regresses spontaneously without therapy.[15,16] Lymphomatoid gastropathy is negative for EBV. T-cell receptor-γ gene rearrangement studies also show no evidence of a clonal process.[16]

GASTRITIS WITH INTRAEPITHELIAL LYMPHOCYTOSIS

Lymphocytic Gastritis

Lymphocytic gastritis is characterized by accumulation of small, mature T lymphocytes in the foveolar epithelium with variably increased lymphoplasmacytic inflammation in the lamina propria (Fig. 6). Endoscopic findings range from normal to enlarged folds, nodules, and/or erosions predominantly in the gastric body. Lymphocytic gastritis may occur in isolation as an idiopathic condition, but may occur in patients with celiac disease and *H pylori* gastritis.[18] Less common associations include Crohn's disease, human immunodeficiency virus infection, lymphoma, inflammatory polyps, and Menetrier-like gastropathy.

Scattered intraepithelial lymphocytes (IELs) are normally present in the gastric epithelium, although they number <25 per 100 epithelial cells. Numbers of IELs tend to be higher in idiopathic cases (mean: 80 per 100 epithelial cells) than celiac disease– (mean: 64) and *H pylori*–associated cases (mean: 48).[19] Cases associated with *H pylori* infection tend to show focally, rather than diffusely, increased IELs accompanied by a superficial band of inflammation in the lamina propria, occasional neutrophils, and scattered eosinophils.[19] Those related to celiac disease show diffusely increased IELs with evenly dispersed inflammation in the lamina propria and rare granulocytes; inflammation is more pronounced in the antrum.[19] Idiopathic cases are histologically similar to celiac disease–associated cases, but tend to show more plasmacytic inflammation in the lamina propria and foveolar hyperplasia.[19]

GASTRITIS WITH EOSINOPHIL-RICH INFLAMMATION

Eosinophilic Gastritis and Gastroenteritis

Eosinophils are normally present in the gastric mucosa, ranging up to approximately 10 per HPF. They are usually dispersed in the lamina propria and do not infiltrate the epithelium. Eosinophilic gastritis is defined as increased eosinophils with an average density of ≥127 eosinophils/mm^2 in at least 5 separate fields (≥30 peak eosinophils/×400 HPF) in the absence of known causes of mucosal eosinophilia (Fig. 7).[20] Most cases represent a manifestation of eosinophilic gastroenteritis, which is a systemic hypersensitivity disorder that can affect any part of the gastrointestinal tract, including the pancreaticobiliary system, although gastric involvement is most common.[21] Patients present in childhood or as young adults with

Fig. 5. (*A*) Lymphomatoid gastropathy shows a diffuse infiltration of medium-sized to large atypical lymphoid cells with an NK-cell phenotype with positive cytoplasmic CD3 (*B*), CD56 (*C*), and granzyme B (*D*) stains (H&E, original magnification, [*B–D*] ×10).

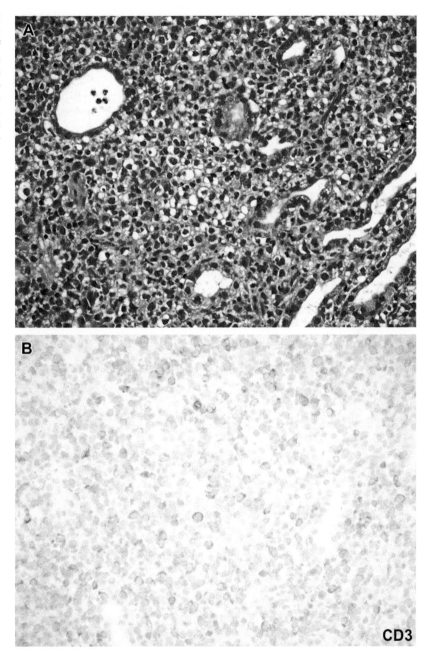

malabsorptive symptoms and failure to thrive, often with an atopic history and peripheral eosinophilia. Other symptoms include nausea, vomiting, abdominal pain, bloating, weight loss, and/or diarrhea.[22] Endoscopic abnormalities include mucosal nodularity, pseudopolyps, hypertrophic gastric folds, and/or vesicles.[6,22] The disease is exquisitely sensitive to systemic

corticosteroid therapy and, in fact, failure to respond to treatment may suggest an alternative diagnosis.

Mucosal findings include an overall increase in lamina propria eosinophils, often with clustering, and intraepithelial aggregates of eosinophils. Gastric pseudopolyps, luminal eosinophilic abscesses, and extension of eosinophils into the

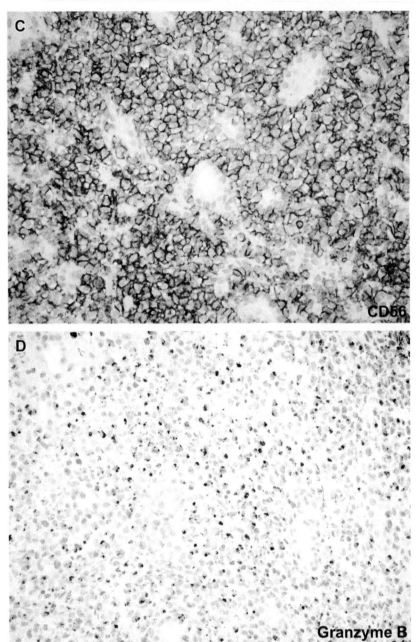

Fig. 5. (*continued*).

muscularis mucosae and submucosa are characteristic.[22] Although mucosal, mural, and serosal forms of disease have been described, most patients with mural and/or serosal involvement also have mucosal eosinophilia. In fact, eosinophils confined to the bowel wall or serosa should prompt concern for another disorder. Patients with subserosal involvement tend to have ascites with high eosinophil counts. The distribution of eosinophils can be patchy, so extensive sampling of the gastric mucosa may be required.[6]

Eosinophilic gastroenteritis is a diagnosis of exclusion; increased eosinophils in the gastric mucosa can be associated with a variety of other etiologies that need to be excluded before establishing a

Fig. 6. Lymphocytic gastritis with increased small T lymphocytes in the surface and foveolar epithelium as well as the expansion of the lamina propria (H&E, original magnification, ×10).

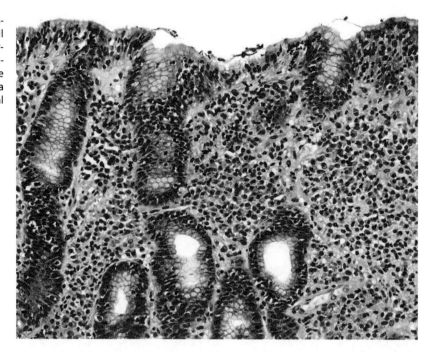

diagnosis. Several food and drug allergies, systemic connective tissue disorders, collagen vascular diseases, vasculitides, Crohn's disease, *H pylori* infection, and even gastric cancer and lymphoma can all be associated with mucosal eosinophilia. Parasitic infection, such as *Strongyloides*, elicits a variably dense eosinophilic response in biopsy samples, whereas *Anisakis* can cause mural and serosal eosinophilia as parasites infiltrate the gastric wall (**Fig. 8**).

Fig. 7. Marked eosinophil-rich infiltrates expand the superficial lamina propria in a case of eosinophilic gastritis (H&E, original magnification, ×4).

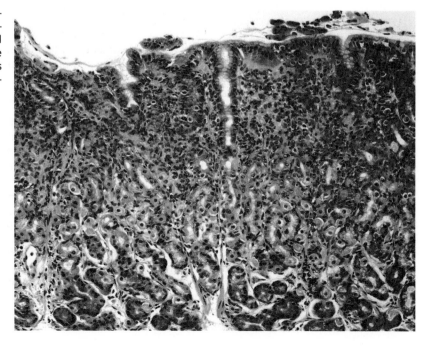

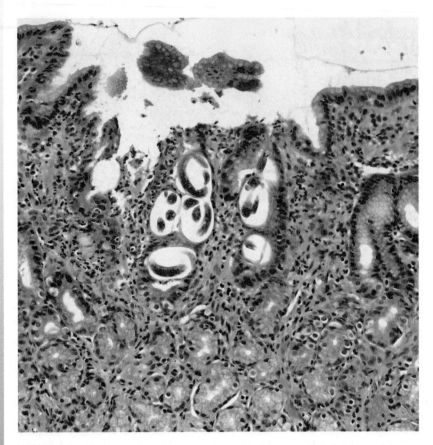

Fig. 8. Gastric Strongyloides in an immunosuppressed patient shows a very limited inflammatory response associated with larvae (H&E, original magnification, ×10).

GASTRITIS WITH PREDOMINANTLY NEUTROPHILIC INFLAMMATION

Acute Suppurative (Phlegmonous) Gastritis

Phlegmonous gastritis is caused by local or disseminated bacterial infection and, by definition, unaccompanied by intramural air. It is mainly caused by *Streptococcus* spp, particularly *Streptococcus pyogenes*, but *Staphylococcus* spp, *Haemophilus influenzae*, *Klebsiella pneumoniae*, *Enterococcus* spp, *Clostridium* spp, and other organisms have been implicated.[23] Symptoms include intense epigastric pain, nausea, vomiting, diarrhea, and/or hematemesis accompanied by edematous and erythematous gastric folds with fibrinopurulent discharge. Extensive mucosal injury with neutrophil-rich infiltrates, submucosal neutrophilic abscesses, and bacterial organisms are characteristic and may be accompanied by extensive mucosal and mural necrosis.[6] Immunosuppression is a major risk factor, but some patients may present without any risk factors. Phlegmonous gastritis has also been reported following endoscopic resection.[24] The mortality rate is high (27%), so early treatment with broad-spectrum antibiotic therapy and possible surgery are important.

Emphysematous Gastritis

Emphysematous gastritis is a severe form of phlegmonous gastritis characterized by intramural gas formation and systemic toxicity. Risk factors include ingestion of corrosive substances, alcohol abuse, diabetes mellitus, use of immunosuppressive agents, dialysis, and recent abdominal surgery or gastroenteritis.[25] Various gas-forming bacterial organisms have been implicated, including *Clostridium* spp, *Escherichia coli*, *Streptococcus* spp, *Klebsiella* spp, *Enterococcus* spp, *Staphylococcus* spp, *Enterobacter* spp, and *Pseudomonas aeruginosa*. Fungal organisms including *Candida* spp and *Mucor* spp may also be encountered.[26] Endoscopy reveals erythema, erosions, nodularity, and necrosis. Computerized tomography is a sensitive and specific modality for detecting intramural gas and determining its extent.[26] Biopsies typically show cystically dilated glands with diffuse neutrophilic inflammation, bacterial organisms, ulcers, hemorrhage, and/or necrosis. The mortality rate is quite high, and treatment consists of broad-spectrum antibiotics, supportive care, and/or possible surgery.[26]

Doxycycline-Induced Gastritis

Doxycycline is used to treat acne, urinary tract infection, pelvic inflammatory disease, and Lyme disease. Thus, many patients with doxycycline-related gastric injury are young adults, although older debilitated patients and those with gastric dysmotility are also at risk.[27,28] Doxycycline is acidic in solution and can cause caustic mucosal injury in the esophagus and stomach. Patients present with odynophagia and epigastric/retrosternal pain due to multiple, superficial linear ulcerations. Gastric biopsies show acute erosive gastritis with neutrophilic inflammation in glandular epithelium and coagulative necrosis of the mucosa and capillary walls (Fig. 9).[28,29] Discontinuation of the medication typically leads to the resolution of the mucosal lesions.

GASTRITIS WITH GRANULOMATOUS INFLAMMATION

CROHN'S DISEASE

Isolated gastric Crohn's disease was once thought to be uncommon, but recent data suggest that 34% to 83% of patients who ultimately prove to have Crohn's disease have either endoscopic or histologic evidence of the disease, particularly in the pediatric population[30,31] (Fig. 10). Endoscopic findings include nodularity, antral fold thickening, friability, loss of vascular pattern, and aphthous or linear ulcers. Granulomata are more common in the antrum; they tend to be small, superficial, and loose (Fig. 11A). The background mucosa may show diffuse chronic gastritis similar to H pylori–associated injury or, more commonly, focally enhanced gastritis.[30,32] The latter appears as focal lymphohistiocytic inflammation involving a few foveolae/glands with or without neutrophils (see Fig. 11B). Focally enhanced gastritis is not a specific diagnostic marker of Crohn's disease; it can be seen in up to 20.8% of children with ulcerative colitis.[33]

SARCOIDOSIS

Gastric sarcoidosis accounts for 1% to 22% of granulomatous gastritis cases and presents either as an isolated finding or part of a multisystem disease.[31] Symptoms are nonspecific and include pain, dyspepsia, early satiety, and/or weight loss. Endoscopy may demonstrate nodularity, erosions, and/or rigidity of gastric wall.[34] Although the diagnosis requires correlation with clinical findings and exclusion of other granulomatous diseases, the presence of compact, non-necrotic granulomata in an otherwise normal mucosa, and detection of

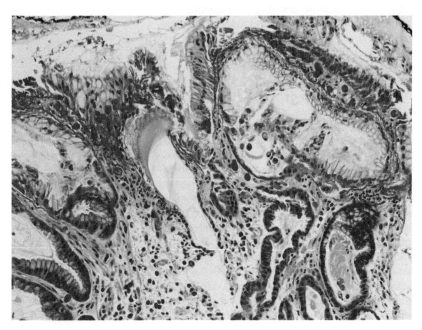

Fig. 9. Doxycycline-induced gastritis characterized by acute erosive gastritis with neutrophilic inflammation, erosion, and/or ulceration (H&E, original magnification, ×10).

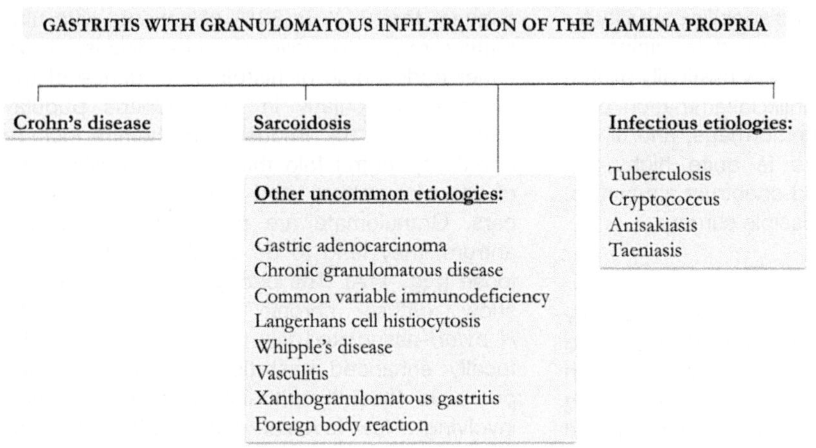

GASTRITIS WITH GRANULOMATOUS INFILTRATION OF THE LAMINA PROPRIA

Crohn's disease   Sarcoidosis   Infectious etiologies:

                                                        Tuberculosis
                         Other uncommon etiologies: Cryptococcus
                                                        Anisakiasis
                         Gastric adenocarcinoma   Taeniasis
                         Chronic granulomatous disease
                         Common variable immunodeficiency
                         Langerhans cell histiocytosis
                         Whipple's disease
                         Vasculitis
                         Xanthogranulomatous gastritis
                         Foreign body reaction

Fig. 10. Differential diagnosis of gastritis with granulomatous infiltration in the lamina propria.

extragastric granulomatous disease are highly suggestive (**Fig. 12**).

INFECTIOUS GASTRITIS

Gastric tuberculosis usually occurs in immunocompromised patients or patients from endemic areas, typically without concomitant pulmonary disease.[6,31] Gastric biopsy is an adequate and rapid diagnostic tool, because the presence of necrotizing granulomata is highly suggestive of tuberculosis and a differentiating feature from Crohn's disease. Other characteristic features include large (400 μm in diameter), confluent granulomata, peri-granulomatous lymphoid cuff, submucosal location, and disproportionate submucosal compared with mucosal inflammation.[35] The diagnosis is confirmed by detection of acid-fast bacilli using special stains, culture, and/or PCR.

Fungal and parasitic infections, including cryptococcus, anisakiasis, and taeniasis, can cause granulomatous gastritis. Cryptococcal infection can present as either a disseminated disease or an isolated finding, and may be detected using mucicarmine-stained sections.[36] Granulomatous inflammation of anisakiasis is accompanied by edema, marked eosinophilia surrounding central abscesses, and/or granulation tissue that can produce an inflammatory mass, mimicking eosinophilic gastroenteritis.[6]

Once Crohn's disease, sarcoidosis, and infections have been excluded, the differential diagnosis of granulomatous gastritis includes several uncommon entities. Rare cases of invasive gastric adenocarcinoma may be accompanied by granulomatous gastritis. Chronic granulomatous disease,[37] common variable immunodeficiency,[38] Langerhans cell histiocytosis,[39] Whipple's disease,[40] vasculitis (including granulomatosis with polyangiitis),[41,42] and xanthogranulomatous gastritis can all elicit granulomatous inflammation accompanied by variable amounts of chronic inflammation in the lamina propria. Impacted food, surgical material, and drugs (ie, antacids containing magnesium, aluminum, and silicon) also can elicit a giant cell–rich reaction in the gastric mucosa.[31]

GASTRITIS WITH LIMITED LAMINA PROPRIA INFLAMMATION

GASTRITIS WITH VIRAL INCLUSIONS

Cytomegalovirus-Associated Gastritis

Reactivation of cytomegalovirus (CMV) occurs in immunocompromised patients. It usually causes nonspecific symptoms and endoscopic findings, although pediatric patients can develop foveolar hyperplasia similar to Menetrier's disease[43] (**Fig. 13**). Infected cells are typically neutral mucin-containing foveolar-type or pyloric-type cells that contain homogeneous eosinophilic intranuclear inclusions and/or granular basophilic intracytoplasmic inclusions (**Fig. 14**).[6] Immunohistochemistry can confirm the diagnosis.

Herpes Simplex Virus–Associated Gastritis

Most patients with Herpes Simplex Virus (HSV)-associated gastritis are immunocompromised patients who present with hematemesis, mucosal

Fig. 11. (*A*) The antral biopsy from a patient with Crohn's disease demonstrates an ill-formed granuloma (H&E, original magnification, ×10). (*B*) Focally enhanced gastritis affects a few adjacent glands (H&E, original magnification, ×10).

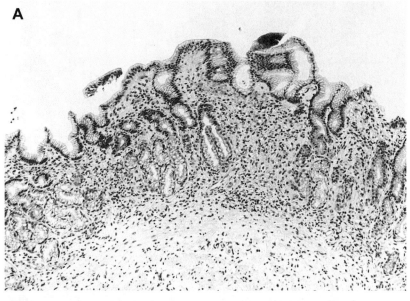

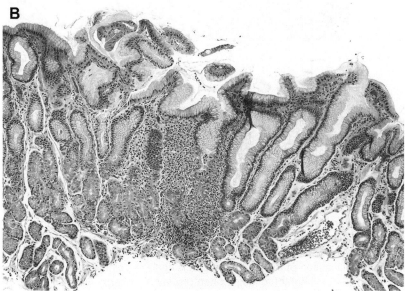

congestion, shallow ulcers, and edema.[44] Biopsies contain single and clumped epithelial cells that contain either ground-glass nuclear inclusions or eosinophilic intranuclear inclusions surrounded by halos. Infection may be accompanied by marked reactive foveolar hyperplasia.[44]

GASTRITIS WITH HEMORRHAGE AND/OR NECROSIS

Caustic Gastritis

Caustic gastritis results from ingestion of acidic or alkaline agents and leads to severe gastric injury.

The antrum is most commonly affected, but extent and severity of disease vary depending on the ingested agent.[45] Endoscopic findings include diffuse mucosal edema, hemorrhage, coagulative necrosis, and deep ulcers.[45,46] Bleach, detergent, and ammonia usually cause mild injury that responds to medical treatment, whereas ingestion of stronger acidic or alkaline agents can result in perforation, scarring, and/or stricture.[45,46]

Ulcero-Hemorrhagic Gastritis

Acute ulcero-hemorrhagic gastritis is an important cause of hematemesis, especially in patients with

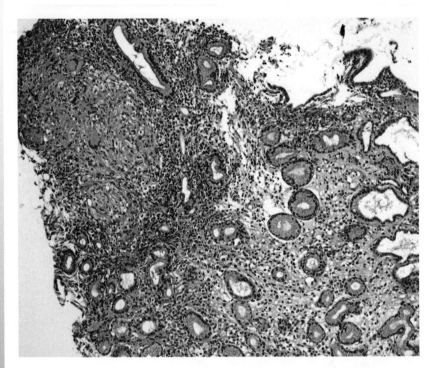

Fig. 12. Gastric sarcoidosis shows a compact, noncaseating granuloma (H&E, original magnification, ×10).

a history of nonsteroidal anti-inflammatory drug (NSAID) use, alcohol abuse, portal hypertension, and/or physiologic stress resulting from life-threatening conditions. An edematous and hyperemic gastric mucosa with multiple petechiae or diffuse hemorrhage is characteristic.[6,31] Histologic changes include mucosal edema, congestion, erosions, and/or hemorrhage of the lamina propria, without significant inflammation.[47] Foveolar hyperplasia with a thickened muscularis mucosae and fibromuscularization of the lamina propria is characteristic (**Fig. 15**). Intact foveolae often display a

mild degree of serration and are lined by mucin depleted epithelial cells; glands show ischemic-type changes with mucin depletion. Severe injury can result in deep ulcers with transmural necrosis.[6,31]

REACTIVE (CHEMICAL) GASTROPATHY

Reactive gastropathy results from mucosal irritants including bile reflux, NSAIDs, and alcohol.[31,48] The disease is quite common: long-term NSAID users have a 50% chance of

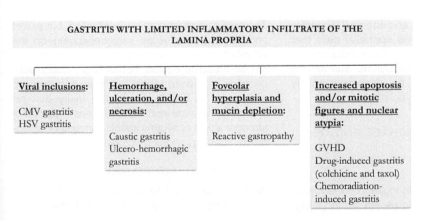

GASTRITIS WITH LIMITED INFLAMMATORY INFILTRATE OF THE LAMINA PROPRIA			
Viral inclusions:	**Hemorrhage, ulceration, and/or necrosis:**	**Foveolar hyperplasia and mucin depletion:**	**Increased apoptosis and/or mitotic figures and nuclear atypia:**
CMV gastritis HSV gastritis	Caustic gastritis Ulcero-hemorrhagic gastritis	Reactive gastropathy	GVHD Drug-induced gastritis (colchicine and taxol) Chemoradiation-induced gastritis

Fig. 13. Differential diagnosis of gastritis with limited inflammation in the lamina propria.

Fig. 14. In CMV gastritis, infected cells show characteristic eosinophilic intranuclear inclusions (surrounded by a clear halo, arrow) and/or granular basophilic intracyto-plasmic inclusions. These changes can be seen in the epithelial, endothelial, and stromal cells (H&E, original magnification, ×20).

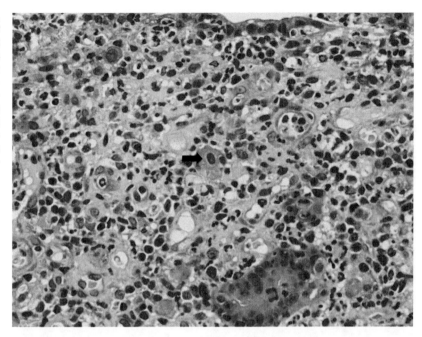

developing gastric erosions and a 10% to 30% incidence of gastric ulcers.[49] Characteristic features include foveolar hyperplasia with a corkscrew appearance likely resulting from increased surface exfoliation, mucin depletion in foveolar epithelium, nuclear enlargement, and hyperchromasia (**Fig. 16**).[6,31,50] Smooth muscle fibers in the lamina propria and superficial mucosal congestion with edema are common findings.[51,52] Scattered eosinophils are often present in the lamina propria; neutrophils are generally lacking unless erosions are also present.

Fig. 15. Acute ulcero-hemorragic gastritis demonstrates erosion with the residual glands displaying regenerative changes with basophilic epithelium (H&E, original magnification, ×4).

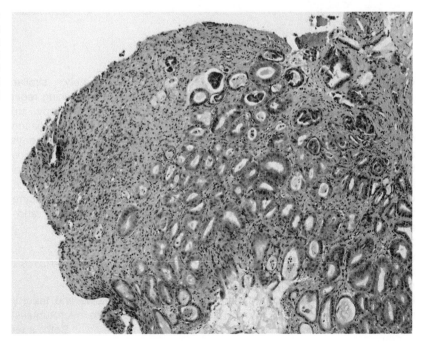

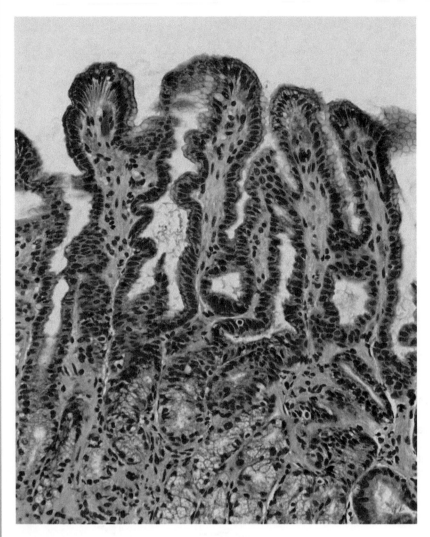

Fig. 16. Reactive gastropathy shows foveolar hyperplasia, tortuosity of the gastric crypts, and mucin depletion (H&E, original magnification, ×20).

GASTRITIS WITH INCREASED APOPTOSIS AND/OR ATYPICAL MITOTIC FIGURES

Graft-Versus-Host Disease

Graft-versus-host disease (GVHD) can happen as early as 1 to 2 months following allogeneic bone marrow transplantation and occurs when immunocompetent donor T cells target antigens on recipient epithelial cells.[6,31,53] Symptoms include nausea, vomiting, dyspepsia, anorexia, and/or food intolerance, but endoscopic findings are usually minimal. Diagnostic features include scattered necrotic epithelial cells and apoptotic cellular debris that are most pronounced in the neck region, while sparing the surface epithelium. Glands are often dilated and contain granular eosinophilic debris without substantial inflammation in the lamina propria (**Fig. 17**).

Unfortunately, similar changes can result from conditioning regimens using radiation and/or chemotherapy during the peritransplant period. For this reason, biopsies should be obtained at least 20 days after transplantation. Of note, severe GVHD with gland destruction or complete loss of epithelium is uncommonly encountered in gastric biopsies; these findings may result from cytoreductive regimens that involve radiation and chemotherapy, or CMV infection.[6,31,54,55]

Drug-Induced Gastritis Due to Colchicine and Taxol

Colchicine and taxol inhibit tubulin polymerization into microtubules and lead to mitotic arrest.[27,56,57] Both agents can cause identical

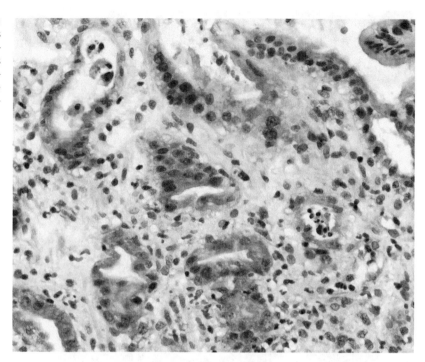

Fig. 17. GVHD often shows dilated glands with granular eosinophilic debris as well as single epithelial cell necrosis/apoptosis in the neck region (H&E, original magnification, ×20).

morphologic alterations in the gastrointestinal tract that can be detected within 2 weeks of drug administration. These include epithelial cell injury associated with increased mitotic activity and mitotic figures arrested in metaphase that appear as "ring" mitoses (**Fig. 18**). Apoptotic debris is readily identified in gastric pits and glands, particularly in the antrum.[56] Of note, features of mitotic arrest are routinely observed in patients who receive taxol and related agents; their detection in biopsy samples is expected and clinically inconsequential. However, ring mitotic figures are observed only in association with high levels of colchicine and, thus, their presence in biopsy samples is a reflection of drug toxicity.

Chemoradiation-Induced Gastritis

Ionizing radiation and chemotherapeutic agents, such as mitomycin C, 5-fluoro-2-deoxyuridine, and floxuridine, can cause substantial nuclear abnormalities in proliferating epithelia of the gastrointestinal tract.[58–60] These changes are usually confined to deep glands and are often accompanied by similar changes in endothelial cells and fibroblasts (**Fig. 19**). Mucin depletion, cell necrosis, erosions, and ulcers are common; radiation may cause endothelial proliferation and/or fibrinoid necrosis of vascular walls.

GASTRITIS CHARACTERIZED BY CRYSTAL OR PIGMENT DEPOSITION

IRON PILL GASTRITIS

Iron-induced injury can be detected after taking iron tablets[61] (**Fig. 20**). The patients can be either asymptomatic or complain of epigastric discomfort, nausea, and/or vomiting. Upper endoscopy may show erythema, small hemorrhage, erosions, and/or ulcerations. Biopsies typically display features of reactive gastropathy associated with gold-brown pigment deposits in the superficial mucosa (**Fig. 21**). Erosions with brown-black crystalline material may be seen in older patients with decreased saliva production who spend more time in the recumbent position.[27,62] These changes should be differentiated from gastric siderosis due to systemic iron overload or hemochromatosis, which tends to show more prominent deposition in the basal glandular epithelium, rather than the lamina propria.[63]

GASTRIC MUCOSAL CALCINOSIS

Gastric mucosal calcinosis reflects accumulation of aluminum phosphate secondary to antacid use or sucralfate therapy in patients with organ transplantation or chronic renal failure.[64] Deposits appear as dark pink to purple, partially calcified,

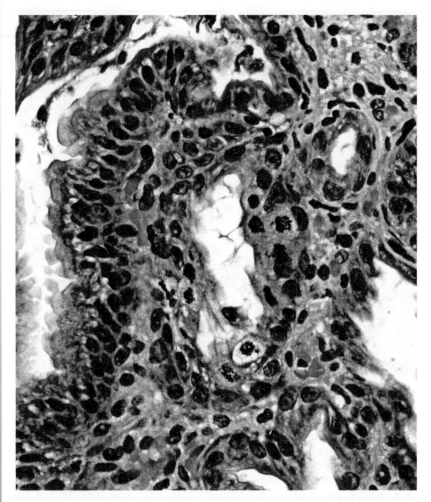

Fig. 18. The presence of arrested mitotic figures is characteristic in drug-induced gastritis due to colchicine and taxol (H&E, original magnification, ×40).

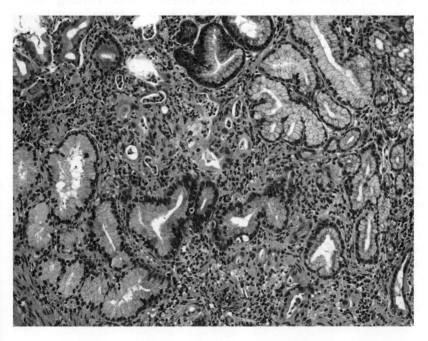

Fig. 19. Chemoradiation may induce significant nuclear atypia, but the change is typically confined to the base of glands (H&E, original magnification, ×4).

Fig. 20. Differential diagnosis of gastritis with crystal or pigment deposition.

GASTRITIS WITH CRYSTAL OR PIGMENT DEPOSITION

Iron-pilled gastritis:	Gastric mucosa calcinosis:	Lanthanum carbonate:	Kayexalate in sorbitol:
Golden brown pigment in a background of reactive gastropathy-type changes	Dark pink to purple, partially calcified, refractile crystals just beneath the surface epithelium	Fine, granular, brownish material in the cytoplasm of histiocytes	Slightly basophilic, rhomboid or triangular in shape with a characteristic mosaic pattern

Fig. 21. (A) The deposition of golden brown pigment is characteristic in iron-pilled gastritis, and an iron stain (B) is confirmatory (H&E, original magnification, [A, B] ×10).

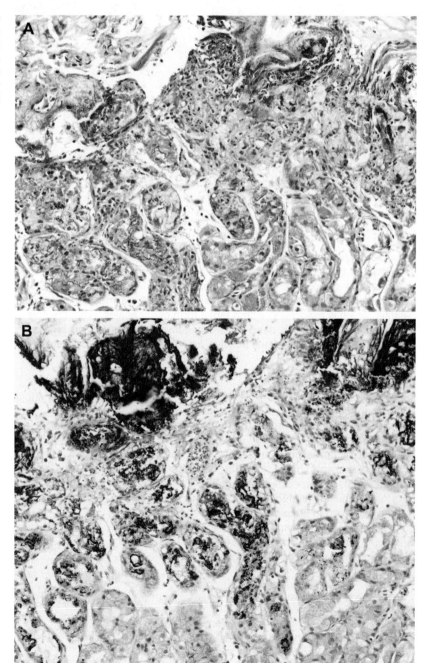

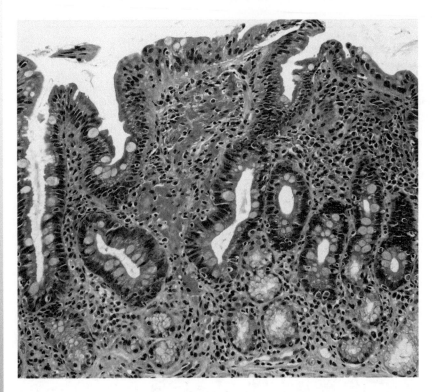

Fig. 22. Lanthanum carbonate is characterized by fine, granular, brownish material deposited within the cytoplasm of histiocytes (H&E, original magnification, ×10).

refractile crystals located subjacent to the surface epithelium at the tips of foveolae.[64] The mucosal changes and deposits are not dissimilar from those recently reported as OsmoPrep-associated gastritis, which is associated with a tablet form of sodium phosphate.[65] The deposits are negative for iron and Alizarin stains but positive for Von-Kossa stain.

LANTHANUM CARBONATE

Lanthanum carbonate is a phosphate-binding agent used to treat hyperphosphatemia in dialysis patients.[66,67] It is poorly absorbed, and gastric deposition is common. More than 85% of dialysis patients have mucosal deposits.[66] Fine, granular, brown material is located in histiocytes or multinucleated giant cells, but can also be observed in areas of erosion and the superficial mucosa, raising the possibility that lanthanum carbonate adheres to erosions and is subsequently entrapped in macrophages[66,67] (Fig. 22).

KAYEXALATE IN SORBITOL

Kayexalate is used to treat hyperkalemia in patients with acute or chronic renal failure, and is usually delivered in sorbitol.[68] The sorbitol carrier is directly toxic to the gastrointestinal mucosa and can cause severe ulcers, perforation, or even death. The crystals are basophilic, rhomboid, or triangular in shape, and have a characteristic internal mosaic pattern that may be likened to fish scales. The crystals are red on Periodic acid-Schiff/Alcian blue and acid-fast stains, and blue with Diff-Quik stain.[68]

REFERENCES

1. Krasinskas AM, Abraham SC, Metz DC, et al. Oxyntic mucosa pseudopolyps: a presentation of atrophic autoimmune gastritis. Am J Surg Pathol 2003; 27:236–41.
2. Torbenson M, Abraham SC, Boitnott J, et al. Autoimmune gastritis: distinct histological and immunohistochemical findings before complete loss of oxyntic glands. Mod Pathol 2002;15:102–9.
3. Coati I, Fassan M, Farinati F, et al. Autoimmune gastritis: pathologist's viewpoint. World J Gastroenterol 2015;21:12179–89.
4. Solcia E, Fiocca R, Villani L, et al. Morphology and pathogenesis of endocrine hyperplasias, precarcinoid lesions, and carcinoids arising in chronic atrophic gastritis. Scand J Gastroenterol Suppl 1991; 180:146–59.
5. Greenstein DB, Wilcox CM, Schwartz DA. Gastric syphilis. Report of seven cases and review of the literature. J Clin Gastroenterol 1994;18:4–9.

6. Lauwers GY, Fujita H, Nagata K, et al. Pathology of non-*Helicobacter pylori* gastritis: extending the histopathologic horizons. J Gastroenterol 2010;45:131–45.

7. Chen CY, Chi KH, George RW, et al. Diagnosis of gastric syphilis by direct immunofluorescence staining and real-time PCR testing. J Clin Microbiol 2006;44:3452–6.

8. Ma C, Park JY, Montgomery EA, et al. A comparative clinicopathologic study of collagenous gastritis in children and adults: the same disorder with associated immune-mediated diseases. Am J Surg Pathol 2015;39:802–12.

9. Kamimura K, Kobayashi M, Sato Y, et al. Collagenous gastritis: review. World J Gastrointest Endosc 2015;7:265–73.

10. Arnason T, Brown IS, Goldsmith JD, et al. Collagenous gastritis: a morphologic and immunohistochemical study of 40 patients. Mod Pathol 2015;28:533–44.

11. Kamimura K, Kobayashi M, Narisawa R, et al. Collagenous gastritis: endoscopic and pathologic evaluation of the nodularity of gastric mucosa. Dig Dis Sci 2007;52:995–1000.

12. Vakiani E, Arguelles-Grande C, Mansukhani MM, et al. Collagenous sprue is not always associated with dismal outcomes: a clinicopathological study of 19 patients. Mod Pathol 2010;23:12–26.

13. Chen ZM, Shah R, Zuckerman GR, et al. Epstein-Barr virus gastritis: an underrecognized form of severe gastritis simulating gastric lymphoma. Am J Surg Pathol 2007;31:1446–51.

14. Owens SR, Walls A, Krasinskas AM, et al. Epstein-Barr virus gastritis: rare or rarely sampled? A case report. Int J Surg Pathol 2011;19:196–8.

15. Takeuchi K, Yokoyama M, Ishizawa S, et al. Lymphomatoid gastropathy: a distinct clinicopathologic entity of self-limited pseudomalignant NK-cell proliferation. Blood 2010;116:5631–7.

16. Mansoor A, Pittaluga S, Beck PL, et al. NK-cell enteropathy: a benign NK-cell lymphoproliferative disease mimicking intestinal lymphoma: clinicopathologic features and follow-up in a unique case series. Blood 2011;117:1447–52.

17. Takata K, Noujima-Harada M, Miyata-Takata T, et al. Clinicopathologic analysis of 6 lymphomatoid gastropathy cases: expanding the disease spectrum to CD4-CD8+ cases. Am J Surg Pathol 2015;39:1259–66.

18. Wu TT, Hamilton SR. Lympocytic gastritis: association with etiology and topology. Am J Surg Pathol 1999;23:153–8.

19. Cui I, Chen Z, Panarelli N, et al. Patterns of lymphocytic gastritis may reflect the underlying etiology. Mod Pathol 2016;29(suppl. 2):167A.

20. Collins MH. Histopathology associated with eosinophilic gastrointestinal diseases. Immunol Allergy Clin North Am 2009;29:109–17.

21. Rothenberg ME. Eosinophilic gastrointestinal disorders (EGID). J Allergy Clin Immunol 2004;113:11–28.

22. Cianferoni A, Spergel JM. Eosinophilic esophagitis and gastroenteritis. Curr Allergy Asthma Rep 2015;15:58.

23. Kim GY, Ward J, Henessey B, et al. Phlegmonous gastritis: case report and review. Gastrointest Endosc 2005;61:168–74.

24. Lee BS, Kim SM, Seong JK, et al. Phlegmonous gastritis after endoscopic mucosal resection. Endoscopy 2005;37:490–3.

25. Allan K, Barriga J, Afshani M, et al. Emphysematous gastritis. Am J Med Sci 2005;329:205–7.

26. Huang CT, Liao WY. Emphysematous gastritis: a deadly infectious disease. Scand J Infect Dis 2009;41:317–9.

27. Parfitt JR, Driman DK. Pathological effects of drugs on the gastrointestinal tract: a review. Hum Pathol 2007;38:527–36.

28. Leber A, Stal J. Simultaneous esophageal and gastric ulceration due to doxycycline ingestion: case report and review of the literature. Gastroenterology Res 2012;5:236–8.

29. Chuang JY, Brown I, Conway L, et al. Doxycycline induced gastritis and oesophageal ulcer. Pathology 2016;48:S121.

30. Polydorides AD. Pathology and differential diagnosis of chronic, noninfectious gastritis. Semin Diagn Pathol 2014;31:114–23.

31. Srivastava A, Lauwers GY. Pathology of non-infective gastritis. Histopathology 2007;50:15–29.

32. Xin W, Greenson JK. The clinical significance of focally enhanced gastritis. Am J Surg Pathol 2004;28:1347–51.

33. Sharif F, McDermott M, Dillon M, et al. Focally enhanced gastritis in children with Crohn's disease and ulcerative colitis. Am J Gastroenterol 2002;97:1415–20.

34. Kaneki T, Koizumi T, Yamamoto H, et al. Gastric sarcoidosis–a single polypoid appearance in the involvement. Hepatogastroenterology 2001;48:1209–10.

35. Pulimood AB, Amarapurkar DN, Ghoshal U, et al. Differentiation of Crohn's disease from intestinal tuberculosis in India in 2010. World J Gastroenterol 2011;17:433–43.

36. Washington K, Gottfried MR, Wilson ML. Gastrointestinal cryptococcosis. Mod Pathol 1991;4:707–11.

37. Varma VA, Sessions JT, Kahn LB, et al. Chronic granulomatous disease of childhood presenting as gastric outlet obstruction. Am J Surg Pathol 1982;6:673–6.

38. Washington K, Stenzel TT, Buckley RH, et al. Gastrointestinal pathology in patients with common variable immunodeficiency and X-linked agammaglobulinemia. Am J Surg Pathol 1996;20:1240–52.

39. Groisman GM, Rosh JR, Harpaz N. Langerhans cell histiocytosis of the stomach. A cause of

granulomatous gastritis and gastric polyposis. Arch Pathol Lab Med 1994;118:1232–5.

40. Ectors N, Geboes K, Wynants P, et al. Granulomatous gastritis and Whipple's disease. Am J Gastroenterol 1992;87:509–13.

41. Temmesfeld-Wollbrueck B, Heinrichs C, Szalay A, et al. Granulomatous gastritis in Wegener's disease: differentiation from Crohn's disease supported by a positive test for antineutrophil antibodies. Gut 1997;40:550–3.

42. O'Donovan C, Murray J, Staunton H, et al. Granulomatous gastritis: part of a vasculitic syndrome. Hum Pathol 1991;22:1057–9.

43. Eisenstat DD, Griffiths AM, Cutz E, et al. Acute cytomegalovirus infection in a child with Ménétrier's disease. Gastroenterology 1995;109:592–5.

44. Jun DW, Kim DH, Kim SH, et al. Ménétrier's disease associated with herpes infection: response to treatment with acyclovir. Gastrointest Endosc 2007;65:1092–5.

45. Poley JW, Steyerberg EW, Kuipers EJ, et al. Ingestion of acid and alkaline agents: outcome and prognostic value of early upper endoscopy. Gastrointest Endosc 2004;60:372–7.

46. García Díaz E, Castro Fernández M, Romero Gómez M, et al. Upper gastrointestinal tract injury caused by ingestion of caustic substances. Gastroenterol Hepatol 2001;24:191–5.

47. Wolfe MM, Lichtenstein DR, Singh G. Gastrointestinal toxicity of nonsteroidal antiinflammatory drugs. N Engl J Med 1999;340:1888–99.

48. Owen DA. Gastritis and carditis. Mod Pathol 2003; 16:325–41.

49. Laine L. Nonsteroidal anti-inflammatory drug gastropathy. Gastrointest Endosc Clin N Am 1996;6:489–504.

50. Lauwers GY, Furman J, Michael LE, et al. Cytoskeletal and kinetic epithelial differences between NSAID gastropathy and Helicobacter pylori gastritis: an immunohistochemical determination. Histopathology 2001;39:133–40.

51. Dixon MF, O'Connor HJ, Axon AT, et al. Reflux gastritis: distinct histopathological entity? J Clin Pathol 1986;39:524–30.

52. Sobala GM, O'Connor HJ, Dewar EP, et al. Bile reflux and intestinal metaplasia in gastric mucosa. J Clin Pathol 1993;46:235–40.

53. Weisdorf DJ, Snover DC, Haake R, et al. Acute upper gastrointestinal graft-versus-host disease: clinical significance and response to immunosuppressive therapy. Blood 1990;76:624–9.

54. Washington K, Bentley RC, Green A, et al. Gastric graft-versus-host disease: a blinded histologic study. Am J Surg Pathol 1997;21:1037–46.

55. Snover DC, Weisdorf SA, Vercellotti GM, et al. A histopathologic study of gastric and small intestinal graft-versus-host disease following allogeneic bone marrow transplantation. Hum Pathol 1985;16: 387–92.

56. Iacobuzio-Donahue CA, Lee EL, Abraham SC, et al. Colchicine toxicity: distinct morphologic findings in gastrointestinal biopsies. Am J Surg Pathol 2001; 25:1067–73.

57. Hruban RH, Yardley JH, Donehower RC, et al. Taxol toxicity. Epithelial necrosis in the gastrointestinal tract associated with polymerized microtubule accumulation and mitotic arrest. Cancer 1989;63: 1944–50.

58. Doria MIJ, Doria LK, Faintuch J, et al. Gastric mucosal injury after hepatic arterial infusion chemotherapy with floxuridine. A clinical and pathologic study. Cancer 1994;73:2042–7.

59. Petras RE, Hart WR, Bukowski RM. Gastric epithelial atypia associated with hepatic arterial infusion chemotherapy. Its distinction from early gastric carcinoma. Cancer 1985;56:745–50.

60. Berthrong M, Fajardo LF. Radiation injury in surgical pathology. Part II. Alimentary tract. Am J Surg Pathol 1981;5:153–78.

61. Abraham SC, Yardley JH, Wu TT. Erosive injury to the upper gastrointestinal tract in patients receiving iron medication: an underrecognized entity. Am J Surg Pathol 1999;23:1241–7.

62. Haig A, Driman DK. Iron-induced mucosal injury to the upper gastrointestinal tract. Histopathology 2006;48:808–12.

63. Marginean EC, Bennick M, Cyczk J, et al. Gastric siderosis: patterns and significance. Am J Surg Pathol 2006;30:514–20.

64. Greenson JK, Trinidad SB, Pfeil SA, et al. Gastric mucosal calcinosis. Calcified aluminum phosphate deposits secondary to aluminum-containing antacids or sucralfate therapy in organ transplant patients. Am J Surg Pathol 1993;17: 45–50.

65. Matsukuma K, Gui D, Olson KA, et al. OsmoPrep-associated gastritis: a histopathologic mimic of iron pill gastritis and mucosal calcinosis. Am J Surg Pathol 2016;40:1550–6.

66. Goto K, Ogawa K. Lanthanum deposition is frequently observed in the gastric mucosa of dialysis patients with lanthanum carbonate therapy: a clinicopathologic study of 13 cases, including 1 case of lanthanum granuloma in the colon and 2 nongranulomatous gastric cases. Int J Surg Pathol 2016;24:89–92.

67. Makino M, Kawaguchi K, Shimojo H, et al. Extensive lanthanum deposition in the gastric mucosa: the first histopathological report. Pathol Int 2015; 65:33–7.

68. Abraham SC, Bhagavan BS, Lee LA, et al. Upper gastrointestinal tract injury in patients receiving kayexalate (sodium polystyrene sulfonate) in sorbitol: clinical, endoscopic, and histopathologic findings. Am J Surg Pathol 2001;25: 637–44.

Practical Approach to the Flattened Duodenal Biopsy

Thomas C. Smyrk, MD

KEYWORDS

- Celiac disease • Intraepithelial lymphocytes • Collagenous sprue • Tropical sprue
- Common variable immunodeficiency

Key points

- Duodenal intraepithelial lymphocytosis is necessary but not specific for a diagnosis of celiac disease.

- The pathology report for a damaged duodenum should include the number of intraepithelial lymphocytes and an assessment of villous injury. The latter can be done descriptively or using published classification systems.

- By paying attention to other histologic features (makeup of lamina propria infiltrate, subepithelial collagen) you may be alerted to a diagnosis other than celiac disease.

ABSTRACT

Celiac disease features duodenal intraepithelial lymphocytosis with or without villous atrophy. Lymphocytosis without villous atrophy will be proven to represent celiac disease in 10% to 20% of cases. The differential diagnosis is broad: *Helicobacter pylori* gastritis, NSAID injury and bacterial overgrowth are considerations. Lymphocytosis with villous atrophy is very likely to be celiac disease, but there are mimics to consider, including collagenous sprue, tropical sprue, drug injury, and common variable immunodeficiency. Histologic clues to a diagnosis other than celiac disease include paucity of plasma cells, excess of neutrophils, granulomas, and relative paucity of intraepithelial lymphocytes.

Duodenal inflammation and villous injury are nonspecific findings. Even when clinical and laboratory findings are known, the diagnosis will be descriptive more often than definitive. This review focuses on celiac disease and other conditions that tend to flatten duodenal mucosa, but it is worth emphasizing at the start that duodenal biopsies should be assessed systematically. Develop a system and stick to it, or you will certainly miss an important finding at some point.

A SYSTEMATIC APPROACH TO DUODENAL BIOPSIES

Scan the entire specimen at low power, looking for focal lesions and assessing villous architecture (**Fig. 1**). Dysplasia, heterotopia, and other abnormal proliferations can all be limited to part of one fragment and are easy to miss if you leave the ×4 objective too quickly. Celiac disease can be patchy too. A definitive opinion about architecture may not be possible at this point, but you should be able to get a feeling for "flat or nearly flat" versus "normal or nearly normal."

Celiac disease sometimes involves only the most proximal part of the duodenum, and biopsy of the duodenal bulb is considered essential to the clinical workup.[1,2] The bulb biopsy might come in a separate container, but usually it will

The author has nothing to disclose.
Department of Pathology, Mayo Clinic, Hilton 11, 200 First Street Southwest, Rochester, MN 55902, USA
E-mail address: Smyrk.thomas@mayo.edu

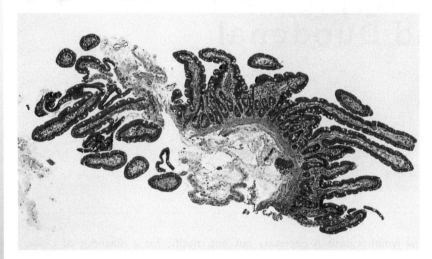

Fig. 1. Normal duo-denum. The orientation is not perfect, but it is good enough to assure one that villous architecture is preserved (H&E, original magnification, ×40).

be mixed with 4 to 6 fragments from the second part of the duodenum. Villi tend to be a bit broader and blunter in the bulb, so watch for that fragment and be careful about making too much of apparent atrophy.

At medium power, look at the mucosal surface for organisms, *Giardia* and *Cryptosporidium* being the main considerations. Then assess the epithelium, which normally has a mix of entero-cytes and goblet cells, with Paneth cells popu-lating the crypts. Healthy enterocytes are columnar and have a brush border; a change to cuboidal cells indicates injury. Mucinous metaplasia commonly accompanies peptic injury and is common in the duodenal bulb. Loss of goblet cells and/or Paneth cells are clues to auto-immune enteropathy, but it is easy to miss the absence of something that is not consciously sought. Apoptotic bodies should be rare; more than 1 or 2 in a biopsy raise consideration for medication effect, viral infection, or graft-versus-host disease.

Duodenal epithelium always has intraepithelial lymphocytes (IELs) distributed along the sides of the villi, usually approximately 10 IELs per 100 epithelial cells (Fig. 2).[3,4] Normal duodenal

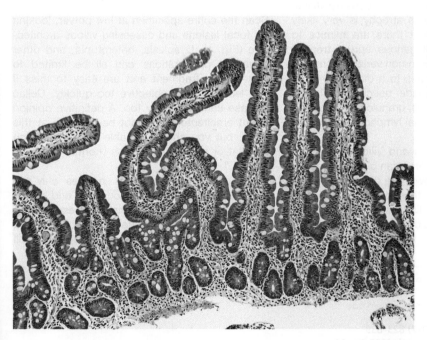

Fig. 2. Normal duo-denum. The 3 well-oriented villi show a villus-crypt ratio of 3:1. IELs are not increased (H&E, original magnifica-tion, ×100).

epithelium does not contain eosinophils or neutrophils; their presence may shift the focus of your diagnosis, so do not assume that all intraepithelial inflammatory cells are equal. As in the colon, subepithelial collagen should be slender (3–5 μm) and even.

Normal lamina propria is dominated by plasma cells, with minor populations of lymphocytes, eosinophils, mast cells, and mesenchymal elements. Histiocytes are generally inconspicuous; clumps or sheets of histiocytes should prompt consideration for special stains to rule out infection. Eosinophils are always present, but density may vary; one study in children found a mean of 9.6 eosinophils per high-power field, with a range up to 26.[5] There may be an association between dyspepsia and increased mucosal eosinophils,[6,7] but I am generally reluctant to diagnose increased eosinophils if they do not form sheets or clumps, or infiltrate surface and gland epithelium, or involve the submucosa.

Duodenal biopsies usually have submucosa at the deep margin. Always look carefully for material suggestive of amyloid. The submucosa is also the place to pick up subtle infiltration by adenocarcinoma of the bile duct or pancreas, which may take the form of 1 or 2 atypical glands (Box 1).

CELIAC DISEASE: HISTOLOGY, REPORTING, SPECIAL SITUATIONS, DIFFERENTIAL DIAGNOSIS

HISTOLOGY

Celiac disease always has increased intraepithelial lymphocytes, currently defined as more than 30 IELs per 100 epithelial cells.[3,4] In celiac disease and other conditions characterized by duodenal lymphocytosis, IELs occupy both the sides and tips of villi, or show a tip-heavy distribution (Fig. 3). Clusters of IELs at the tips of villi are always an abnormal finding.[8] Assessing IELs in the duodenum need not be tedious. Many examples of intraepithelial lymphocytosis will be apparent as you go through your routine: the surface epithelium looks too blue even at medium power. In that case, focus on a few well-preserved areas and consider the IEL-to-epithelial cell ratio: is it 1:1, slightly below 1:1, or above 1:1? Although increasing IEL counts seem to correlate with increasing villous injury, there is no need to do exhaustive counts on obvious cases. At the other extreme, many biopsies will be obviously normal, with only scattered IELs along the sides of villi. Borderline cases require some extra time, but 2 efficient methods have been endorsed in published guidelines[1]: one is to count IELs per 20 enterocytes at the tips of 5 villi[9] and the other is to count IELs per 50 enterocytes along the sides of 2 villi.[10] I prefer the latter method; IELs at the villus tip are sometimes the first clue to an abnormality, but limiting the count only to the tip may miss some cases of duodenal lymphocytosis. Fig. 4 illustrates a duodenal biopsy with minimally increased IELs.

Duodenal IELs are almost exclusively T cells, and can be decorated nicely with antibodies against CD3 (Fig. 5). Villanacci and colleagues,[11] representing the Italian division of the International Academy of Pathology, argue that the IEL count should always be done with the help of immunohistochemistry. My sense is that few US pathologists do this; my own experience is that a good hematoxylin-eosin stain is sufficient for counting IELs. I use immunohistochemistry only as an adjunct on difficult cases; mostly that means on the rare days when our histology laboratory gives me slides with chatter artifact. Up-front use of immunohistochemistry for CD3 and CD8 does not seem to increase the likelihood of detecting an abnormal IEL count.[12]

Duodenal enterocytes often look damaged in celiac disease, especially when there is villous atrophy.[13] They become cuboidal and more basophilic. The lamina propria has increased cellularity, with plasma cells predominating. Brown and colleagues[13] documented an increase in mucosal eosinophils that seems to parallel increasing villous damage. Neutrophils are not usually considered a feature of celiac disease, but Brown and colleagues[13]

Box 1
Key features to evaluate when assessing duodenal biopsy sample

Scan the entire sample at low power

Identify focal lesions, assess villous architecture, identify duodenal bulb

Mucosal surface

Giardia, cryptosporidium

Surface epithelium, damaged epithelium, foveolar metaplasia, intraepithelial inflammation, thickened collagen

Lamina propria

Plasma cells present, eosinophils evenly distributed, neutrophils rare or absent

Submucosa

Amyloid, deep inflammation, granulomas

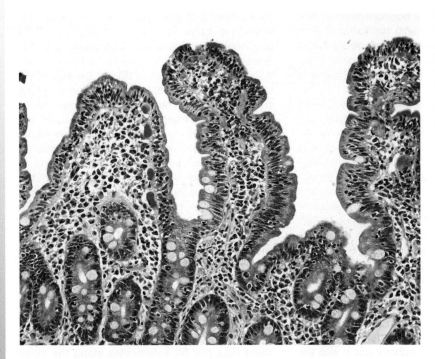

Fig. 3. Three villi with an obvious increase in IELs. I did not count these, but there appear to be as many IELs as epithelial cells, so I would report 100 IELs per 100 epithelial cells (H&E, original magnification, ×200).

found at least focal neutrophil groups (more than 5 in a cluster) in 41% of their patients with celiac disease, and multifocal collections in 15%; crypt abscesses were seen in only 1.3% of cases.

The villus-crypt ratio in the second part of the duodenum should be 3:1 and may be as much as 5:1. This assessment depends on good tissue orientation, generally defined as at least 3 consecutive villi and their associated crypts visible along their entire length. There are advocates for placing duodenal biopsies on a substrate in the endoscopy suite as the best way to achieve proper orientation.[11] Our institution does not follow that advice, and I think we are typical in that regard. Perfect orientation is difficult to come by in routinely processed biopsies, but with multiple tissue fragments sectioned multiple times, areas of adequate orientation usually can be found. Remember that abnormal IELs are more important to the diagnosis of celiac disease than abnormal villi: if you get the IEL right, the appropriate clinical workup will follow regardless of what you say about villous architecture.

SPECIAL SITUATIONS IN CELIAC DISEASE

Ultra-short Celiac Disease

As many as 10% of patients with newly diagnosed celiac disease may have villous atrophy confined to the duodenal bulb.[14] The interpretation of bulb biopsies is complicated by the presence of Brunner glands, peptic injury, and lymphoid follicles, but those distractors can be overcome by being aware that one of the fragments on your slide likely came from the bulb. You may need to relax your criteria for normal villous architecture here, relying on increased IELs as the primary reason to suspect celiac disease, but prospective studies show that moderate to severe atrophy is recognizable in bulb biopsies.[15]

Collagenous Sprue

This is a descriptive diagnosis with several possible etiologies, but is often a complication of celiac disease, so is discussed here. The defining characteristics are villous atrophy and a thickened band of subepithelial collagen (Fig. 6). "Thickened" does not seem to have a uniform definition, but cases reported under this rubric generally have at least patchy areas more than 10 μm thick. Fraying of the band, with wrapping around capillaries, is also a typical feature. Many examples of otherwise typical celiac disease have with focal, minimal thickening of collagen; Brown and colleagues[13] recognized this feature in 45% of their celiac biopsies, although only 4 of their 150 patients had collagen thickness greater than 10 μm. Note the absence of increased IELs in

Fig. 4. (*A*) Increased IELs with normal villous architecture (H&E, original magnification, ×100). (*B*) There is slight tip accentuation, particularly in the left-hand villus (H&E, original magnification, ×200).

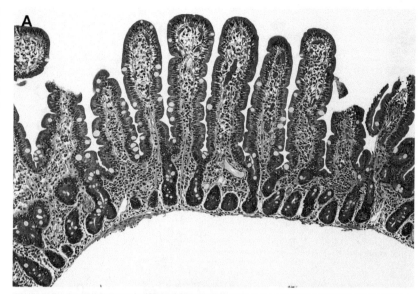

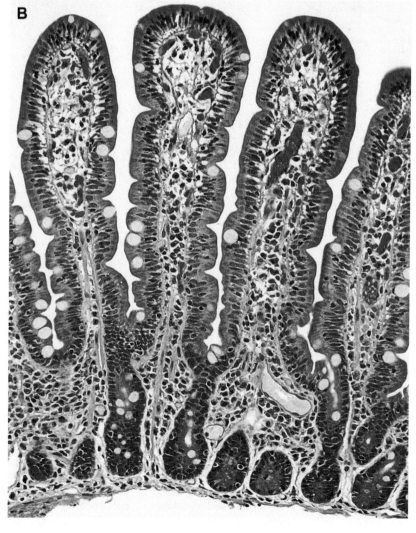

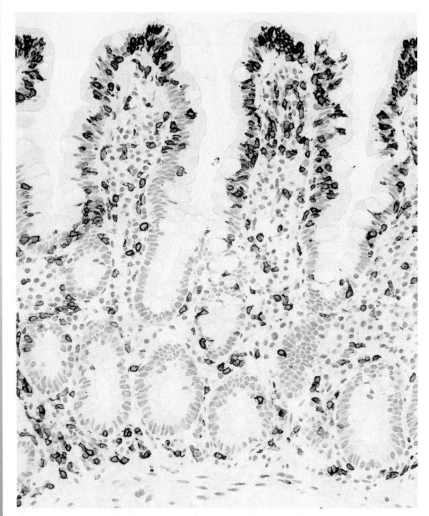

Fig. 5. Immunohistochemical stain for CD3 highlights many IEL in a tip-heavy distribution. I use this stain sparingly, except as part of the workup for refractory celiac disease (CD3, original magnification, ×200).

the definition for collagenous sprue; villous atrophy and increased collagen without increased IELs suggests a cause other than celiac disease.

Collagenous sprue has a reputation as a condition refractory to treatment; this may be undeserved. Rubio-Tapia and colleagues[16] described a series of 30 patients, reporting total villous atrophy in 20 and subtotal atrophy in 10. Collagen thickness ranged from 18 to 95 μm; abnormal collagen was diffuse in 23 patients and patchy in 7. IELs were increased in 21 patients. Celiac disease was the most common underlying risk factor (11 patients). Vakiani and colleagues[17] collected 19 patients with collagenous sprue; 17 had celiac disease and 9 of those were classified as refractory. Eight patients responded to gluten-free diet and 10 responded to immunomodulatory therapy.

Investigators from the Cleveland Clinic described 21 patients, all of whom had symptomatic improvement with gluten-free diet, corticosteroids, or both.[18]

Treated Celiac Disease

All patients with confirmed celiac disease should be on gluten-free diet for life. Because serologic markers for celiac disease are gluten-dependent, they are expected to decline within months of eliminating gluten from the diet. Mucosal healing takes longer: a median of 3 years in one US study.[19] Some adults fail to completely heal despite negative serology and absence of symptoms.[20,21] For that reason, American College of Gastroenterology (ACG) guidelines say that follow-up biopsy "could be

Fig. 6. A subtle case of collagenous sprue. (*A*) Slight villous atrophy and focally thickened subepithelial collagen. (*B*) IELs are not increased, therefore this example of collagenous sprue is not celiac disease (H&E, original magnification, [*A*] ×100 [*B*] ×200).

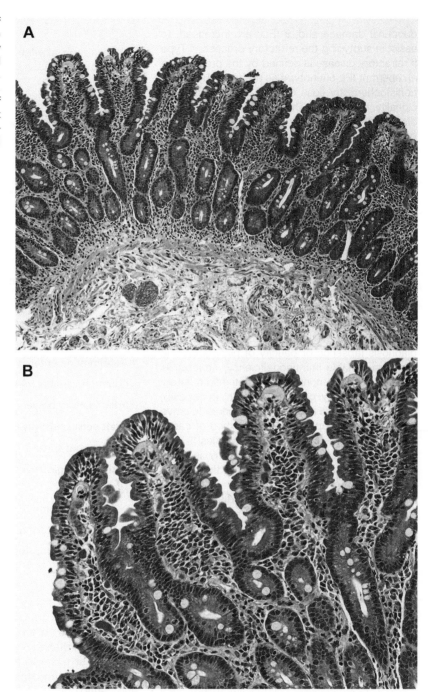

considered" after 2 years on gluten-free diet to assess mucosal healing.[2] The role of the pathologist here is the same as for any other duodenal biopsy: report the number of IELs, describe the state of the villi, and note any other features of interest.

Refractory Celiac Disease

Persistent symptoms or laboratory abnormalities despite 6 to 12 months of gluten-free diet raise consideration for refractory celiac disease.[2] Here, the role of the pathologist is to confirm ongoing duodenal damage and, if IELs are increased, to assist in subtyping the refractory process.[22] Type II refractory disease is defined by the presence of an aberrant IEL phenotype as assessed by immunohistochemistry (loss of CD8) or tests of T-cell clonality, or both.[23,24] The IELs in Type I refractory disease are positive for both CD3 and CD8 and do not have clonal rearrangements of T-cell receptors.

DIFFERENTIAL DIAGNOSIS

The differential diagnosis for celiac disease will vary depending on whether villous architecture is preserved or altered. Increased IELs with normal villous architectures is a relatively common finding in duodenal biopsies, which has been well-covered in recent years.[25,26] A minority (10%–20%) of biopsies with this finding will represent new cases of celiac disease.[27] Box 2 lists proposed associations with this histologic finding. There are a few histologic clues that could narrow the differential diagnosis (absence or paucity of plasma cells in common variable immunodeficiency; neutrophils and erosions in nonsteroidal anti-inflammatory drug (NSAID) injury; granulomas in Crohn disease), but in general it will take a clinical workup to arrive at a diagnosis. Approximately one-third of cases are idiopathic, even in prospective studies.[28]

Increased IELs with villous atrophy is likely to be celiac disease, at least in the United States and Europe. Box 3 lists other considerations, some of which are discussed as follows.

Box 2
Possible causes of increased intraepithelial lymphocytes (IELs) with preserved villous architecture

Celiac disease

Helicobacter pylori gastritis

Giardiasis

Cryptosporidiosis

Nonsteroidal anti-inflammatory drug (NSAID) injury

Small intestinal bacterial overgrowth

Hypersensitivity cow's milk, soy, cereals

Autoimmune conditions (thyroiditis, rheumatoid arthritis)

Immune deficiency (immunoglobulin A deficiency, common variable immunodeficiency)

Inflammatory bowel disease

Box 3
Other causes of villous atrophy with or without increased IEL

Infection
  Tropical sprue
  Small bowel bacterial overgrowth
  Giardiasis
  Tuberculosis
  Whipple disease
  Acquired immune deficiency syndrome enteropathy

Medication injury
  NSAID
  Angiotensin II inhibitors
  Mycophenolate mofetil
  Chemotherapy agents
  Monoclonal antibodies

Autoimmune enteropathy

Common variable immunodeficiency

Inflammatory bowel disease

Graft-versus-host disease

Collagenous sprue

Eosinophilic gastroenteritis

Neoplasia
  T-cell lymphoma
  Type II refractory celiac disease
  Systemic mastocytosis

Tropical Sprue

This acquired disorder is characterized by chronic diarrhea among individuals with residence in or travel to tropical regions (30° north or south of the equator). It is treatable (oral folate and antibiotics) and does not respond to gluten-free diet, so it is a coup to be able to suggest the correct diagnosis on biopsy. Unfortunately, there are no unique histologic features in the duodenum. In my experience, tropical sprue has at least partly preserved villi in the face of marked intraepithelial lymphocytosis, sometimes with prominent eosinophils or patchy neutrophils in the lamina propria (Fig. 7).

A recent series from Australia supported the idea that villous architecture is partly preserved,

Fig. 7. Tropical sprue. (*A*) Markedly increased IELs with partial villous atrophy. Tropical sprue does not usually make the mucosa flat. (*B*) Active cryptitis in tropical sprue (H&E, original magnification, [*A*] ×200 [*B*] ×200).

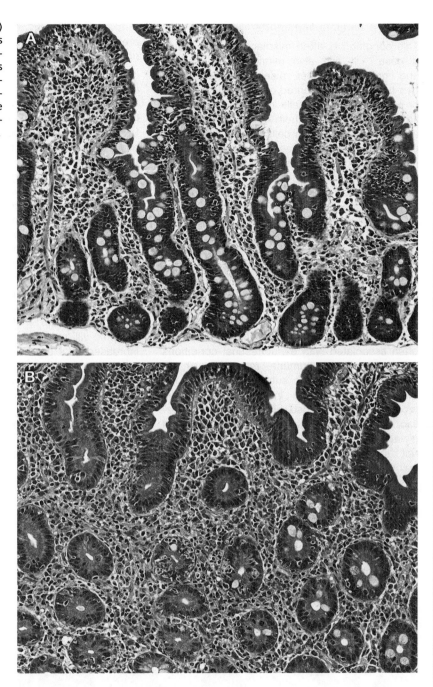

none of the 12 cases had flat mucosa, but IEL counts were similar to those seen in a comparison series of patients with celiac disease.[29] The investigators also found that lamina propria eosinophils were more numerous in tropical sprue compared with celiac disease, and neutrophils were less common. The B12 and folate deficiencies associated with tropical sprue can produce megaloblastoid changes in duodenal epithelium. Tropical sprue affects the entire small bowel, so the best histologic clue to the proper diagnosis is villous atrophy with increased IELs in an ileal biopsy. In the end, tropical sprue is a clinicopathologic diagnosis, depending on travel history, histology, negative celiac serology, absence of response to gluten-free diet, and rapid response to appropriate treatment.

Common Variable Immunodeficiency

This condition is often misdiagnosed as celiac disease.[30] It can also mimic Crohn disease and graft-versus-host disease. One-half to two-thirds of documented cases show absence or paucity of plasma cells in the lamina propria, so you will not miss them if you remember to always look for plasma cells (Fig. 8). ("Paucity" could be defined as having to work hard to find plasma cells; the huge numbers of plasma cells in celiac disease are impossible to miss.) Other histologic clues include lymphoid aggregates, increased crypt apoptosis, increased intraepithelial neutrophils, small mucosal granulomas, and giardiasis or cytomegalovirus infection.[30–32] In one series of 20 patients, 1 patient had increased subepithelial collagen.[30]

Autoimmune Enteropathy

This intractable diarrhea with villous atrophy is often associated with extraintestinal conditions reflecting altered immune regulation or, in children, with systemic autoimmune disease.[33] Villous atrophy is an invariable feature; in most cases, the mucosa is flat. In contrast to celiac disease, the surface epithelium does not always have increased IEL. Characteristic but not invariable features include neutrophils in crypt epithelium, increased apoptosis, and absence of goblet and Paneth cells

(Fig. 9).[34,35] Serum anti-enterocyte antibodies are detected in 80% to 90% of patients but are not entirely specific.

Medication Injury

NSAIDs are well-known as a possible cause of increased IELs. NSAID injury can also produce foveolar metaplasia, ulcers, and erosions. Villous atrophy is not usually a feature of NSAID injury to the duodenum.

Antihypertensive drugs classed as angiotensin II receptor inhibitors have recently emerged as an important mimic of celiac disease.[36] Olmesartan is the subject of most reports, but I have seen a few examples associated with losartan, and a recent review documented cases associated with valsartan, irbesartan, and telmisartan.[37] This is a very gratifying diagnosis to make, because these patients can be quite ill; 14 of 22 patients in the original series required hospitalization for malabsorptive symptoms.[36] Atrophic villi are a nearly invariable feature, but increased IELs are not. In fact, only 61 of 100 reported cases reviewed by Choi and McKenna[38] showed increased IELs. Increased neutrophils were seen in 15 of 22 patients in another series from the Mayo clinic; biopsies from 7 of those patients had thickened subepithelial collagen layers as well (Fig. 10).[36] Lymphocytic gastritis, collagenous gastritis, and collagenous colitis can all be seen if other sites are biopsied.

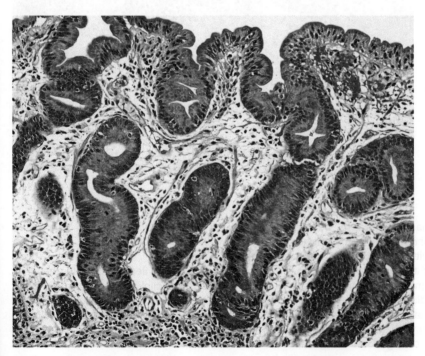

Fig. 8. Common variable immunodeficiency, showing flat mucosa devoid of plasma cells. Note the absence of goblet cells and Paneth cells; autoimmune enteropathy can coexist with common variable immunodeficiency (H&E, original magnification, ×200).

Fig. 9. Two examples of autoimmune enteropathy. (A) Partial villous atrophy with minimally increased IELs and a few intraepithelial neutrophils. Paneth cells and goblet cells are absent. Apoptotic bodies are increased (H&E, original magnification, ×200). (B) Nearly flat mucosa with just of few IEL. Goblet cells are present (H&E, original magnification, ×200).

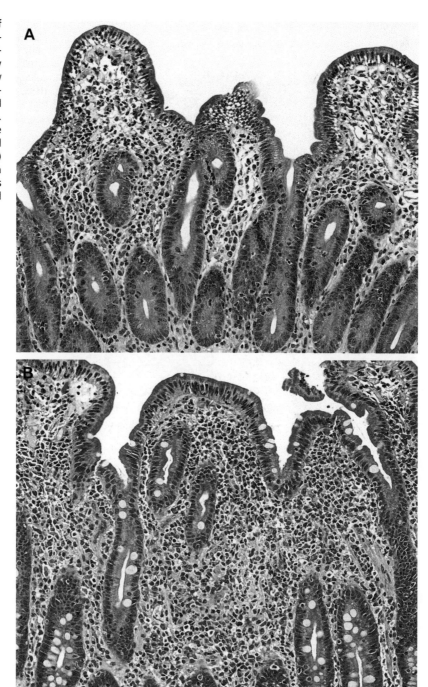

Pathologists are used to thinking about mycophenolate mofetil as a possible confounder in a biopsy submitted to rule out graft-versus-host disease, but villous blunting also has been described in association with this agent.[39] Absence of IELs, increased crypt apoptosis, and the presence of dilated damaged crypts should prevent confusion with celiac disease.

There is a growing literature on the topic of enterocolitis related to immunotherapy with monoclonal antibodies. Among the checkpoint inhibitors, anti-cytotoxic T-lymphocyte–associated antigen 4 antibodies (ipilimumab and tremelimumab) had had the most frequent gastrointestinal toxicity. In one series of 39 patients with enterocolitis, 18 had duodenal biopsies; 10 of those

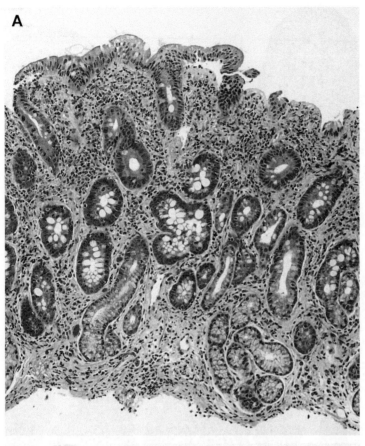

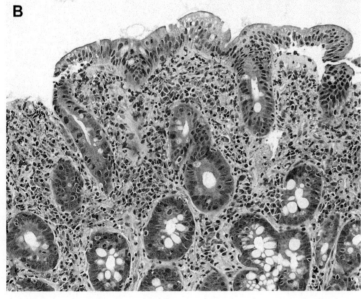

Fig. 10. Olmesartan injury. (*A*) Flat mucosa with increased eosinophils (H&E, original magnification, ×100). (*B*) Thickened subepithelial collagen. IELs are not increased (H&E, original magnification, ×200).

showed chronic duodenitis with patchy villous atrophy and increased lamina propria eosinophils; IELs were not mentioned.[40] In an earlier description of 5 patients on this therapy, one of whom had a duodenal biopsy, Oble and colleagues[41] described increased IELs, villous blunting, erosion, increased eosinophils, and scattered neutrophils. Anti-PD-1 and anti-PD-L1 checkpoint inhibitors (nivolumab, pembrolizumab) have been associated with colitis in 1% to 2% of patients.[42] I have not seen reports or morphologic descriptions of enteritis in patients using these therapies.

Idelalisib, a selective inhibitor of phosphatidylinositol 3-kinase delta, may cause significant gastrointestinal toxicity in more than 40% of patients receiving it.[43] In a series of 8 such patients who had small bowel biopsies, Louie and colleagues[43] noted increased apoptosis in all 8, acute inflammation in 5, increased IEL in 6, and at least mild villous blunting in 7.

Traditional chemotherapies can also damage the duodenum. Villous atrophy is common, but active inflammation predominates and dilated, damaged crypts lined by cells with bizarre cytologic change are characteristic (Fig. 11).

Small Intestinal Bacterial Overgrowth

An increase in the number of bacteria in the upper small bowel, or a change in the type of bacteria at that location, can cause chronic diarrhea and (sometimes) abnormal histology. Lappinga and colleagues[44] noted villous atrophy in 16 of 67 biopsies from patients with documented bacterial overgrowth, and found 22 cases to show increased IELs. I know of no histologic clues that would lead one to suspect small intestinal bacterial overgrowth. It has been proposed that bacterial overgrowth potentiates NSAID-related small bowel injury.[45]

Inflammatory Bowel Disease

Ulcerative colitis and Crohn disease can both cause inflammation in the upper gastrointestinal tract, sometimes including duodenitis with architectural distortion.[46,47] Neutrophils can be a helpful clue; cryptitis and crypt abscesses are very unusual in celiac disease. There also may be crypt distortion, with shortening and branching of crypts (Fig. 12). Mucosal and submucosal granulomas are helpful if present (Box 4).

THE PATHOLOGY REPORT

Based on histology alone, it is rarely possible to specifically diagnose of any of the conditions discussed here. The diagnosis line will typically be descriptive and will be followed by a comment listing possible etiologies, perhaps favoring one above others. Gradations in histologic severity can be communicated descriptively, or by applying one of several classification systems.[48,49]

Fig. 11. Oxaliplatin-based chemotherapy has produced villous atrophy and marked reactive epithelial change (H&E, original magnification, ×100).

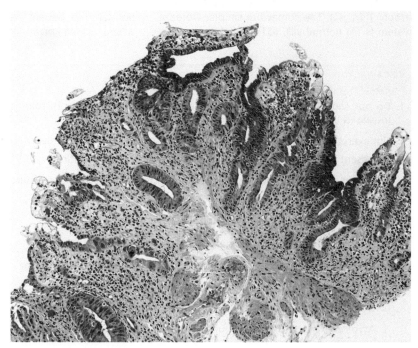

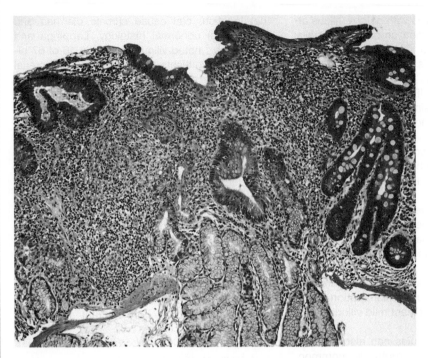

Fig. 12. Crohn disease of the duodenum. The mucosa is flat, but IELs are not increased. There are abundant neutrophils in lamina propria and crypts, with a crypt abscess just left of center. This patient also had active chronic ileitis with granulomas (H&E, original magnification, ×200).

Both the modification of Marsh by Oberhuber and colleagues[48] and the Corazza system[49] were developed for celiac disease and both require increased IELs, but the categories of villous injury could be adapted to other conditions as well. Briefly, the modified Marsh system is as follows: (1) normal villi without crypt hyperplasia, (2) normal villi with crypt hyperplasia, (3a) partial villous atrophy, (3b) subtotal villous atrophy, (3c) total villous atrophy (**Fig. 13**). The somewhat simpler Corazza system is (A) normal villi, (B1) partial or subtotal villous atrophy, (B2) total villous atrophy. Clinical guidelines allow either a descriptive diagnosis or a system-based one[1]; practices vary regionally, with the choice of reporting style often the result of negotiation between pathologists and clinicians at a given institution.

One of the most embarrassing moments of my professional life (and there have been a few) involved a duodenal biopsy that I had called normal. The patient went to another institution, where a well-known gastrointestinal pathologist

---

Box 4
Key points to consider when diagnosing celiac disease

1. Do not suggest celiac disease if IELs are not increased. Other histologic features may vary, but increased IELs are invariable.

2. Not everything with increased IELs is celiac disease. Some clues to other conditions:

   a. Absent or sparse plasma cells: common variable immunodeficiency (CVID)

   b. Villous atrophy without increased IELs: drug injury, autoimmune enteropathy

   c. Too many neutrophils: drug injury, autoimmune enteropathy, tropical sprue

   d. Too many eosinophils: eosinophilic gastroenteritis, drug injury

   e. Increased subepithelial collagen: collagenous sprue, drug injury

   f. Absence of Paneth cells and/or goblet cells: autoimmune enteropathy

   g. Increased apoptosis: autoimmune enteropathy, drug injury, CVID

   h. Granulomas: CVID, infection, Crohn disease

   i. Atypical or monotonously regular cells in lamina propria: T-cell lymphoma, systemic mastocytosis

Fig. 13. Various degrees of mucosal injury in celiac disease. (*A*) Partial villous atrophy (Marsh 3a). (*B*) subtotal villous atrophy (Marsh 3b). (*C*) Total villous atrophy (Marsh 3C) (H&E, original magnification, [*A- C*] ×100).

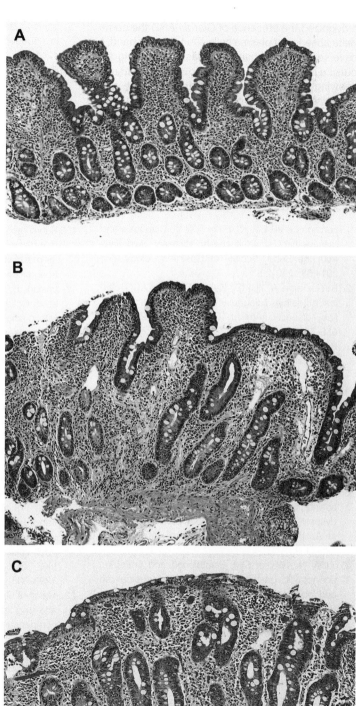

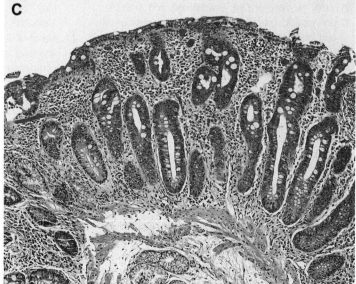

recognized the presence of *Giardia* AND the complete absence of plasma cells. On the other hand, I have several times had the pleasure of calling an outside pathologist or clinician to suggest, without knowing anything about the history, that the patient was likely taking olmesartan, and that a dramatic recovery would ensue if the drug were stopped. A systematic approach to duodenal biopsies will give you the chance to make gratifying contributions to patient care, and avoid a few pitfalls.

REFERENCES

1. Ludvigsson JF, Bai JC, Biagi F, et al. Diagnosis and management of adult coeliac disease: guidelines from the British Society of Gastroenterology. Gut 2014;63:1210–28.
2. Rubio-Tapia A, Hill ID, Kelly PC, et al. ACG clinical guidelines: diagnosis and management of celiac disease. Am J Gastroenterol 2013;108: 656–76.
3. Hayat M, Cairns A, Dixon MF, et al. Quantitation of intraepithelial lymphocytes in human duodenum: what is normal? J Clin Pathol 2002;55:393–4.
4. Veress B, Franzen L, Bodin L, et al. Duodenal intraepithelial lymphocyte count revisited. Scand J Gastroenterol 2000;39:138–44.
5. DeBrosse CW, Case JW, Putnam PE, et al. Quantity and distribution of eosinophils in the gastrointestinal tract of children. Pediatr Dev Pathol 2006;9: 210–8.
6. Walker MM, Aggarwal KR, Shim LSE, et al. Duodenal eosinophilia and early satiety in functional dyspepsia: confirmation of a positive association in an Australian cohort. J Gastroenterol Hepatol 2014; 29:474–9.
7. Talley NJ, Walker MM. Established and emerging eosinophilic gastrointestinal diseases: seeing red and looking ahead. Dig Dis Sci 2016;61:2453–5.
8. Goldstein NS. Proximal small-bowel mucosal villous intraepithelial lymphocytes. Histopathology 2004; 44:199–205.
9. Jarvinen TT, Collin P, Rasmussen M, et al. Villous tip intraepithelial lymphocytes as markers of early-stage coeliac disease. Scand J Gastroenterol 2004;39: 428–33.
10. Walker MM, Murray JA, Ronkainen J, et al. Detection of celiac disease and lymphocytic enteropathy by parallel serology and histopathology in a population-based study. Gastroenterology 2010; 139:112–9.
11. Villanacci V, Ceppa P, Tavani E, et al. Coeliac disease: the histology report. Dig Liver Dis 2011;43S: S385–95.
12. Hudacko R, Zhou XK, Yantiss RK. Immunohistochemical stains for CD3 and CD8 do not improve detection of gluten-sensitive enteropathy in duodenal biopsies. Mod Pathol 2013;26: 1241–5.
13. Brown IS, Smith J, Rosty C. Gastrointestinal pathology in celiac disease. A case series of 150 consecutive newly diagnosed patients. Am J Clin Pathol 2002;138:42–9.
14. Mooney PD, Kurien M, Evans KE, et al. Clinical and immunologic features of ultra-short celiac disease. Gastroenterology 2016;150:1125–34.
15. Evans KE, Aziz I, Cross SS, et al. A prospective study of duodenal bulb biopsy in newly diagnosed and established adult celiac disease. Am J Gastroenterol 2011;106:1837–42.
16. Rubio-Tapia A, Talley NJ, Gurudu SR, et al. Gluten-free diet and steroid treatment are effective therapy for most patients with collagenous sprue. Clin Gastroenterol Hepatol 2010;8:344–8.
17. Vakiani E, Agruelles-Grande C, Mansukhani MM, et al. Collagenous sprue is not always associated with dismal outcomes: a clinicopathological study of 19 patients. Mod Pathol 2010;23:12–26.
18. Lan N, Shen B, Yuan L, et al. Comparison of clinical features, treatment, and outcomes of collagenous sprue, celiac disease, and collagenous colitis. J Gastroenterol Hepatol 2017;32:120–7.
19. Rubio-Tapia A, Rahim MW, See JA, et al. Mucosal recovery and mortality in adults with celiac disease after treatment with a gluten-free diet. Am J Gastroenterol 2010;105:1412–20.
20. Wahab PJ, Meijer JW, Mulder CJ. Histologic follow-up of people with celiac disease on a gluten-free diet: slow and incomplete recovery. Am J Clin Pathol 2002;118:459–63.
21. Lanzini A, Lanzarotto F, Villanacci V, et al. Complete recovery of intestinal mucosa occurs very rarely in adult coeliac patients despite adherence to gluten-free diet. Aliment Pharmacol Ther 2009;29: 1299–308.
22. Malamut G, Afchain P, Verkarre V, et al. Presentation and long-term follow-up of refractory celiac disease: comparison of type I with type II. Gastroenterology 2009;136:81–90.
23. Rubio-Tapia A, Kelly D, Lahr BD, et al. Clinical staging and survival in refractory celiac disease: a single center experience. Gastroenterology 2009;136: 99–107.
24. Patey-Mariaud De Serre N, Cellier C, Jabri B, et al. Distinction between coeliac disease and refractory sprue: a simple immunohistochemical method. Histopathology 2000;37:70–7.
25. Brown I, Mino-Kenudson M, Deshpande V, et al. Intraepithelial lymphocytosis in architecturally preserved proximal small intestinal mucosa. An increasing diagnostic problem with a wide differential diagnosis. Arch Pathol Lab Med 2006;130: 1020–5.

26. Hammer STG, Greenson JK. The clinical significance of duodenal lymphocytosis with normal villous architecture. Arch Pathol Lab Med 2013;137:1216–9.

27. Shmidt E, Smyrk TC, Boswell CL, et al. Increasing duodenal intraepithelial lymphocytosis found at upper endoscopy: time trends and associations. Gastrointest Endosc 2014;80:105–11.

28. Aziz I, Evans KE, Hopper AD, et al. A prospective study into the aetiology of lymphocytic duodenosis. Aliment Pharmacol Ther 2010;32:1392–7.

29. Brown IS, Bettington A, Bettngton M, et al. Tropical sprue: revisiting an underrecognized disease. Am J Surg Pathol 2014;38:666–72.

30. Daniels JA, Lederman HM, Maitra A, et al. Gastrointestinal tract pathology in patients with common variable immunodeficiency (CVID). Am J Surg Pathol 2007;31:1800–12.

31. Jorgensen SF, Reims HM, Frydenlnd D, et al. A cross-sectional study of the prevalence of gastrointestinal symptoms and pathology in patients with common variable immunodeficiency. Am J Gastroenterol 2016;111:1467–75.

32. Lougaris V, Ravelli A, Villanacci V, et al. Gastrointestinal pathologic abnormalities in pediatric and adult-onset common variable immunodeficiency. Dig Dis Sci 2015;60:2384–9.

33. Gentile NM, Murray JA, Pardi DS. Autoimmune enteropathy: a review and update of clinical management. Curr Gastroenterol Rep 2012;14:380–5.

34. Akram S, Murray JA, Pardi DS, et al. Adult autoimmune enteropathy: Mayo Clinic Rochester experience. Clin Gastroenterol Hepatol 2007;5:1282–90.

35. Montalto M, D'Onofrio F, Santoro L, et al. Autoimmune enteropathy in children and adults. Scand J Gastroenterol 2014;44:1029–36.

36. Rubio-Tapia A, Herman ML, Ludvigsson JF, et al. Severe spruelike enteropathy associated with olmesartan. Mayo Clin Proc 2012;87:732–8.

37. Burbure N, Lebwohl B, Arguelles-Grande C, et al. Olmesartan-associated sprue-like enteropathy: a systematic review with emphasis on histopathology. Hum Pathol 2016;50:127–34.

38. Choi E-YK, McKenna BJ. Olmesartan-associated enteropathy. A review of clinical and histologic findings. Arch Pathol Lab Med 2015;139:1242–7.

39. Parfitt JR, Jayakumar S, Driman DK. Mycophenolate mofetil-related gastrointestinal mucosal injury: variable injury patterns, including graft-versus-host disease-like changes. Am J Surg Pathol 2008;32:1367–72.

40. Marthey L, Mateus C, Mussini C, et al. Cancer immunotherapy with anti CTLA-4 monoclonal antibodies induces an inflammatory bowel disease. J Crohns Colitis 2016;10(4):395–401.

41. Oble DA, Mino-Kenudson M, Goldsmith J, et al. Alpha-CTLA-4 mAb-associated panenteritis. A histologic and immunohistochemical analysis. Am J Surg Pathol 2008;32:1130–7.

42. Naidoo J, Page DB, Li BT, et al. Toxicities of the anti-PD-1 and anti-PD-L1 immune checkpoint antibodies. Ann Oncol 2015;26(12):2375–91.

43. Louie CY, DiMaio MA, Matsukuma KE, et al. Idelalisib-associated enterocolitis. Clinocopathologic features and distinction from other enterocolitides. Am J Surg Pathol 2015;39:1653–60.

44. Lappinga PJ, Abraham SC, Murray JA, et al. Small intestinal bacterial overgrowth. Histopathologic features and clinical correlates in an underrecognized entity. Arch Pathol Lab Med 2010;134:264–70.

45. Muraki M, Fujiwara Y, Machida H, et al. Role of small intestinal bacterial overgrowth in severe small intestinal damage in chronic non-steroidal anti-inflammatory drug users. Scand J Gastroenterol 2014;49:267–73.

46. Lin J, McKenna BJ, Appelman HD. Morphologic findings in upper gastrointestinal biopsies of patients with ulcerative colitis. Am J Surg Pathol 2010;34:1672–7.

47. Turner D, Griffiths AM. Esophageal, gastric, and duodenal manifestations of IBD and the role of upper endoscopy in IBD diagnosis. Curr Gastroenterol Rep 2009;11:234–7.

48. Oberhuber G, Granditsch G, Vogelsang H. The histopathology of coeliac disease: time for a standardized report scheme for pathologists. Eur J Gastroenterol Hepatol 1999;11:1185–94.

49. Corazza GR, Villanacci V, Zambelli C, et al. Comparison of the interobserver reproducibility with different histologic criteria used in celiac disease. Clin Gastroenterol Hepatol 2007;5:838–43.

Chronic Colitis in Biopsy Samples
Is It Inflammatory Bowel Disease or Something Else?

Eun-Young Karen Choi, MD[a],*, Henry D. Appelman, MD[b]

KEYWORDS

• Chronic colitis in biopsies • Ulcerative colitis • Crohn colitis

---

Key points

- Ulcerative colitis is a diffuse chronic distorting inflammation that typically involves the rectum and any amount of colon proximal to the rectum.
- Ulcerative colitis has many possible combinations of histologic features, depending on whether the disease is clinically active or quiescent and its response or lack of response to treatment.
- Crohn colitis is generally a patchy intense inflammation that is easiest to diagnose when there is proven Crohn disease involving the terminal ileum.
- Chronic colitides other than ulcerative and Crohn colitis occasionally falls into the histologic differential diagnosis, but they usually can be separated by clinical and morphologic features.

ABSTRACT

Chronic colitis, regardless of type, is defined histologically by chronic inflammation, mainly plasmacytosis, in the lamina propria. Specific diagnosis of chronic colitides in biopsies can be challenging for practicing pathologists. This article focuses on discussing specific histologic features in biopsies of the inflammatory bowel diseases (IBDs), including ulcerative colitis, Crohn colitis, and colitis of indeterminate type. It also offers suggestions as to how to separate the IBDs from other chronic colitides, such as lymphocytic colitis, collagenous colitis, diverticular disease–associated colitis, diversion colitis, and chronic colitides that are due to drugs. Normal histology in colon biopsies is also briefly discussed.

OVERVIEW

Inflammatory bowel diseases are a group of chronic inflammations of the colon and small intestine that include ulcerative colitis and Crohn disease. The etiologies are not fully understood, but they are thought to be a combination of genetic and environmental factors as well as abnormal immune responses. Inflammatory bowel diseases are diagnosed mostly on

---

Disclosure Statement: The authors have nothing to disclose.
[a] Department of Pathology, University of Michigan, 5231B Medical Science I, 1301 Catherine Street, SPC 5602, Ann Arbor, MI 48109-5602, USA; [b] Department of Pathology, University of Michigan, 5220 Medical Science I, 1301 Catherine Street, SPC 5602, Ann Arbor, MI 48109-5602, USA
* Corresponding author.
E-mail address: ekchoi@med.umich.edu

Surgical Pathology 10 (2017) 841–861
http://dx.doi.org/10.1016/j.path.2017.07.005
1875-9181/17/© 2017 Elsevier Inc. All rights reserved.

endoscopic and clinical grounds, but pathologists are asked to confirm these impressions by histologic evaluation. This discussion covers the histologic findings of ulcerative colitis, Crohn disease, and other types of chronic colitis in biopsies.

NORMAL COLON HISTOLOGY

It is imperative for pathologists to be familiar with the histologic appearance of normal colonic mucosa (**Box 1**). The small intestine and the colon normally have low-grade lamina propria chronic inflammation that is part of the mucosal immune system. This inflammation is mostly composed of plasma cells with scattered lymphocytes and eosinophils, but no neutrophils, and the lamina propria of the right colon is more cellular than that of the left (**Fig. 1**). The change in cellularity from more intense proximally to less intense distally may be related to the luminal contents, which are more liquid and perhaps more antigenic on the right. The epithelium lining the uniform, evenly spaced crypts and covering the mucosal surface have a mixture of goblet and absorptive cells that also vary in number from the right to the left side. Absorptive cells are more numerous on the right side where water and electrolyte absorption occurs, whereas goblet cells are more numerous on the left side. Paneth cells are normal in the right colon but are generally not found distal to the hepatic flexure.

INFLAMMATORY BOWEL DISEASE

ULCERATIVE COLITIS

According to traditional teaching, ulcerative colitis is a chronic and diffuse mucosal disease that involves the rectum and any length of colon proximal to that. It is uniform throughout the length of involved colon, meaning that it is not patchy or segmental in distribution. Terminal ileal disease, commonly referred to as "backwash ileitis," sometimes accompanies colonic inflammation, but only in continuity with an inflamed right colon. For all intents and purposes, every patient with ulcerative colitis has endoscopic disease.

In classic ulcerative colitis, the rectum and variable lengths of more proximal colon have a characteristic combination of histologic findings, including lamina propria chronic inflammation and architectural distortion (**Box 2**). Plasmacytosis, the hallmark of chronic injury in the gastrointestinal tract, is required for a biopsy diagnosis of ulcerative colitis. This plasmacytosis is most intense superficially, but commonly extends down to the base of mucosa, a change that has been termed "basal plasmacytosis" (**Fig. 2**A). Although plasma cells can be normally found at the base in the right colon, they are not present in high numbers. Eosinophilia (see **Fig. 2**B) may accompany plasmacytosis, and hyperplastic lymphoid follicles also may be found at the base of the mucosa.

Crypt architectural distortion is another indicator of chronicity when it accompanies lamina propria chronic inflammation, but it is not always seen at the time of initial presentation, especially in children.[1,2] Distortion results from destruction and repair of epithelial structures, and includes surface contour changes, including villiform and undulating contours, loss of crypts (atrophy), and variations in crypt size, shape, and orientation (**Fig. 3**A–C). Sometimes distorted crypts are shaped as animals, continents, musical instruments, Hebrew letters, or even Dr Seuss characters (see **Fig. 3**D). It should be

---

Box 1
Key features: normal colon

Right side: darker at low magnification because there are

- More plasma cells in the lamina propria, some at base of mucosa

- More absorptive cells in the crypts

- Fewer goblet cells in the crypts

Left side: lighter at low magnification because there are

- Fewer plasma cells in the lamina propria, rare at base of mucosa

- Fewer absorptive cells in the crypts

- More goblet cells in the crypts

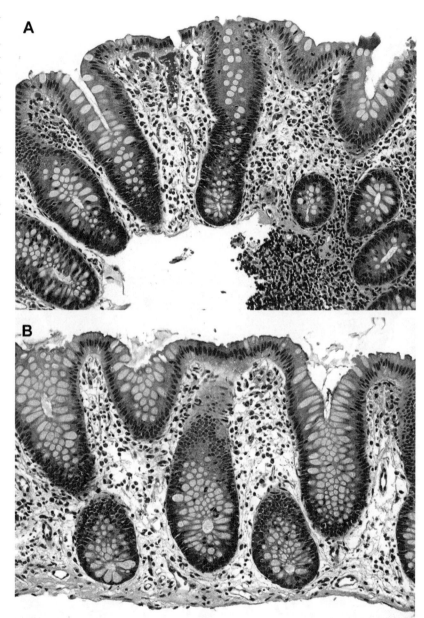

Fig. 1. Comparison between normal right and left colon. The right colon (*A*) has more cellularity in the lamina propria than the left colon (*B*). In the right colon, the crypts have fewer goblet cells and more absorptive cells. The overall result is that the normal right colon looks darker at lower power than the left. On both sides, the crypts are uniform and evenly spaced (H&E, Original magnification, [*A, B*] ×200).

Box 2
Key features: full-blown ulcerative colitis in biopsies

Chronic inflammation

- Plasmacytosis in the lamina propria that often extends to the base of mucosa ("basal plasmacytosis")

- Variable eosinophilia

Active damage (activity)

- Neutrophils in crypt epithelium (cryptitis)

- Epithelial destruction by neutrophils (crypt ulcers, crypt abscesses)

Prior damage and repair

- Crypt and surface architectural distortion

- Left colon Paneth cell metaplasia

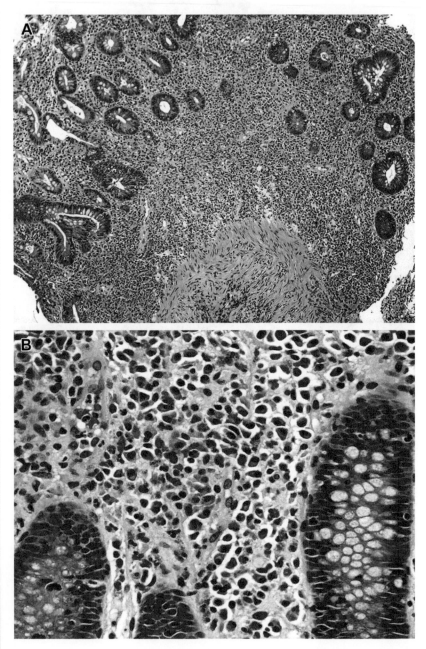

Fig. 2. Ulcerative colitis. (*A*) Chronic inflammation in the lamina propria characterized by plasmacytosis. The plasma cells extend to the base of the mucosa, termed "basal plasmacytosis." (*B*) Eosinophils mixed with plasma cells, a common finding in ulcerative colitis (H&E, Original magnification, [*A*] ×100 [*B*] ×400).

noted that a distorted but noninflamed mucosa is an indication of prior mucosal injury, but it is not diagnostic of any type of chronic colitis. Another abnormality commonly seen with chronic mucosal injury is an alteration in the Paneth cell population, including hyperplasia on the right side where Paneth cells normally exist and metaplasia throughout the rest of the colon in areas where Paneth cells are normally absent (Fig. 4).

Ulcers are often found in ulcerative colitis. After all, the disease is named ulcerative colitis for a reason! These ulcers have various endoscopic appearances including aphthous, longitudinal, and geographic ulcers. Aphthous ulcers usually occur over lymphoid follicles and may

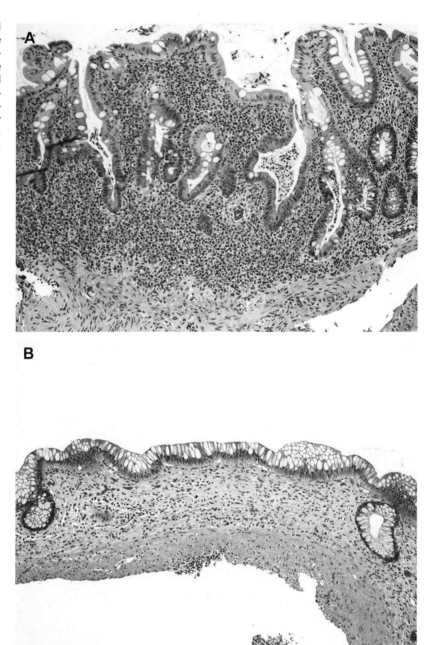

Fig. 3. Architectural distortion in ulcerative colitis. (*A*) Crypt distortion. No 2 crypts are the same size, shape, and orientation. (*B*) Architectural distortion characterized by loss or atrophy of crypts (H&E, Original magnification, [*A, B*] ×100).

be so small they can be entirely sampled with biopsy forceps. Endoscopists generally biopsy intact mucosa at the ulcer edges, because biopsies of ulcer beds may not be as informative as the adjacent mucosa with regard to the etiology of the ulcer. Islands of mucosa and submucosa surrounded by ulcers are dragged into the lumen, presumably by the colonic motility forces, resulting in inflammatory pseudopolyps, which may form large masses with chronically inflamed and severely distorted mucosa (Fig. 5A, B). Inflammatory pseudopolyps of quiescent colitis undergo remodeling with loss of distortion and inflammation. Grossly, these may appear to be nodular, pedunculated, or filiform, like worms or stalks of polyps without heads. Microscopically, they usually are seen in cross section as round structures composed of relatively normal

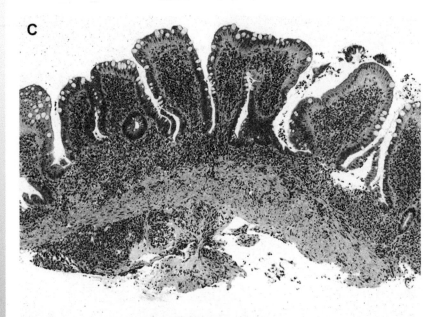

Fig. 3. (continued). (*C*) Villiform surface distortion. (*D*) Animal crypt distortion, a rabbit-shaped crypt with pus in its abdomen (H&E, Original magnification [*C*] ×100 [*D*] ×200).

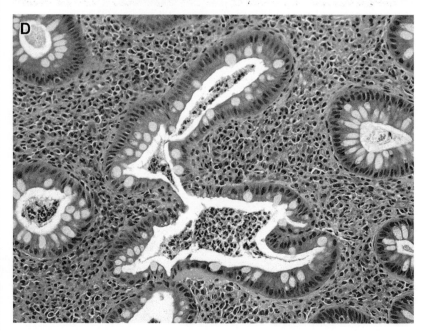

mucosa surrounding a core of hypercellular muscularis mucosae and altered submucosa with an increased number of ganglion cells and small blood vessels (see Fig. 5C).

Activity is usually, but not always, seen at initial presentation. Histologically, activity refers to neutrophils in the tissue, especially crypt epithelium, which can produce cryptitis, crypt ulcers, and crypt abscesses (Fig. 6). The presence of a crypt abscess indicates a nearby ulcer in that crypt, as that is the mode of migration of neutrophils into the crypt lumen. Larger abscesses result from destruction of crypts and adjacent lamina propria. Epithelial regeneration follows the outlines of these complex abscesses, leading to distortion. Epithelial atypia due to reactive or regenerative change can occur and may mimic dysplasia.

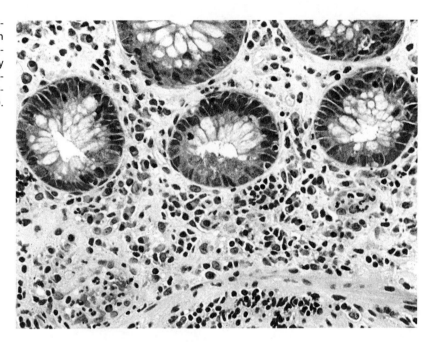

Fig. 4. Paneth cell metaplasia in the left colon in ulcerative colitis. Paneth cells are not normally found distal to the hepatic flexure (H&E, Original magnification ×400).

Activity is not required for the diagnosis of ulcerative colitis. In fact, the disease may be totally quiescent in treated patients. Is it important from a clinical standpoint to mention histologic activity? Gastroenterologists generally treat patients based on clinical findings, not histologic activity. There are, however, studies that suggest histologic activity has prognostic importance. In a study from 1991, activity was found to predict an increased incidence of relapse following treatment.[3] In more recent studies, the severity of active inflammation in surveillance biopsies was reported to correlate with an increased risk of neoplastic progression, including carcinoma and dysplasia.[4–6] What is fascinating is that the criteria for scoring activity differed among these studies, but they all came to similar conclusions (Table 1). The results of these studies suggest that reporting activity may be helpful in stratifying patients for surveillance, but we are not aware of its current use in clinical practice.

There are some unusual scenarios that challenge diagnosis. In one scenario, there is diffuse chronic colitis identical to ulcerative colitis, with the exception of a normal rectum. In some cases, treatment results in rectal healing, such that it appears endoscopically and histologically normal. Another scenario is distal colitis identical to ulcerative colitis with patches of proximal inflammation, especially endoscopic inflammation around the appendiceal orifice (ie, "cecal red patch").[7] Although not a classic presentation, this combination of distal colitis and proximal inflamed patches with a normal terminal ileum is known to occur in ulcerative colitis and is not Crohn colitis. In a third scenario, the colitis is typical of ulcerative colitis, but has scattered mucosal granulomas. In some practices, this is designated as Crohn colitis because of the granulomas. However, occasional mucosal granulomas occur in ulcerative colitis, especially in association with ruptured crypts and extruded mucus into the lamina propria (Fig. 7).

CROHN COLITIS

In contrast to ulcerative colitis, only some patients with Crohn disease have disease limited to the colon. The traditional teaching is that Crohn colitis is a patchy or segmental transmural chronic disease involving any part of the colon. Microscopic changes in biopsies of endoscopically abnormal mucosa are likely to include multifocal intense chronic inflammation with plasma cells extending into submucosa, patchy architectural distortion, and active inflammation with crypt injury (Fig. 8A, B). There may be accompanying aphthous ulcers and occasional granulomas.[8] Random biopsies of endoscopically normal colon in patients with Crohn disease also can contain microscopic

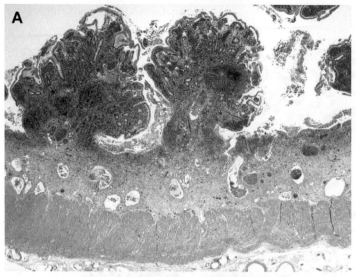

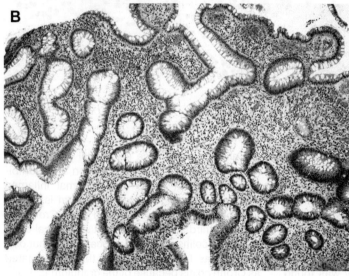

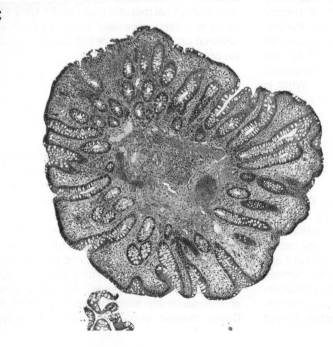

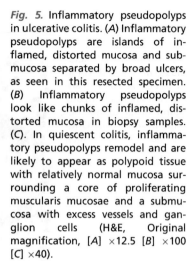

Fig. 5. Inflammatory pseudopolyps in ulcerative colitis. (*A*) Inflammatory pseudopolyps are islands of inflamed, distorted mucosa and submucosa separated by broad ulcers, as seen in this resected specimen. (*B*) Inflammatory pseudopolyps look like chunks of inflamed, distorted mucosa in biopsy samples. (*C*). In quiescent colitis, inflammatory pseudopolyps remodel and are likely to appear as polypoid tissue with relatively normal mucosa surrounding a core of proliferating muscularis mucosae and a submucosa with excess vessels and ganglion cells (H&E, Original magnification, [*A*] ×12.5 [*B*] ×100 [*C*] ×40).

Fig. 6. Activity in ulcerative colitis. (*A*) Cryptitis (*left side*) characterized by neutrophils migrating through and destroying crypt epithelium. Crypt ulcer (*right side*) with loss of crypt epithelium on the bottom and exudate extending from the ulcer into the dilated crypt, which is lined by regenerating epithelium. (*B*) Large crypt ulcer on the left with pus filling and distending the crypt. Multiple adjacent crypts with pus in the lumens, "crypt abscesses," some of which are lined by epithelium with enlarged, hyperchromatic, and stratified nuclei that can mimic dysplasia (H&E, Original magnification [*A*] ×400 [*B*] ×200).

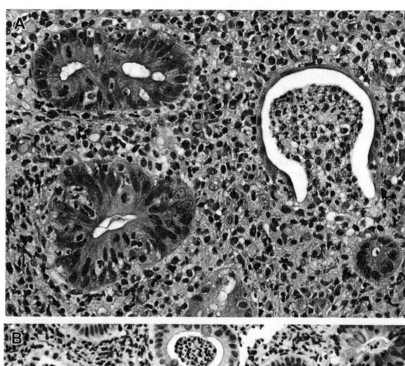

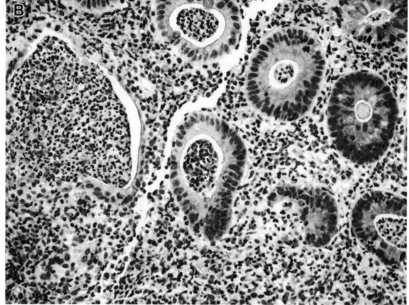

inflammation, crypt injury, and even occasional granulomas (see **Fig. 8**C).

A biopsy diagnosis of Crohn colitis can be made when there is intense patchy chronic colitis in a patient who also has clinical and histologic evidence of Crohn ileitis. Although Crohn ileitis is a transmural disease with chronic mucosal injury, deep penetrating ulcers, transmural lymphoid aggregates, and structural abnormalities including strictures and fistulas, biopsies cannot pick up the transmural findings. A set of mucosal changes in biopsies of the terminal ileum that are almost pathognomonic of Crohn disease include ulcers, especially aphthous ulcers, lamina propria chronic inflammation, mucous gland metaplasia (ie, "pyloric gland metaplasia" or "ulcer-associated cell lineage"), profound architectural distortion with striking alteration in size, shape, and number of crypts and villi, and increased number of goblet cells in surface epithelium (**Fig. 9**A, B). There may be misplaced Paneth cells, and irregular expansion of the muscularis mucosae can be

Table 1
Three classification schemes for histologic activity in ulcerative colitis

Study	Inflammation Scores and Definitions
Rutter et al,[4] 2004	0 = normal (no inflammation) 1 = chronic inflammation only 2 = mild (cryptitis without crypt abscesses) 3 = moderate (few crypt abscesses) 4 = severe (numerous crypt abscesses)
Gupta et al,[5] 2007	0 = no intraepithelial neutrophils (normal, inactive, quiescent) 1 = mild (neutrophils in <50% of crypts, no ulcers or erosions) 2 = moderate (neutrophils in >50% of crypts, no ulcers or erosions) 3 = severe (erosion or ulcer)
Rubin et al,[6] 2013	0 = normal (no inflammation or distortion) 1 = quiescent disease (distortion or chronic mucosal inflammation) 2 = increased lamina propria granulocytes, but not in epithelium 3 = intraepithelial granulocytes without crypt abscesses 4 = crypt abscesses in <50% of crypts 5 = crypt abscesses in >50% or crypts or erosion or ulcer

seen if biopsies are sufficiently deep (see **Fig. 9**C). Granulomas are not required for the diagnosis of Crohn disease, although their presence makes the diagnosis easier. When most of these changes are present, it is highly likely that the patient has Crohn disease. Medication-related injury, particularly due to nonsteroidal anti-inflammatory drugs, has been reported to result in similar changes, although they tend to be milder and less extensive.[9] Ulcerative colitis also can involve the terminal ileum ("backwash ileitis"), but it virtually never has all of these changes.

Without terminal ileal involvement, establishing a biopsy diagnosis of Crohn colitis is challenging. Some of the changes of chronic ileitis, such as mucous gland metaplasia and expansion of muscularis mucosae, are almost never seen in Crohn colitis. Small mucosal granulomas without other inflammatory changes are insufficient for the diagnosis.

Some cases diagnosed as Crohn colitis may have overlapping features with ulcerative colitis. For example, diffuse pancolitis identical to ulcerative colitis with concurrent ileal findings typical of Crohn disease are almost always diagnosed as Crohn ileocolitis by our clinical colleagues. Furthermore, clinical findings may take precedence over endoscopic and histologic findings. Patients with diffuse pancolitis identical to ulcerative colitis who lack small bowel disease but have perianal disease or rectal sparing are commonly diagnosed as Crohn colitis by the gastroenterologists (**Box 3**).

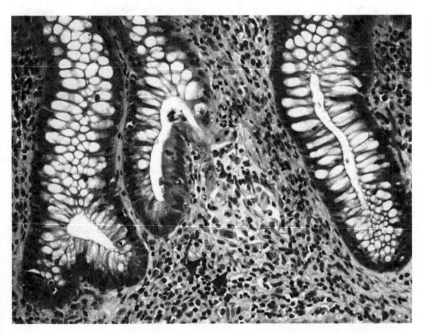

Fig. 7. A granuloma (*arrowheads*) surrounds a point of crypt rupture in a patient with ulcerative colitis (H&E, Original magnification ×200).

Fig. 8. Crohn colitis. (*A*) Biopsy of right colon. On the left side of the photo, there is intense active and chronic inflammation that extends through the muscularis mucosae into the submucosa. In contrast, the mucosa on the right is relatively normal. (*B*) An aphthous ulcer with regenerative surface epithelium to the right of center. (*C*) Granulomas in endoscopically normal mucosa without accompanying intense inflammation. These may be a marker of Crohn disease elsewhere, but they are not diagnostic of Crohn colitis (H&E, Original magnification [*A*] ×100 [*B*, *C*] ×200).

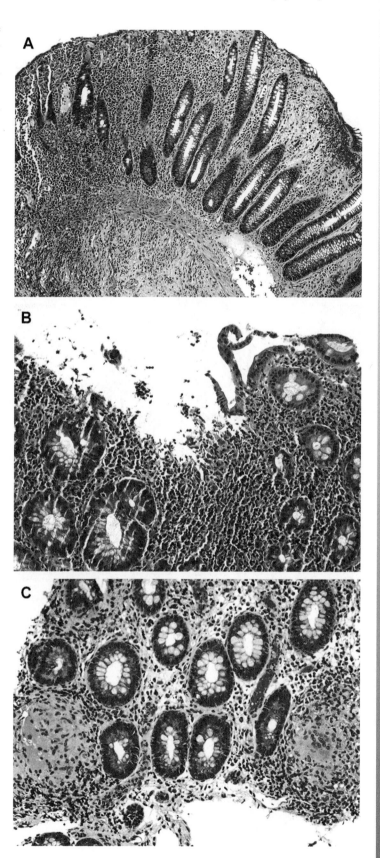

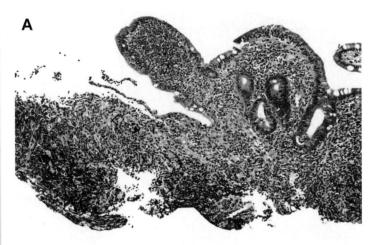

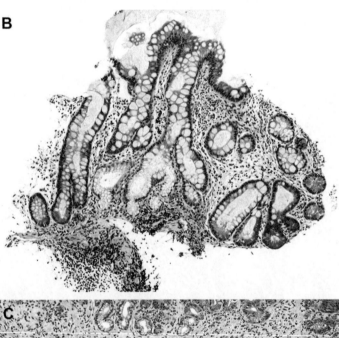

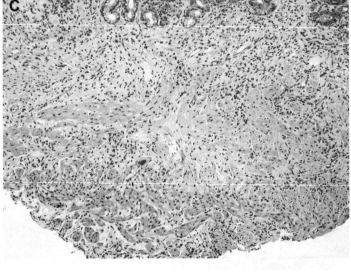

Fig. 9. Crohn ileitis in biopsies. (*A*) Architectural distortion in the form of a club-shaped villus, chronic inflammation in the lamina propria, and an aphthous ulcer on the left with a strip of partially detached regenerating surface epithelium. (*B*) Architectural distortion with irregular shapes and sizes of crypts, many of which have too many Paneth cells, some extending high, and mucous gland metaplasia at the base. (*C*) Irregular expansion of the muscularis mucosae can sometimes be seen in biopsies (H&E, Original magnification [*A, B*] ×100 [*C*] ×40).

> **Box 3**
> **Key features: Crohn colitis in biopsies**
>
> Any chronic inflammation in the colon in a patient with proven small bowel Crohn disease may be considered Crohn colitis.
>
> When there is no small bowel Crohn disease, then Crohn colitis is difficult to diagnose from biopsies with confidence.
>
> Crohn colitis is likely to be a multifocal intense chronic destructive inflammation in biopsies of endoscopically abnormal mucosa. Histologic changes may include lamina propria plasmacytosis extending into the submucosa, mild active cryptitis and ulcers (including aphthous ulcers).
>
> Biopsies of endoscopically normal colon may have microscopic foci of inflammation, but this is not diagnostic of Crohn colitis.
>
> The presence of isolated granulomas in the colon is insufficient to diagnose Crohn colitis.
>
> There are cases that look identical to ulcerative colitis on biopsies that our clinical colleagues designate as Crohn colitis based on nonbiopsy clinical issues, such as perianal disease and rectal sparing, both of which are considered to be typical Crohn features.

INDETERMINATE COLITIS

Some chronic colitides have clinical, endoscopic, and microscopic features that are not clearly diagnostic of either ulcerative colitis or Crohn colitis. These are usually characterized by patchy chronic lamina propria inflammation, variable crypt distortion, and activity resembling ulcerative colitis without terminal ileal or diffuse rectal disease. Although there are recommendations that the diagnosis of "indeterminate colitis" be limited to resected specimens,[8] we feel that in such situations, the indeterminate designation is appropriate when assessing biopsy samples.

EFFECT OF TREATMENT ON INFLAMMATORY BOWEL DISEASE

The goal of ulcerative colitis treatment is endoscopic and histologic restitution of the colonic mucosa (Fig. 10A, B). During treatment, the various histologic features may resolve at different rates, leading to patches of persistent chronic inflammation and/or distortion that are surrounded by entirely normal mucosa (see Fig. 10C). In general, most cases of patchy chronic colitis reflect long-standing treated ulcerative colitis, rather than Crohn colitis. Based on long-term follow-up studies involving patients with proven ulcerative colitis on surveillance, we know this trend toward normal mucosa is more likely to occur when ulcerative colitis remains quiescent for long periods as a result of treatment.[10–12] Not only can treated disease be patchy, but there may be changes in its extent. Ulcerative pancolitis may incompletely resolve such that active disease is limited to the rectum, or alternatively, the rectal mucosa undergoes healing with persistent inflammation of the more proximal colon. Severely abnormal mucosa can revert to normal over a period of several months. Thus, pathologists must be cognizant of the fact that histologic features of ulcerative colitis change with time and treatment (Box 4).

We have few data regarding the response of Crohn colitis to treatment, but it is conceivable that histologic disease also varies with time and treatment. Cases of Crohn colitis with diffuse distribution usually have a histologic response to treatment similar to that of ulcerative colitis. It is difficult, however, to follow histologic changes of healing in Crohn colitis when there is patchy disease distribution, as the original areas of inflammation may not be re-biopsied in subsequent colonoscopies.

DIFFERENTIAL DIAGNOSIS OF CHRONIC COLITIS

Chronic colitides can be divided into 3 types: (1) the ulcerating and distorting types, (2) the nonulcerating and nondistorting types, and (3) the types that are not predictable (Box 5). Classic inflammatory bowel diseases fall into the first group, whereas the microscopic colitides, lymphocytic and collagenous colitis, comprise the second group. The third group includes diverticular disease–related colitis, diversion colitis, and many of the drug-induced chronic colitides. Although this classification system works well for most forms of chronic colitis, we probably see several cases a week that we cannot confidently classify because they do not follow the rules. These are unnamed chronic colitides, which perhaps one day will be named.

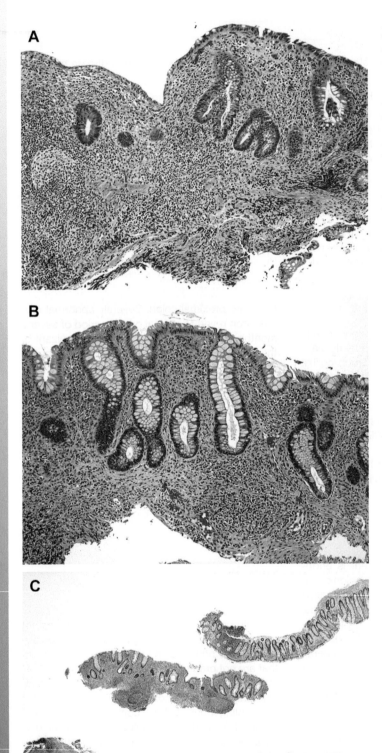

Fig. 10. Histologic changes with treatment in ulcerative colitis. (A) Severe ulcerative colitis, before treatment, with distortion, atrophy, plasmacytosis (including basal plasmacytosis), and a lymphoid follicle on the left. (B) Partially treated ulcerative colitis with persistent plasmacytosis but milder crypt architectural distortion than before treatment. The goal of treatment is restitution of normal mucosa. (C) Patchy chronic inflammation in a set of biopsies from a single segment of colon during treatment. The patchiness may lead one to suspect Crohn disease, but this distribution is common in ulcerative colitis during treatment (H&E, Original magnification [A, B] ×100 [C] ×12.5).

Box 4
Key features: treatment-related changes in ulcerative colitis

The goal of treatment is restitution of normal mucosa.

Biopsy changes during treatment:

- Activity subsides

- Plasmacytosis recedes

- Architecture gradually returns to normal

As the mucosa heals, there may be persistent plasmacytosis and distortion that are less intense than in the full-blown situation with no or very little activity.

Sometimes, as a result of treatment, ulcerative colitis will appear endoscopically and histologically patchy.

For all colitis biopsies, diagnosis is easiest when the biopsies are accompanied by clinical history and endoscopic findings because such information tells us what questions we need to answer and what correlations we need to make. At our institution, we are very fortunate that every endoscopic biopsy is sent to us accompanied by a copy of the endoscopy report. Unfortunately, many practicing pathologists receive endoscopic biopsies with very little clinical and endoscopic information, and in too many cases, no information at all.

THE NONDISTORTING, NONULCERATING COLITIDES

These colitides almost always occur in patients with chronic, watery diarrhea. The mucosa is endoscopically normal or has minimal changes, such as patchy erythema. Lymphocytic and collagenous colitis are the only 2 currently named nondistorting, nonulcerating colitides.[13–15] Both have increased lamina propria cellularity with numerous plasma cells, surface intraepithelial inflammatory cells, and no significant crypt or surface architectural distortion. The surface epithelium tends to be disorganized with diminished cytoplasmic maturation, and the nuclei are stratified instead of being uniformly lined up at the bases of the cells. These epithelial changes presumably reflect cell injury.

In lymphocytic colitis, the lamina propria is expanded by chronic inflammation from top to bottom with numerous plasma cells, so biopsies are very blue at low power (Fig. 11A). There is also prominent lymphocytosis involving both the surface and superficial crypt epithelium (see Fig. 11B).

Collagenous colitis is so named because of the deposition of a layer of collagen beneath the surface basement membrane, which commonly has an irregular lower border with thin collagen fibers

---

Box 5
Differential diagnosis: chronic colitides

Ulcerating and distorting colitides: the inflammatory bowel diseases

- Ulcerative colitis

- Crohn colitis

- Indeterminate colitis

Nonulcerating and nondistorting colitides: the microscopic colitides

- Lymphocytic colitis

- Collagenous colitis

Chronic colitides with variable histologic features

- Diverticulosis disease–associated colitis

- Diversion colitis

- Drug-associated colitis

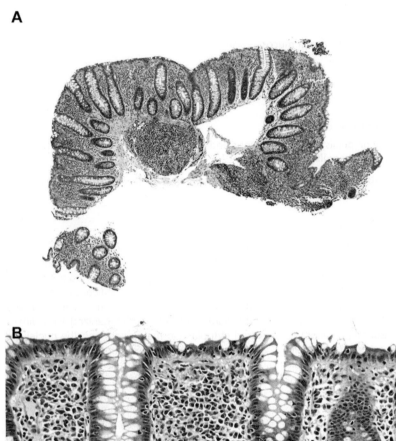

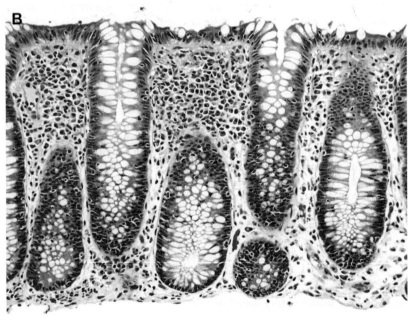

Fig. 11. The microscopic colitides. (*A*) Biopsies of lymphocytic colitis look blue at low power because of the dense chronic inflammation in the lamina propria. (*B*) Surface and crypt epithelial lymphocytosis in lymphocytic colitis.

extending into the superficial lamina propria (see **Fig. 11**C, D). This collagen layer traps inflammatory cells, karyorrhectic debris, and small capillaries, which we refer to as "trapillaries." The subepithelial collagen is thick enough to be seen on hematoxylin-eosin (H&E) stain in most cases, but for borderline cases, a trichrome stain may be needed. Detachment of surface epithelium is a frequent finding in collagenous colitis, and there is often an increased number of lamina propria eosinophils. Surface intraepithelial lymphocytosis is generally less pronounced than in lymphocytic colitis, and the lymphocytes are usually accompanied by scattered intraepithelial eosinophils. Lymphocytic cryptitis is usually not a prominent feature. Paneth cell metaplasia can be seen in collagenous colitis,[16] but it hardly ever occurs in lymphocytic colitis. Occasional cases of both collagenous and lymphocytic colitis can have tiny foci of inflammatory bowel diseaselike change including distortion and neutrophilic cryptitis.[17,18]

Fig. 11. (*continued*). (*C*) Biopsies of full-blown collagenous colitis have a thick subsurface collagen layer that can be seen on H&E. The hypercellular lamina propria is below this layer and often has increased number of eosinophils. Intraepithelial lymphocytes and scattered eosinophils are in surface and crypt epithelium (H&E, Original magnification [*A*] ×40 [*B, C*] ×200). (*D*) A trichrome stain highlights the irregularly thickened subsurface collagen layer with entrapped capillaries ("trapillaries") and inflammatory cells (Trichrome stain, Original magnification, [*D*] ×200).

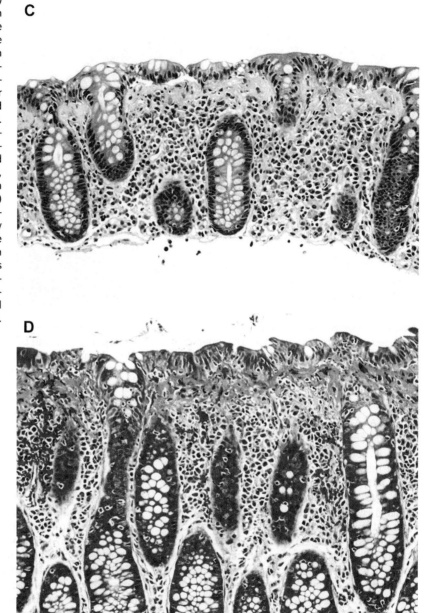

CHRONIC COLITIDES WITH VARIABLE HISTOLOGIC FEATURES

Diverticular Disease–Associated Colitis

A small subset of patients who have diverticulosis have mild chronic mucosal inflammation that is limited to the diverticular segment, usually the sigmoid colon where diverticula are most common.[19] It is a segmental colitis, and thus has also been named segmental colitis associated with diverticulosis. Endoscopists generally see some abnormalities such as erythema or granularity, but the microscopic features resemble those of inflammatory bowel disease. Most cases have low-grade plasmacytosis with scattered dilated crypts, or focal crypt abscesses in biopsy samples, simulating a mild form of ulcerative colitis (Fig. 12). Occasional cases contain small non-necrotic granulomas, transmural inflammation, lymphoid aggregates, and fibrosis that mimic Crohn colitis.[20] Pathologists can confirm a clinical impression of diverticular disease–associated colitis if

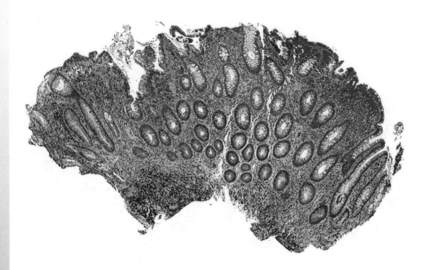

Fig. 12. Diverticular disease–associated colitis. Histologic findings may vary. In this example, there is chronic lamina propria inflammation without significant architectural distortion. Correlation with endoscopic findings to determine if the distribution of colitis is limited to the segment with diverticular disease is necessary to make the diagnosis (H&E, Original magnification, ×40).

biopsies from the segment affected by diverticular disease have chronic colitis and the biopsies of mucosa immediately proximal and distal to the diseased segment are normal. This means the rectum is usually spared. The pathogenesis of this colitis is poorly understood.

Diversion Colitis

Diversion colitis occurs in colonic segments diverted from the fecal stream. The precise mechanism is not known, but the prevailing theory is that it results from a lack of exposure to short-chain fatty acids and changes in the gut microbiota. We most commonly encounter diversion colitis in Hartmann pouch (rectal stump) biopsies from patients who have undergone partial colectomy for complicated diverticulitis, or a total abdominal colectomy for severe ulcerative pancolitis. These patients require a 2-stage surgical approach that initially results in a rectal stump and end colostomy or ileostomy. A colorectal anastomosis (or ileoanal anastomosis in the case of ulcerative colitis) is performed later to reestablish continuity. The most characteristic feature of a diverted colonic segment is diffuse nodular lymphoid hyperplasia with linear arrays of large follicles, some of which contain prominent germinal centers, in the deep mucosa and superficial submucosa (**Fig. 13**). Other diversion-related features include crypt and mucosal atrophy, crypt branching, and diffusely increased plasma cell–rich inflammation in the lamina propria. These features often occur in the absence of symptoms and, thus, are considered by some to be diversion-related changes rather than diversion colitis.[21,22] Other cases have variably severe

neutrophilic activity with cryptitis, crypt abscesses, or erosions, in which case the findings resemble ulcerative proctitis. Prominent lymphoid hyperplasia also can be seen in the distal colorectum of patients with ulcerative colitis, so it may not be possible to determine if such inflammatory changes in a Hartmann pouch of a patient with ulcerative colitis are diversion-related, ulcerative colitis, or both. Diversion-related inflammatory changes typically regress on reestablishment of the fecal stream.

Drug-Associated Chronic Colitis

Various drugs, including chemotherapeutic and immunotherapeutic medications, have been associated with chronic colitis. The most well-known is colitis due to mycophenolate mofetil, an immunosuppressant commonly used in patients with solid organ transplants, and in some cases patients with bone marrow transplantation. Mycophenolate mofetil usually produces an acute injury resembling acute graft-versus-host disease with crypt epithelial apoptosis and hypocellular lamina propria. We have, however, seen patients on long-term therapy whose colonic biopsies have chronic inflammation with plasmacytosis accompanied by heterogeneous crypt morphology including dilated crypts, and small crypts lined by regenerative epithelium mixed with normal crypts[23,24] (**Fig. 14**A). Ipilimumab and nivolumab, 2 checkpoint inhibitors that activate the immune system, are used to treat metastatic melanoma and other malignancies. Both agents can cause chronic colitis characterized by mild plasmacytosis, cryptitis, and crypt epithelial cell apoptosis[25–27] (see **Fig. 14**B). Idelalisib, a phosphoinositide 3-kinase

Fig. 13. Diversion colitis. (*A*) A resected Hartmann pouch contains a row of lymphoid follicles at the mucosal-submucosal junction. (*B*) Hyperplastic lymphoid nodules accompanied by low-grade plasmacytosis in the lamina propria of biopsy from a Hartmann pouch (H&E, Original magnification, [*A*] ×20 [*B*] ×100).

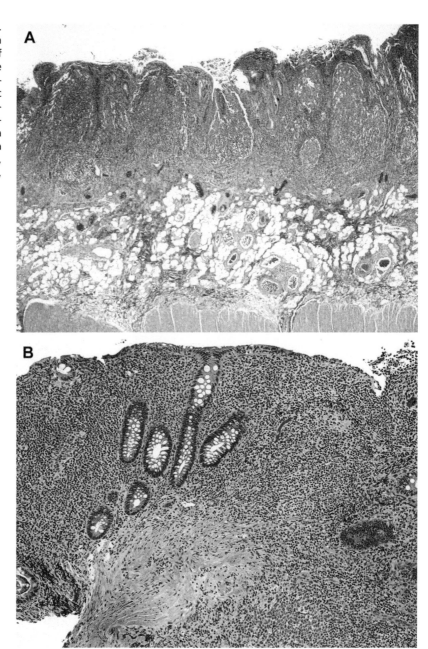

inhibitor used to treat low-grade lymphomas, can cause a lymphocytic colitis pattern of injury associated with numerous apoptotic crypt epithelial cells.[28,29] In these situations, the treating clinician may presumptively treat symptomatic patients with discontinuation of the suspected drug and administration of corticosteroids before obtaining colonic biopsies. Together with other variables, such as duration of exposure to the offending drug and concomitant medications, the morphologic features in biopsy samples may differ from those described in literature. We will likely encounter more examples of medication-associated colitis with the advent of new immunotherapy drugs.

Infection and Unclassified Colitides

There are very few colonic infections that become chronic. Most bacterial infections are acute and self-limited. The exception is certain sexually transmitted infections, such as syphilis and

A

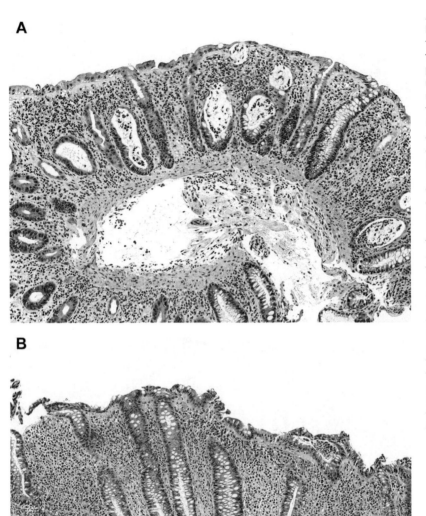

B

Fig. 14. Drug-induced colitis. (*A*) Left colon biopsy from a patient with a renal transplant who complained of chronic diarrhea while taking mycophenolate mofetil for immunosuppression. Dilated crypts lined by attenuated epithelium and filled with mucin and pus are mixed with crypts lined by regenerating epithelium and normal crypts. The lamina propria has plasmacytosis. (*B*) Colon biopsy from a patient treated with ipilimumab and nivolumab immunotherapy for metastatic melanoma who developed diarrhea and was presumptively treated with steroids before this biopsy. Histologic findings resembled ulcerative colitis with intense plasmacytosis in the lamina propria and active cryptitis, but no significant crypt distortion (H&E, Original magnification, [*A, B*] ×100).

chlamydia, both of which can result in a localized chronic proctitis characterized by marked plasmacytosis. Often, the degree of inflammation is disproportionate to the extent and severity of architectural distortion, which is typically mild compared with inflammatory bowel disease.[30] In countries where gastrointestinal infections are endemic, some species of *Shigella* and *Salmonella* can cause chronic diseases. However, these infections are so uncommon in developed societies that they are unlikely to account for a substantial number of chronic colitis cases, unless there is a clinical suspicion for infection in an individual.

SUMMARY

The named chronic colitides have recognizable microscopic features. Specific diagnosis of any chronic colitis is best made when microscopic changes are correlated with endoscopic and clinical findings.

REFERENCES

1. Markowitz J, Kahn E, Grancher K, et al. Atypical rectosigmoid histology in children with newly diagnosed ulcerative colitis. Am J Gastroenterol 1993;88(12): 2034–7.
2. Robert ME, Tang L, Hao LM, et al. Patterns of inflammation in mucosal biopsies of ulcerative colitis: perceived differences in pediatric populations are limited to children younger than 10 years. Am J Surg Pathol 2004;28(2):183–9.
3. Riley SA, Mani V, Goodman MJ, et al. Microscopic activity in ulcerative colitis: what does it mean? Gut 1991;32(2):174–8.
4. Rutter M, Saunders B, Wilkinson K, et al. Severity of inflammation is a risk factor for colorectal neoplasia in ulcerative colitis. Gastroenterology 2004;126(2):451–9.
5. Gupta RB, Harpaz N, Itzkowitz S, et al. Histologic inflammation is a risk factor for progression to colorectal neoplasia in ulcerative colitis: a cohort study. Gastroenterology 2007;133(4):1099–105, [quiz: 1340–1].
6. Rubin DT, Huo D, Kinnucan JA, et al. Inflammation is an independent risk factor for colonic neoplasia in patients with ulcerative colitis: a case-control study. Clin Gastroenterol Hepatol 2013;11(12):1601–8.e1-4.
7. D'Haens G, Geboes K, Peeters M, et al. Patchy cecal inflammation associated with distal ulcerative colitis: a prospective endoscopic study. Am J Gastroenterol 1997;92(8):1275–9.
8. Magro F, Langner C, Driessen A, et al. European consensus on the histopathology of inflammatory bowel disease. J Crohns Colitis 2013;7(10):827–51.
9. Lengeling RW, Mitros FA, Brennan JA, et al. Ulcerative ileitis encountered at ileo-colonoscopy: likely role of nonsteroidal agents. Clin Gastroenterol Hepatol 2003;1(3):160–9.
10. Bernstein CN, Shanahan F, Anton PA, et al. Patchiness of mucosal inflammation in treated ulcerative colitis: a prospective study. Gastrointest Endosc 1995;42(3):232–7.
11. Kleer CG, Appelman HD. Ulcerative colitis: patterns of involvement in colorectal biopsies and changes with time. Am J Surg Pathol 1998;22(8):983–9.
12. Kim B, Barnett JL, Kleer CG, et al. Endoscopic and histological patchiness in treated ulcerative colitis. Am J Gastroenterol 1999;94(11):3258–62.
13. Lazenby AJ, Yardley JH, Giardiello FM, et al. Lymphocytic ("microscopic") colitis: a comparative histopathologic study with particular reference to collagenous colitis. Hum Pathol 1989;20(1):18–28.
14. Munch A, Langner C. Microscopic colitis: clinical and pathologic perspectives. Clin Gastroenterol Hepatol 2015;13(2):228–36.
15. Lazenby AJ, Yardley JH, Giardiello FM, et al. Pitfalls in the diagnosis of collagenous colitis: experience with 75 cases from a registry of collagenous colitis at the Johns Hopkins hospital. Hum Pathol 1990; 21(9):905–10.
16. Goff JS, Barnett JL, Pelke T, et al. Collagenous colitis: histopathology and clinical course. Am J Gastroenterol 1997;92(1):57–60.
17. Ayata G, Ithamukkala S, Sapp H, et al. Prevalence and significance of inflammatory bowel disease-like morphologic features in collagenous and lymphocytic colitis. Am J Surg Pathol 2002;26(11): 1414–23.
18. Chang F, Deere H, Vu C. Atypical forms of microscopic colitis: morphological features and review of the literature. Adv Anat Pathol 2005;12(4):203–11.
19. Harpaz N, Sachar DB. Segmental colitis associated with diverticular disease and other IBD look-alikes. J Clin Gastroenterol 2006;40(Suppl 3):S132–5.
20. Gledhill A, Dixon MF. Crohn's-like reaction in diverticular disease. Gut 1998;42(3):392–5.
21. Glotzer DJ, Glick ME, Goldman H. Proctitis and colitis following diversion of the fecal stream. Gastroenterology 1981;80(3):438–41.
22. Roe AM, Warren BF, Brodribb AJ, et al. Diversion colitis and involution of the defunctioned anorectum. Gut 1993;34(3):382–5.
23. Lee S, de Boer WB, Subramaniam K, et al. Pointers and pitfalls of mycophenolate-associated colitis. J Clin Pathol 2013;66(1):8–11.
24. Liapis G, Boletis J, Skalioti C, et al. Histological spectrum of mycophenolate mofetil-related colitis: association with apoptosis. Histopathology 2013; 63(5):649–58.
25. Oble DA, Mino-Kenudson M, Goldsmith J, et al. Alpha-CTLA-4 mAb-associated panenteritis: a histologic and immunohistochemical analysis. Am J Surg Pathol 2008;32(8):1130–7.
26. Gonzalez RS, Salaria SN, Bohannon CD, et al. PD-1 inhibitor gastroenterocolitis: case series and appraisal of 'immunomodulatory gastroenterocolitis'. Histopathology 2016;70(4):558–67.
27. Verschuren EC, van den Eertwegh AJ, Wonders J, et al. Clinical, endoscopic, and histologic characteristics of ipilimumab-associated colitis. Clin Gastroenterol Hepatol 2016;14(6):836–42.
28. Louie CY, DiMaio MA, Matsukuma KE, et al. Idelalisib-associated enterocolitis: clinicopathologic features and distinction from other enterocolitides. Am J Surg Pathol 2015;39(12):1653–60.
29. Weidner AS, Panarelli NC, Geyer JT, et al. Idelalisib-associated colitis: histologic findings in 14 patients. Am J Surg Pathol 2015;39(12):1661–7.
30. Voltaggio L, Montgomery EA, Ali MA, et al. Sex, lies, and gastrointestinal tract biopsies: a review of selected sexually transmitted proctocolitides. Adv Anat Pathol 2014;21(2):83–93.

The Differential Diagnosis of Acute Colitis: Clues to a Specific Diagnosis

 CrossMark

Jose Jessurun, MD

KEYWORDS

- Acute colitis • Infectious colitis • Drug-induced colitis • Hemorrhagic colitis
- Pseudomembranous colitis • Ischemic colitis

Key points

- Colonic biopsy specimens from patients with acute colitis are usually obtained in patients with a prolonged clinical course or who do not respond as expected to treatment.

- Five basic histologic patterns are identified: acute colitis, focal active colitis, pseudomembranous colitis, hemorrhagic colitis, and ischemic colitis.

- These patterns are associated with certain etiologic considerations that influence therapeutic decisions.

- Acute colitis patterns should be differentiated from those associated with chronic inflammatory disorders.

ABSTRACT

This review describes a systematic approach to the interpretation of colonic biopsy specimens of patients with acute colitis. Five main histologic patterns are discussed: acute colitis, focal active colitis, pseudomembranous colitis, hemorrhagic colitis, and ischemic colitis. For each pattern, the most common etiologic associations and their differential diagnoses are presented. Strategies based on histologic analysis and clinical considerations to differentiate acute from chronic colitides are discussed.

laboratory findings without need for colonoscopy and mucosal biopsy analysis. For the most part, patients with acute colitic symptoms only undergo endoscopic evaluation if they have a severe or atypical clinical presentation, do not improve within an expected timeframe, or fail to respond to treatment. Pathologists are most helpful when they are able to generate a circumscribed differential diagnosis based on interpretation of inflammatory patterns; descriptive diagnoses, such as "acute and chronic inflammation" or "nonspecific inflammation," do not contribute substantially to patient care. Such designations may be used to describe a variety of circumstances ranging from normal mucosa to inflammatory bowel disease. In this article, a brief review of the normal histology of the colonic mucosa is followed by a discussion of the most frequent histologic patterns of acute colonic injury encountered in biopsy specimens.

OVERVIEW

Most patients with acute colitis are diagnosed and treated based on a combination of clinical and

The author does not have any commercial or financial conflicts of interest.

Department of Pathology and Laboratory Medicine, Weill Cornell Medicine New York, Starr 1031 B, 1300 York Avenue, New York, NY 10065, USA

E-mail address: Joj9034@med.cornell.edu

Surgical Pathology 10 (2017) 863–885
http://dx.doi.org/10.1016/j.path.2017.07.008
1875-9181/17/© 2017 Elsevier Inc. All rights reserved.

HISTOLOGY OF THE NORMAL COLONIC MUCOSA

The colonic mucosa comprises epithelial cells, stromal cells, and "inflammatory" cells. Straight tubular crypts composed of absorptive and goblet cells extend perpendicularly from the surface to the muscularis mucosae. These crypts are evenly spaced resembling test tubes in a rack. Crypts of the left colon and rectum contain many more goblet cells than those of the right colon where absorptive cells predominate (Fig. 1). When cut tangentially, their even distribution can be compared with a pack of cigarettes opened at the top (Fig. 2). Occasional branched crypts may be encountered in an otherwise normal colonic mucosa. Paneth cells are confined to the right colon in adults where their numbers vary from none to a few cells within a single crypt. Because these cells play a role in immune modulation, apoptosis, autophagy, and regeneration, their numbers are probably related to environmental factors. In young children, Paneth cells are normally encountered in the transverse colon and rectum and tend to decrease in number with increasing age.[1] Mitotic figures are confined to the lower third of the crypts. Regenerative crypts may show mitotic figures in the middle or upper thirds of the crypts or more than 2 mitotic figures per crypt in tangentially cut sections.

The lamina propria normally contains plasma cells, eosinophils, lymphocytes, and few histiocytes. The density of these cells and their relative proportions vary considerably among different populations, reflecting environmental and sanitary conditions. The colonic lamina propria from asymptomatic individuals living in underdeveloped countries tends to be more cellular compared with that of those living in developed nations. The number of eosinophils present in the lamina propria is also highly variable. People living in the northern United States tend to have fewer eosinophils than those living in southern states.[2] Eosinophil numbers throughout the colon show slight seasonal variation, which may reflect allergen exposure.[3] The density of all inflammatory cell types is more pronounced in the right colon compared with the distal colorectum. Plasma cells tend to be more abundant in the luminal third of the mucosa and decrease toward the deep mucosa, although this pattern is obscured in the cecum where a transmucosal distribution of plasma cells is frequently present. Mildly increased mononuclear cells in the lamina propria of the proximal colon should not be taken as evidence of a chronic inflammatory disorder if there are no other features that support this interpretation. The superficial regions of the crypts and luminal epithelium normally contains CD3+/CD8+ intraepithelial lymphocytes. Although variable, their number rarely exceed 5 per 100 colonic epithelial cells.

HISTOLOGIC PATTERNS ASSOCIATED WITH ACUTE COLITIS

There are no generally accepted classifications for the histologic patterns encountered in colonic biopsy specimens from patients with acute colitis, although 2 basic patterns may be recognized based on mechanisms of disease: inflammatory and ischemic. Infiltration of the mucosa by inflammatory cells characterizes the former pattern, whereas hypoperfusion explains the ischemic pattern. Decreased perfusion may result from

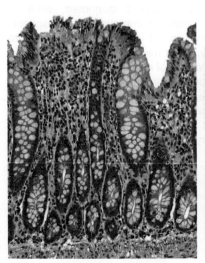 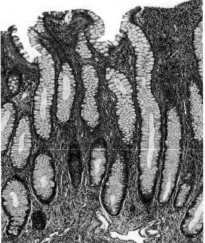

Fig. 1. Normal colonic mucosa. Evenly distributed straight crypts extend from the luminal surface to the muscularis mucosae. Goblet cells are less abundant in the right colon (*left panel*) compared with the sigmoid colon and rectum (*right panel*). Inflammatory cells predominate in the luminal third of the lamina propria. (H&E, original magnification ×100)

Fig. 2. Normal colonic mucosa. On tangential sections, the crypts are evenly sized, rounded, and nonclustered. Mitotic figures, when present, rarely exceed 1 per cross-section. Intraepithelial lymphocytes may be present in the superficial third of the crypts. (H&E, original magnification ×300)

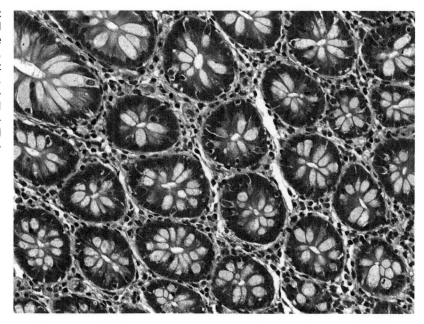

circulatory compromise (ie, low-flow states) or an inflammatory/toxic endothelial injury with, or without, occlusive fibrin thrombi. The latter may be associated with variable amounts of inflammation; thus, these patterns are not mutually exclusive (Box 1).

ACUTE COLITIS (ACUTE SELF-LIMITED COLITIS)

An acute colitis pattern is associated primarily with infections and drug-induced injuries that cause limited injury and show spontaneous resolution after removal of the offending pathogen or medication. For this reason, the terms, *acute colitis* and *acute self-limited colitis*, are often used interchangeably, although the latter does not accurately reflect the clinical evolution of disease.

Some cases of acute colitis persist for several weeks or months, particularly if the etiology is not addressed. In addition, the term, *self-limited*, implies that the injury is mild and that treatment might not be necessary, which is not always the case.

Infectious colitis may result from foodborne pathogens or organisms contaminating water, secretions, and other sources. Foodborne pathogens are usually acquired after ingestion of contaminated dairy, meat, and fish products. Organisms that are more frequently associated with this form of transmission in the United States include *Campylobacter*, *Salmonella*, *Escherichia coli* O157.H7, and Norwalk virus. Nonfoodborne agents include *Shigella*, *Yersinia*, Coxsackie virus, rotavirus, enterovirus, and adenovirus.[4] Most infectious agents produce a patchy colitis and less

---

Box 1
Classification of patterns

Purely inflammatory
Acute colitis

Focal active colitis

Mixed inflammatory/ischemic

With prominent pseudomembranes (pseudomembranous colitis)

With prominent lamina propria hemorrhage (hemorrhagic colitis)

Mostly ischemic

Acute ischemic colitis

frequently a diffuse pancolitis. Although any part of the colon may be involved, infections by certain organisms show a predilection for certain regions. *Campylobacter, Salmonella, Yersinia,* tuberculosis, and amebiasis should be considered when inflammatory changes predominately affect the proximal colon. Sexually transmitted infections, such as herpesvirus, gonorrhea, syphilis, and lymphogranuloma venereum, typically cause proctitis with extension into the distal sigmoid colon in some cases.

HISTOPATHOLOGY

Low-power examination reveals preserved crypt architecture and a patchy or diffuse distribution of inflammatory changes. The lamina propria is often edematous with mixed inflammatory cell infiltrates and abundant neutrophils. The latter infiltrate the crypt epithelium (active cryptitis) forming luminal aggregates (crypt abscesses) that may result in crypt destruction and erosion or ulceration of the mucosa (**Figs. 3** and **4**). Lamina propria hemorrhage may be present. Loss of epithelial cells triggers regeneration manifested by increased mitotic activity and proliferation of immature, mucin-depleted cells without crypt architectural remodeling. Within 2 weeks to 3 weeks, neutrophils decrease in number whereas plasma cells and eosinophils are recruited to the lamina propria (**Fig. 5, Box 2**).

DIFFERENTIAL DIAGNOSIS OF ACUTE COLITIS AND INFLAMMATORY BOWEL DISEASE

Acute colitis is readily distinguished from early-onset inflammatory bowel disease when biopsies are taken shortly after the initial symptoms. Most patients do not undergo colonoscopy during the early phases of the disease, however; only patients with atypical manifestations or those who fail to respond to antibiotic therapy undergo evaluation with mucosal biopsy. In this situation, tissue samples often contain plasma cells, eosinophils, and

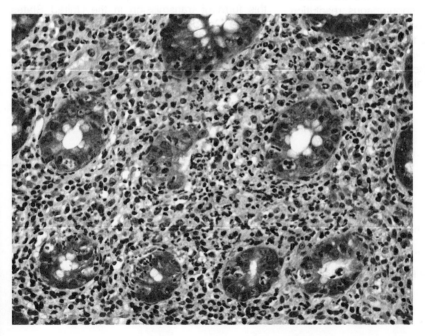

Fig. 3. Acute colitis. The lamina propria is expanded by inflammatory cells, including abundant neutrophils that also infiltrate the crypts. Despite crypt injury, there is no architectural derangement (H&E, original magnification ×300).

Fig. 4. Acute colitis. Neutrophils within crypts (active cryptitis) and crypt abscesses are seen in both acute colitis and active inflammatory bowel disease. Neutrophils within the lamina propria, as seen in this case, are more typical of an acute colitis, particularly if plasma cells are inconspicuous (H&E, original magnification ×400).

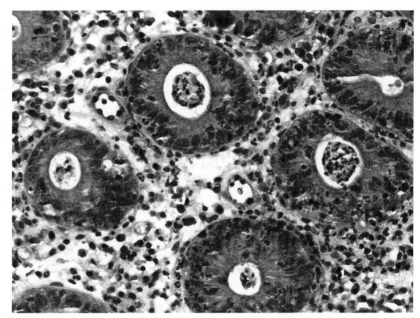

macrophages in combination with a paucity of neutrophils that may make it difficult to distinguish acute colitis from early inflammatory bowel disease. Resolving this diagnostic dilemma is generally possible when histologic findings are interpreted in light of clinical information, as enumerated in **Tables 1** and **2**.[5] Even in its early phases, ulcerative colitis is characterized by dense, transmucosal, plasma cell–rich inflammation in the lamina propria that is generally accompanied by crypt remodeling (**Fig. 6**). On the other hand, the plasma cell–rich inflammation of evolving acute colitis tends to have a patchy distribution and rarely expands the deep lamina propria (**Fig. 7**).

Distinguishing acute colitis from Crohn disease is by far more challenging. *Salmonella* and *Yersinia* primarily affect the ileocecal region and appendix, thereby simulating the distribution of Crohn disease. Similar to Crohn colitis, acute colitis of any etiology frequently shows patchy mucosal involvement. On the other hand, Crohn colitis often produces inconsistent crypt architectural changes and granulomata are usually absent (**Fig. 8**). Features that favor a diagnosis of acute colitis over Crohn disease include the presence of

Fig. 5. Plasma cells and eosinophils are recruited to the colon within weeks of acute colitis onset.

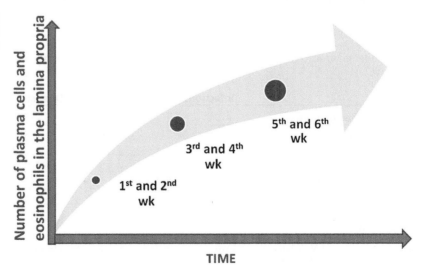

Table 1
Infectious colitis versus early-onset inflammatory bowel disease, clinical and endoscopic differential diagnosis

	Infectious Colitis	Inflammatory Bowel Disease
Onset of symptoms	Sudden	Insidious
Fever	Early	Absent or late
Bowel movements	>6	Fewer
C-reactive protein and erythrocyte sedimentation rate	−/+	+++
Anemia	−	+
Mucosal inflammation	Patchy	Diffuse in ulcerative colitis
Linear ulcers	Rare	Crohn disease
Ileitis	Salmonella Yersinia	Crohn disease

Data from Surawicz CM. What's the best way to differentiate infectious colitis (acute self-limited colitis) from IBD? Inflamm Bowel Dis 2008;14:S157–58.

disproportionately more neutrophils in the lamina propria than in crypts and colonic inflammation unaccompanied by ileal involvement.[5] As discussed in Heewon A. Kwak and John Hart's article, " The Many Faces of Medication-Related Injury in the GI Tract," in this issue, nonsteroidal anti-inflammatory drugs (NSAIDs) can cause acute ileitis and/or colitis with erosions and ulcers similar to those seen in Crohn disease.[6–8] Well-demarcated ulcers in the cecum and ascending colon surrounded by a normal appearing mucosa are typically seen in NSAID-related injury, although any segment of the colon may be affected. Patchy neutrophilic cryptitis, apoptotic crypt epithelial cells, increased intraepithelial lymphocytes, and regenerative changes may be present in variable combinations, whereas lamina propria plasma cells and lymphocytes tend to be sparse. Granulomata are not typically seen in

acute colitis; their presence should suggest an alternative diagnosis. Overt regenerative crypt changes and pyloric metaplasia are generally absent in cases of NSAID-related colitis except when patients receive high doses over an extended period of time.[6,9]

INFECTIOUS CAUSES OF ACUTE COLITIS WITH SPECIAL HISTOLOGIC PATTERNS

Nontyphoid *Salmonella* species are foodborne pathogens that cause acute enterocolitis and, in approximately 5% of patients, septicemia. The 2 most common organisms are *Salmonella enterica* serovar Enteritidis and *S enterica* serovar Typhimurium. Biopsy specimens from patients infected by these enteroinvasive organisms show either a classic acute colitis pattern or a subacute pattern with fewer neutrophils and more plasma cells

Table 2
Histologic features that aid distinction between infectious colitis and types of inflammatory bowel disease

	Infectious Colitis	Crohn Disease	Ulcerative Colitis
Diffuse inflammation	+	+	+++
Patchy/focal inflammation	+++	+++	+
Active cryptitis	+++	+++	+++
Mucosal remodeling	−/+	++/+/−	+++/+
Basal plasmacytosis	−	−	+++
Neutrophils in lamina propria	++	−/+	−

Data from Surawicz CM. What's the best way to differentiate infectious colitis (acute self-limited colitis) from IBD? Inflamm Bowel Dis 2008;14:S157–58.

Fig. 6. Comparative images of acute colitis (*left panel*) and acute presentation of ulcerative colitis (*right panel*). Despite the presence of numerous active lesions, the lamina propria in acute colitis shows fewer inflammatory cells. There is no architectural derangement. By contrast, abundant plasma cells expand the lamina propria and distort crypts even during an acute presentation of ulcerative colitis (H&E, original magnification ×300).

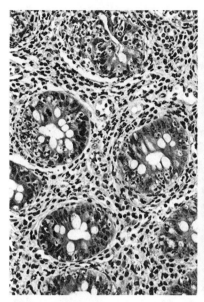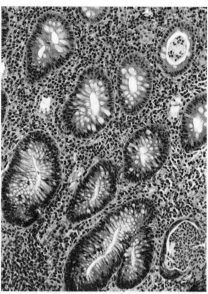

and lymphocytes in the lamina propria, which may be accompanied by crypt architectural distortion.[10] By contrast, the inflammatory response associated with infection by *Salmonella* typhi (*S enterica* subsp enterica serovar Typhi), the causative agent of typhoid fever, may deviate entirely from the acute colitis pattern. Also transmitted by contaminated food and water, this facultative gram-negative bacillus affect 21 million people

worldwide and causes 200,000 deaths per year.[11] Endoscopic examination of the right colon and terminal ileum shows mucosal edema and raised nodules corresponding to hyperplastic Peyer patches. Ulceration of the overlying mucosa causes aphthous ulcers that mimic Crohn disease. More advanced cases show linear or discoid ulcers that may perforate and cause peritonitis (**Fig. 9**).[12] The characteristic microscopic lesions

Fig. 7. Evolving acute colitis. This biopsy was taken 5 weeks after the initial onset of symptoms. The lamina propria shows increased cellularity that is more prominent in the upper (luminal) half of the mucosa. The crypts have a regenerative appearance but preserve their tubular shape (H&E, original magnification ×200).

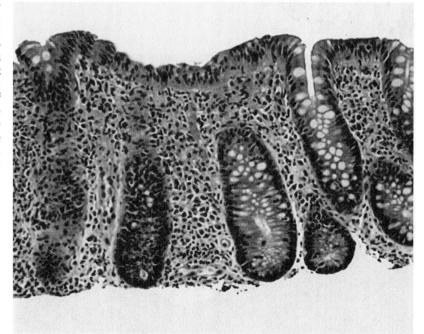

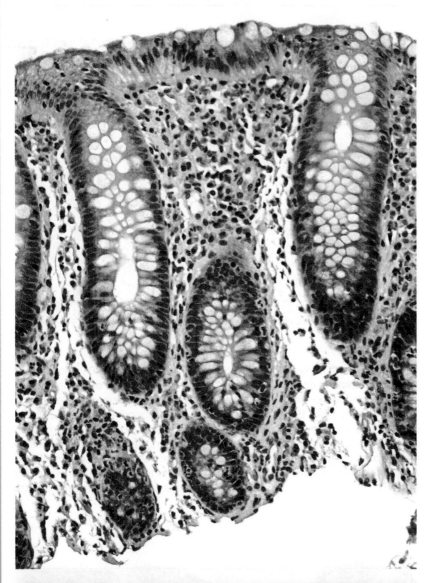

Fig. 8. Active lesions in Crohn disease. Crohn colitis may cause neutrophil-rich crypt injury unassociated with crypt distortion, indistinguishable from an acute colitis. It is imperative to take into consideration the clinical and endoscopic findings before rendering a diagnosis of acute colitis (H&E, original magnification ×200).

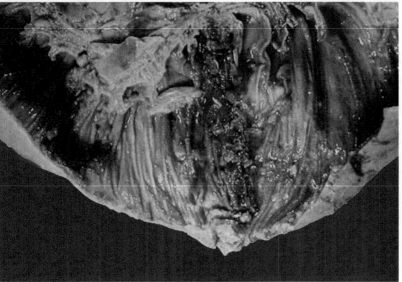

Fig. 9. Typhoid fever. Discoid ulcer in the small intestine.

are typhoid nodules, representing enlarged Peyer patches that contain aggregates of macrophages.[13] These macrophages, referred to as typhoid cells, harbor bacteria and blood cells (Fig. 10). Well-formed granulomata are rare but have been reported.[14] Even in the absence of nodular aggregates, mucosal biopsy specimens can contain numerous macrophages; thus, this inflammatory pattern should raise concern for typhoid fever in patients with acute-onset diarrhea, particularly if the findings are most severe in the terminal ileum and right colon.[13,14]

Histiocytes that show erythrophagocytosis should be differentiated from trophozoites. *Entamoeba histolytica* infects 10% of the world's population and causes 40,000 to 100,000 deaths annually, making it the second leading cause of death due to parasitic disease.[15,16] Most infections are acquired after ingestion of food or water contaminated with feces that contains cysts. Other forms of transmission include oral and anal sex and contaminated endoscopes or enema apparatus.[17] The cecum and ascending colon are most commonly affected and display discrete ulcers separated by a normal-appearing or edematous mucosa.[18] Despite an abundance of tissue necrosis, inflammation is often sparse, consisting of peripherally arranged neutrophils, lymphocytes, and histiocytes around necrotic areas that contain finely granular, eosinophilic material with little nuclear debris.[19–21] This material typically contains a few to multiple rounded trophozoites with pale eosinophilic or bubbly cytoplasm and central nuclei. Trophozoites contain a central or slightly eccentrically located chromatin condensation (karyosome), which appears as a black dot and facilitates distinction from macrophages (Fig. 11). Cytoplasmic red blood cell fragments allow distinction between *E histolytica* and other species.

Yersinia is another organism that shows a predilection to infect the ileocolic region and simulate Crohn disease. These gram-negative coccobacilli have a worldwide distribution; they are a common cause of bacterial enteritis in Europe, but less so in the United States.[22–24] *Yersinia enterocolitica* and *Yersinia pseudotuberculosis* are the 2 species associated with human enteric infections, and both are transmitted mostly by contaminated food and water.[25] Ileitis, appendicitis, mesenteric adenitis, and colitis may occur in isolation, or in various combinations. Similar to *Salmonella* typhi, *Yersinia* is an enteroinvasive organism that primarily involves Peyer patches and the surrounding mucosa. Aphthous and linear ulcers with exudates closely mimic the endoscopic appearance of Crohn disease. Histologic features include an acute colitis/enteritis pattern or lymphoid hyperplasia that may be accompanied by non-necrotic epithelioid granulomata or suppurative granulomata that show central microabscesses (Fig. 12). Although both species may elicit granulomata, suppurative granulomata are more frequently associated with *Y pseudotuberculosis*. Ulcers, fissures, and transmural inflammation also be present, further complicating the differential diagnosis with Crohn disease.[26,27]

For obvious reasons, colonic biopsy specimens of neutropenic patients with acute colitis do not

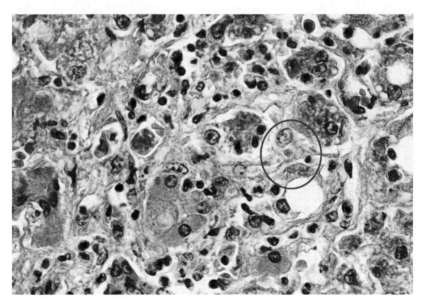

Fig. 10. Typhoid fever. Characteristic histiocyte-rich infiltrates. Some histiocytes show erythrophagocytosis (*circle*) (H&E, original magnification ×400).

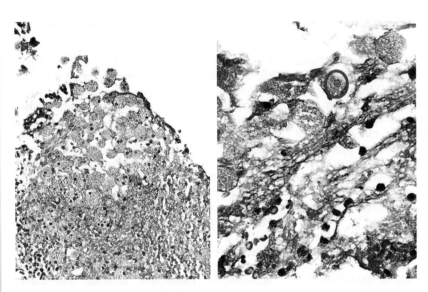

Fig. 11. Amebiasis. Multiple trophozoites of (*Left Panel*) *Entamoeba histolytica.* Notice the close resemblance to histiocytes. (*Right Panel*) One trophozoite has a visible karyosome (*circle*), which helps to distinguish these orgnanisms from inflammatory cells (H&E, original magnification, left ×400, right ×600).

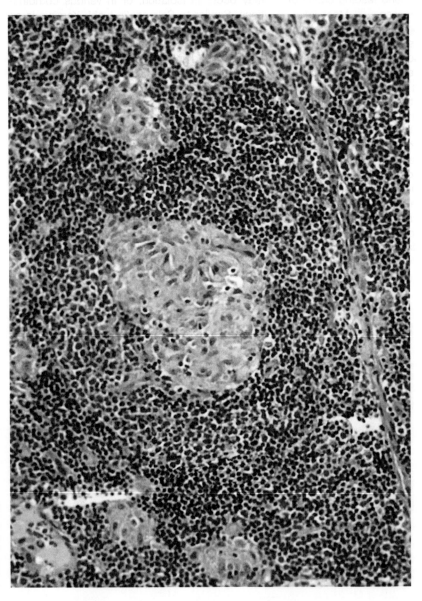

Fig. 12. Yersinia infection. An epithelioid granuloma is seen in a biopsy of the terminal ileum (H&E, original magnification ×400).

show the classical pattern described previously. These patients are prone to develop a life-threatening condition that almost always affects the cecum, which has been termed, *neutropenic typhlitis* (**Fig. 13**). Severe cases may show more extensive involvement of the terminal ileum, other segments of the small bowel, and more distal colon.[28–30] In the absence of neutrophils, the organisms invade a mucosa that may be previously damaged by chemotherapy or complications of stem cell transplantation.[31] The triad of abdominal pain, fever, and diarrhea in patients with unexplained bacteremia with enteric organisms should suggest this condition.[30] Cross-sectional imaging reveals thickening of the cecal wall and right colon with, or without, pneumatosis coli and pericolonic

soft tissue stranding.[31] Histologic examination reveals necrosis, ulcers, edema, hemorrhage, and invasive bacteria that may be accompanied by fungi. Despite severe tissue injury and overwhelming infection, there is a disproportionate scarcity of inflammatory cells (**Fig. 14**).

FOCAL ACTIVE COLITIS

Focal active colitis is an inflammatory pattern that may or may not be clinically relevant. It is mostly encountered in adult patients with infectious colitis, drug-induced gastrointestinal injury, and irritable bowel syndrome.[32–35] Less frequently, it may be a manifestation of inflammatory bowel disease, in particular Crohn disease, or partially treated

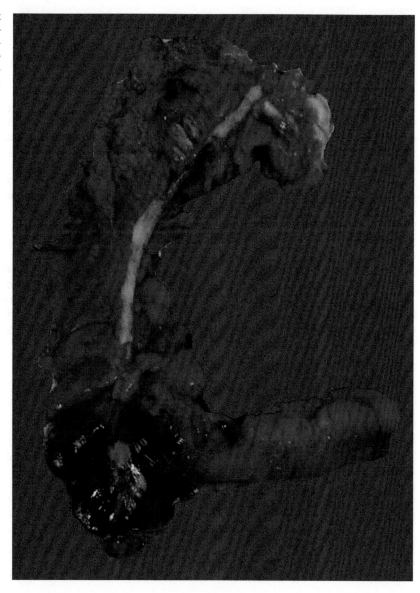

Fig. 13. Neutropenic enterocolitis. Right hemicolectomy showing severe inflammation of the cecum (typhlitis). (*Courtesy of* Dr Luis Muñoz, Aguascalientes, Mexico.)

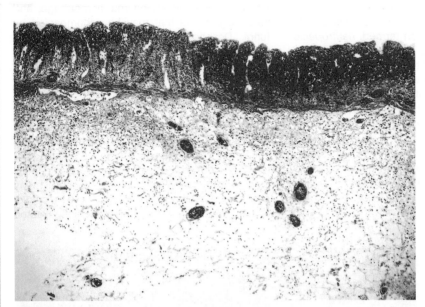

Fig. 14. Neutropenic enterocolitis. Section of the cecum showing mucosal necrosis and hemorrhage, and massive submucosal edema with sparse lymphocytic inflammation (H&E, original magnification ×100). (*Courtesy of* Dr Luis Muñoz, Aguascalientes, Mexico.)

ulcerative colitis.[33] Because irritable bowel syndrome and drug-induced colitis are infrequent among children, a higher number of pediatric patients with this inflammatory pattern in colonic biopsies have inflammatory bowel disease.[36,37] Focal active colitis is occasionally encountered in patients undergoing colonoscopy for reasons other than a suspected inflammatory disorder. Mucosal injury caused by laxatives used for bowel preparation may explain this finding in some cases (**Table 3**).[36]

HISTOPATHOLOGY

Focal active colitis is characterized by neutrophilic cryptitis involving a few contiguous crypts within 1 biopsy fragment, often with increased cellularity of the surrounding lamina propria. The background mucosa displays normal crypt architecture and no Paneth cell metaplasia (**Figs. 15** and **16**). Apoptotic crypt epithelial cells are variably present and, if numerous, may suggest a drug-related injury. Medications should also be suspected when active lesions involve the base of the crypts (**Box 3**).[33]

ACUTE COLITIS WITH ISCHEMIC FEATURES

Three histologic variants of acute colitis with ischemic features are recognized. A mixed inflammatory/ischemic pattern is characteristic of pseudomembranous colitis. Hemorrhagic colitis shows ischemic mucosal injury with extensive hemorrhage in the lamina propria and variable

Table 3
Clinical conditions associated with a focal acute colitis pattern

Author	No. Patients	Infections	Drugs	Iirritable Bowel Syndrome	Incidental	Inflammatory Bowel Disease[a]	Other
Greenson et al,[32] 1997	42, adults	55%[b]	45%[b]	14%	26%	0%	5%
Volk et al,[35] 2997	31, adults	48%	?	?	29%	13%	10%
Xin et al,[36] 2003	31, children	31%	0%	0%	28%	31%	10%
Shetty et al,[33] 2011	90, adults	19%	24%	33%	8%	16%	—

[a] Crohn disease >> ulcerative colitis.
[b] Several patients who were thought to have an acute infectious colitis were also taking NSAID.

Fig. 15. Focal acute colitis. This inflammatory pattern may be easily overlooked because on low-power examination the mucosa has an almost normal appearance. (H&E, original magnification ×50).

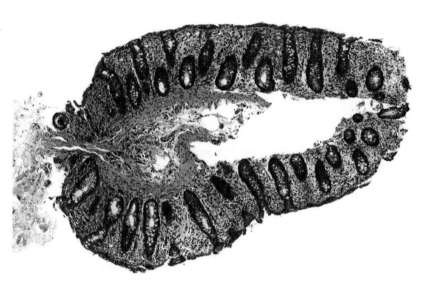

inflammation. The third pattern is purely ischemic with minimal or no inflammation. Proper identification of the predominant pattern is clinically relevant because there is a strong correlation between the histologic features and the underlying etiology.

PSEUDOMEMBRANOUS COLITIS

Pseudomembranous colitis is a pattern of injury typically associated with infection by *Clostridium difficile*, although it is not always caused by this pathogen.[38,39] Other causes include infection with *E coli* O157, *Shigella*, and other Shiga toxin–producing organisms as well as acute ischemia, acute radiation injury, and several drugs. Medications associated with a pseudomembranous colitis include various antibiotics, alosetron, cisplatin, cocaine, cyclosporin A, dextroamphetamine, docetaxel, 5-fluorouracil, gold, glutaraldehyde, NSAID, and paraquat.[38]

Infection by *C difficile* is mostly acquired in a nosocomial setting in the United States, although

Fig. 16. Focal acute colitis. Neutrophilic cryptitis is present in contiguous crypts (*circles*). Other mucosal biopsy specimens from this site were histologically unremarkable (H&E, original magnification ×300).

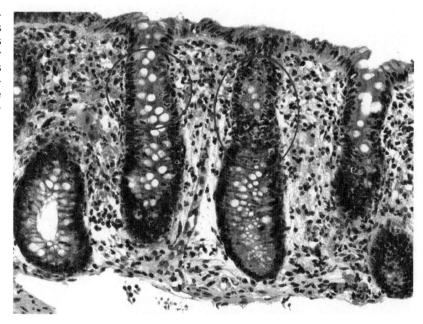

Box 3
Reporting focal active colitis

Diagnosis: Focal active colitis. See note.

Note: This inflammatory pattern is associated with bacterial (*Campylobacter, Salmonella, Shigella, E coli*, and *Yersinia*) and viral infections or drug-induced injury. Other clinical associations include irritable bowel syndrome and inflammatory bowel disease, particularly Crohn disease. In the absence clinical colitis, these changes often remain unexplained and could be related to bowel preparation.

---

it can also be acquired in the community.[40] The incidence of *C difficile* infections has increased recently from 4.5 per 1000 in 2001 to 8.2 per 1000 in 2010.[38] Importantly, the proportion of severe cases has also increased from 7.1% in 1991 to 18.2% in 2003.[40,41] Risk factors for infection include hospitalization, administration of antibiotics, increased age, use of proton pomp inhibitors, contact with carriers of the organism, and comorbid conditions.[42,43] The clinical presentation of *C difficile* infection is variable: some patients are asymptomatic whereas others develop classic pseudomembranous colitis which, when severe, may cause toxic megacolon.[42–44] Because the latter complication has a high mortality, surgical intervention with hemicolectomy or total colectomy may be necessary (**Fig. 17**).[45–47] Cross-sectional imaging may reveal focal or diffuse wall thickening with pericolonic soft tissue stranding. Thickened haustral folds with flocculated oral contrast media or entrapped bowel contents (ie, accordion sign) are highly suggestive, but not pathognomonic, of this condition.[48–50] Diffuse pseudomembranes are commonly encountered at endoscopy and are characterized by elevated yellow-white nodules or plaques that rarely exceed 2 cm in diameter. The intervening mucosa may be normal or show granularity, ulcers, or mucosal edema. In some patients, pseudomembranes may be absent and the mucosa may show nonspecific alterations, such as erythema, friability, or ulcers. Biopsies of these abnormalities should always be taken because histologic examination may reveal a diagnostic inflammatory pattern.[51–54]

Mucosal injury is mediated by 2 toxins: TcdA and TcdB. These molecules cause epithelial cell necrosis, inflammation, and loss of mucosal barrier function. The gold standard tests for infection are the cytotoxin neutralizing assay and the toxigenic culture.[55] The former is based on detection of the cytopathic effect of toxin B on cells and the neutralization of this effect by antitoxin. The latter is based on standard stool cultures that identify both toxigenic and nontoxigenic strains, followed by assays to detect the toxin genes or

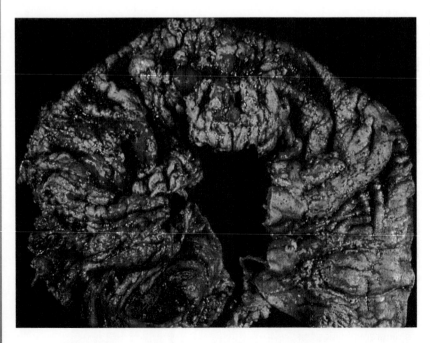

Fig. 17. Pseudomembranous colitis. Colectomy specimen of a patient with severe *Clostridium difficile* colitis who developed toxic megacolon. Notice the diffuse distribution of pseudomembranes.

proteins. Turnaround times for both methods are on the order of several days, which limits their clinical utility.[55,56] In clinical practice, the most commonly used diagnostic tests are enzyme immunoassays for both toxins.[56] More recently, tests based on nucleic acid amplification and glutamate dehydrogenase, an enzyme produced by *C difficile*, detection have been developed. The enzymatic assay detects both toxigenic and nontoxigenic strains; thus, a positive result is followed by an assay to identify the toxins.[57,58] It is recommended that only stools from patients with diarrhea be tested for *C difficile* infection.

HISTOPATHOLOGY

The hallmark feature of pseudomembranous colitis is the presence of laminated pseudomembranes composed of fibrin-rich exudates and mucus with embedded neutrophils and necrotic epithelial cells. On low power, this exudate seems to emanate from the underlying crypts, comparable to a volcanic eruption or a mushroom (Fig. 18). Subjacent crypts are dilated, often filled with sloughed epithelial cells and neutrophils or mucus, and the surface epithelium in contact with the pseudomembrane is either inflamed or necrotic. As the disease progresses, typical ischemic changes develop, first affecting the luminal half of the crypt and then extending to involve whole crypt. The mucosa adjacent to the pseudomembrane may show features of an acute colitis, seem relatively spared, or display variable hemorrhage within the lamina propria. Fibrin

thrombi within capillaries are frequently observed (Fig. 19).

DIFFERENTIAL DIAGNOSIS

A pseudomembranous pattern of injury can occur in noninfectious ischemic colitis. At variance with the diffuse distribution of pseudomembranes in *C difficile* colitis, the lesions in noninfectious ischemia tend to be localized and, on endoscopic examination, the pseudomembranes may appear as large, polypoid masslike lesions (Table 4) (Fig. 20). If the clinical context and endoscopic appearance are not taken into account, mucosal biopsy specimens from these lesions may be misinterpreted as indicative of *C difficile*–associated colitis. Hyalinization of the lamina propria and small, regenerative crypts (withered crypts) with sparse inflammation favor a diagnosis of ischemia (Box 4).[59]

HEMORRHAGIC COLITIS

A well-known cause of hemorrhagic colitis is infection with the Shiga toxin–producing enterohemorrhagic strain of *E coli*, O157:H7. In the United States, this organism accounts for 73,000 clinical apparent infections, 3000 hospitalizations, and 500 deaths annually.[60,61] The organism primarily colonizes the right colon and causes high-volume, nonbloody watery diarrhea that may progress to bloody diarrhea. In approximately 10% of patients, life-threatening extraintestinal complications develop, including

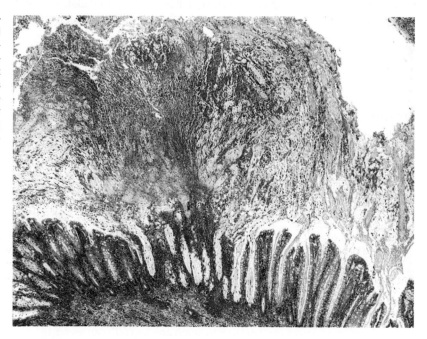

Fig. 18. Pseudomembranos colitis: fibrin and mucin-rich pseudomembrane with layers of inflammatory and necrotic epithelial cells. This appearance is evocative of a volcano eruption or a sprouting mushroom (H&E, original magnification ×100).

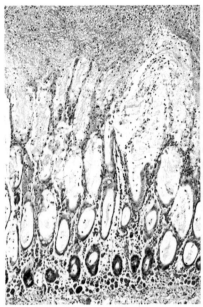 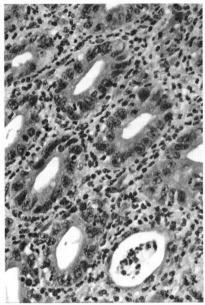

Fig. 19. Pseudomembranous colitis. The pseudomembranes are composed of fibrin-rich exudate with admixed inflammatory cells. The surface epithelium frequently shows ischemic changes, which may extend to the crypts. At variance with an exudate of an ulcer, which appears detached from the mucosa, the pseudomembranes tend to merge with the underlying lamina propria (*left panel*) (H&E, original magnification ×100). The intervening mucosa in this case showed the features on an acute colitis (*right panel*) (H&E, original magnification ×300). In some cases it may be normal or have a hemorrhagic appearance.

hemolytic uremic syndrome and thrombotic thrombocytopenic purpura.[60–62] Unfortunately, there is no satisfactory treatment of this infection because killing the bacteria with antibiotic therapy triggers release of Shiga toxin, which promotes development of hemolytic uremic syndrome.[63] *Klebsiella oxytoca*, a bacterium that was believed for many years to be an innocuous commensal, is another cause of hemorrhagic colitis. Clinical symptoms typically follow antibiotic use, possibly resulting from the organism's capacity to produce β-lactamase. *K oxytoca* typically produces a segmental colitis of the proximal colon that resolves shortly after discontinuation of antibiotic therapy.[64] Other causes of hemorrhagic colitis include *Shigella* infection, noninfectious acute ischemia, and some medications, including several antibiotic agents, alpha-interferon, hyperosmolar medication formulations, and other drugs associated with mucosal ischemia.[65]

HISTOPATHOLOGY

The lamina propria appears hemorrhagic and edematous. Fibrin thrombi within capillaries are commonly observed. Crypts show ischemic injury and/or display a regenerative appearance. There is variable neutrophilic inflammation. Pseudomembranes may be present but are not the predominant feature (**Figs. 21** and **22**) (**Box 5**).

ACUTE ISCHEMIC COLITIS

Hypoperfusion of the colon due to circulatory failure or vascular occlusive diseases is the most frequent cause of ischemic colonic injury. Although this simple explanation accounts for many cases, the multiple etiologies associated with this condition point toward a more complex pathophysiology.[66] Acute ischemic colitis is predominantly

Table 4
Differential diagnosis of *Clostridium difficile* pseudomembranous colitis and ischemia

Feature	*Clostridium difficile*	Ischemia
Diffuse pseudomembranes (endoscopy)	21/22	2/24
Localized process (endoscopy)	1/22	24/24
Polyps or masses (endoscopy)	0/22	7/24
Hyalinization of lamina propria (histology)	0/25	19/24
Microcrypts (histology)	6/25	18/24

Data from Dignan CR, Greenson JK. Can ischemic colitis be differentiated from C difficile colitis in biopsy specimens? Am J Surg Pathol 1997;21:706–10.

Fig. 20. Comparative features of *Clostridium difficile*–related pseudomembranous colitis (*left panel*) and ischemic colitis with pseudomembranes (*right panel*). The diffuse distribution of the lesions favor an infection while localized confluent membranes are typical of ischemia.

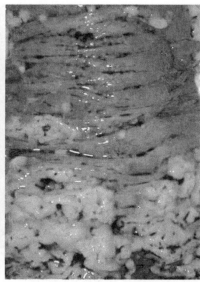

observed in elderly individuals with an incidence of 6.1/person-year to 9.9/person-year.[67,68] The extent of the mucosal injury determines the clinical presentation and is not only related to the severity of the circulatory imbalance but also to the underlying etiology. Conditions associated with an acute ischemic colitis include vascular occlusive disorders, such as thromboemboli, vascular injury during surgery or trauma, vasculitis, and vascular compromise associated with volvulus, intussusception, and serosal adhesions. Nonocclusive etiologies include cardiac failure, shock, sepsis, medications, and infections. Organisms capable of causing mucosal ischemia include those associated with pseudomembranous and hemorrhagic colitis (*Shigella*, *E coli* O157:H7, and *C difficile*), *Campylobacter*, *Salmonella*, cytomegalovirus, and angioinvasive fungi or parasites, such as *Angiostrongylus costaricensis*. Drugs that have been reported associated with ischemic colitis are listed in **Box 6**.[65,66]

Colonoscopy and biopsies are seldom performed in patients presenting with an acute abdomen due to embolic occlusion or intestinal obstruction. Conditions that produce an acute, progressive decrease in blood flow have a less dramatic clinical presentation. The classic scenario is an elderly patient with crampy abdominal pain, bloody stools, and leukocytosis, sometimes preceded by a known cause of transient hypoperfusion.[66] Depending of the severity of the ischemic insult, abdominal imaging may show a nonspecific gas pattern or focal mural thickening (thumbprinting) caused by submucosal hemorrhage and edema. Cross-sectional imaging may be normal or show segmental thickening of the colonic wall and pericolic fat stranding. Because these radiologic findings are similar to those seen in other types of colitis, colonoscopy is frequently performed to confirm the diagnosis and to evaluate the degree of ischemia. Mucosal friability with bleeding, petechial hemorrhages, edema,

---

Box 4
Reporting pseudomembranous colitis

Diagnosis: Pseudomembranous colitis. See note.

Note: This inflammatory pattern is associated with infections primarily caused by *C difficile* and less frequently by other bacteria (*E coli* and *Shigella*). A similar pattern may be caused by ischemia, certain drugs and radiation injury.

Additional annotations according to the endoscopic appearance of the lesions:

The diffuse distribution of the lesions favors an infectious or drug-induced etiology.

The localized distribution of the lesions favors an ischemic etiology.

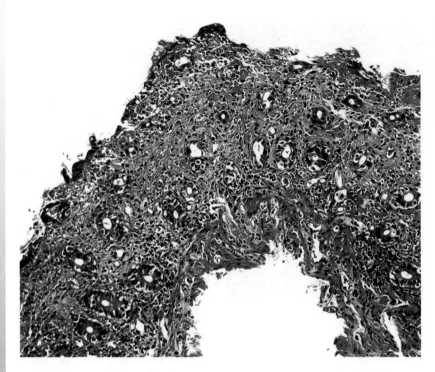

Fig. 21. Hemorrhagic colitis. Diffuse hemorrhage expands the lamina propria. In addition, small crypts (microcrypts) typical of ischemia are also present (H&E, original magnification ×100).

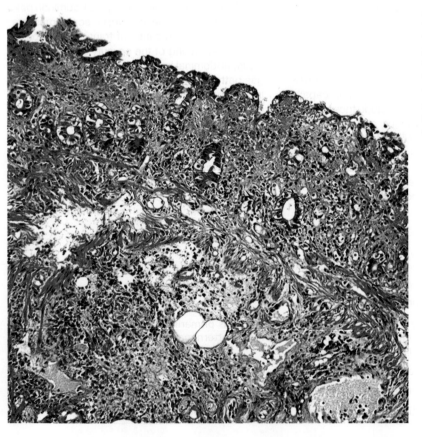

Fig. 22. Hemorrhagic colitis. The hemorrhage extends into the submucosa and is associated with inflammatory cells. Injury to endothelial cells by bacterial toxins rather than an angiitis causes the extensive hemorrhage (H&E, original magnification ×150).

Box 5
Reporting hemorrhagic colitis

Diagnosis: Acute ischemic/hemorrhagic colitis. See note.

Note: This pattern of injury is commonly associated with hypoperfusion due to vascular occlusion/hypovolemia, infections (*E coli* O157 and other serotypes, *Shigella*, and *K oxytoca*) and certain drugs.

---

erythema, erosions, and linear ulcers may be observed in various combinations. In severe cases, there is loss of haustral markings, cyanosis, and gangrene.[69] Although classic teaching suggests a predilection for ischemic injury in watershed areas and the rectosigmoid colon, more recent data suggest that ischemic injury occurs at any location within the colon with a similar frequency.[70]

Box 6
Drugs associated with ischemic colitis

Cocaine

Ergotamine

Estrogens

Alosetron

Alpha-interferon

Amphetamines

Digitalis

Dopamine

Epinephrine and norepinephrine

NSAIDs

Barbiturates

Type I interferons (IFN-α and IFN-β)

Antipsychotics

Vasopressin

Pseudoephedrine

Chlorpromazine

Cyclosporine

Danazol

Diuretics

Flutamide

Glycerin enemas

Phospho-soda solution

Clozapine

Na huang (herbal food supplement)

Tumor necrosis factor α

Serotonergic medications

Data from Cappell MS. Colonic toxicity of administered drugs and chemicals. Am J Gastroenterol 2004;99:1175–90; and FitzGerald JF, Hernandez LO. Ischemic colitis. Clin Colon Rectal Surg 2015;28:93–8.

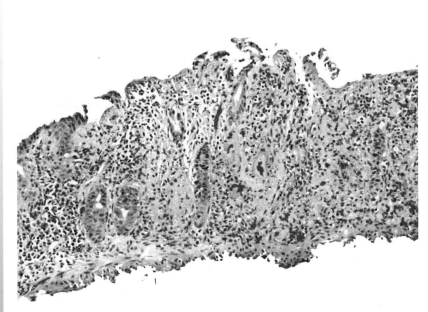

Fig. 23. Ischemic colitis. Injury and detachment of the surface epithelium with preservation of the basal portions of the crypts, and hyalinization and hemorrhage of the lamina propria are characteristic features of ischemia. Inflammatory cells may be present but are not a necessary component of the ischemic pattern (H&E, original magnification ×200).

HISTOPATHOLOGY

Ischemic necrosis first affects the superficial epithelium followed by the luminal third of the crypts. In early ischemia, the basal portions of the crypts are preserved, although total crypt loss develops with progressive injury. Ischemic crypts tend to have a smaller diameter than the nonischemic counterparts, a feature referred to as microcrypts or withering crypts (**Figs. 23** and **24**). As discussed previously, pseudomembranes may be present. Changes within the lamina propria include hyalinization, edema, hemorrhage, and scant inflammation. Focal neutrophilic cryptitis is sometimes observed (**Box 7**).[69]

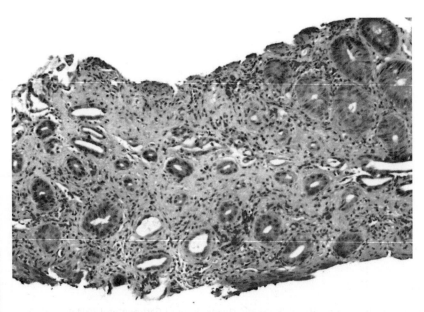

Fig. 24. Ischemic colitis. Tangential section of the colonic mucosa showing a paucicellular lamina propria, injury to crypt epithelium, microcrypts, and hyalinization of the lamina propria (H&E, original magnification ×200).

> **Box 7**
> **Reporting acute ischemic colitis**
>
> Diagnosis: Acute ischemic colitis. See note.
>
> Note: This pattern of injury is commonly associated with hypoperfusion due to vascular occlusion/hypovolemia. Infections (*E coli* O157 and other serotypes, *Shigella*, and *K oxytoca*) and certain drugs are other etiologic considerations.

SUMMARY

Patients presenting with acute colitis benefit from a comprehensive pathology report in which the recognition of few histologic patterns helps identify possible etiologic associations and the formulation of a differential diagnosis. A predominant inflammatory response (acute colitis pattern) is associated with infections and drug injuries. The clinical significance of a focal inflammatory pattern (focal active colitis) varies and etiologic associations differ in pediatric and adult patients. Mixed inflammatory/ischemic patterns, such as those present in pseudomembranous and hemorrhagic colitis, although primarily caused by specific organisms, namely *C difficile* and *E coli* O157:H7, respectively, may also be associated with other infectious and noninfectious etiologies. Finally, a pure ischemic pattern of injury may be related to drug injuries and infections, in addition to disorders causing hypoperfusion.

REFERENCES

1. Pezhouh MK, Chen E, Weinberg AG, et al. Significance of paneth cells in histologically unremarkable rectal mucosa. Am J Surg Pathol 2016;40:968–71.

2. Pascal RR, Gramlich TL, Parker KM, et al. Geographic variations in eosinophil concentration in normal colonic mocosa. Mod Pathol 1997;10:363–5.

3. Polydorides AD, Banner BF, Hannaway PJ, et al. Evaluation of site-specific and seasonal variation in colonic mucosal eosinophils. Hum Pathol 2008;29:832–6.

4. DuPont HL. Approach to the patient with infectious colitis. Curr Opin Gastroenterol 2012;28:39–46.

5. Surawicz CM. What's the best way to differentiate infectious colitis (acute self-limited colitis) from IBD? Inflamm Bowel Dis 2008;14:S157–8.

6. Goldstein NS, Cinenza AN. The histopathology of nonsteroidal anti-inflammatory drug-associated colitis. Am J Clin Pathol 1998;110:622–8.

7. Higuchi K, Umegaki E, Watanabe T, et al. Present status and strategy of NSAIDs-induced small bowel injury. J Gastroenterol 2009;44:879–88.

8. Klein M, Linnemann D, Rosenberg J. Non-steroidal anti-inflammatory drug-induced colopathy. BMJ Case Rep 2011. http://dx.doi.org/10.1136/bcr.10.2010.3436, [pii:bcr1020103436].

9. McCarthy AJ, Lauwers GY, Sheahan K. Iatrogenic pathology of the intestines. Histopathology 2015;66:15–28.

10. Lamps LW. Infective disorders of the gastrointestinal tract. Histopathology 2007;50:55–63.

11. Parry CM, Hien TT, Dougan G, et al. Typhoid fever. N Engl J Med 2002;347:1770–82.

12. Lee JH, Kim JJ, Jung JH, et al. Colonoscopic manifestations of typhoid fever with lower gastrointestinal bleeding. Dig Liver Dis 2004;36:141–6.

13. Kraus MD, Amatya B, Kimula Y. Histopathology of typhoid enteritis: morphologic and immunophenotypic findings. Mod Pathol 1999;12:949–55.

14. Cheung C, Merkeley H, Srigley JA, et al. Ileocecal ulceration and granulomatous ileitis as an unusual presentation of typhoid fever. CMAJ 2012;184(16):1808–10.

15. Stanley SL Jr. Amoebiasis. Lancet 2003;361(9362):1025–34.

16. Walsh J. Prevalence of *Entamoeba histolytica* infection. In: Ravdin JI, editor. Amebiasis: human infection by entamoeba histolytica. New York: John Wiley and Sons; 1988. p. 93–105.

17. Istre GR, Kreiss K, Hopkins RS, et al. An outbreak of amebiasis spread by colonic irrigation at a chiropractic clinic. N Engl J Med 1982;307:339–42.

18. Pittman FE, Hennigar GR. Sigmoidoscopic and colonic mucosal biopsy findings in amebic colitis. Arch Pathol 1974;97:155–8.

19. Variyam EP, Gogate P, Hassan M, et al. Nondysenteric intestinal amebiasis colonic morphology and search for Entamoeba histolytica adherence and invasion. Dig Dis Sci 1989;34(5):732–40.

20. Ralston KS, Petri WA Jr. Tissue destruction and invasion by Entamoeba histolytica. Trends Parasitol 2011;27(6):254–63.

21. Brandt H, Perez-Tamayo R. Pathology of human amebiasis. Hum Pathol 1970;1:351–85.

22. Attwood SEA, Cafferkey MT, Keane FBV. Yersinia infections in surgical practice. Br J Surg 1989;76:499–504.

23. Boqvist S, Pettersson H, Svensson A, et al. Sources of sporadic Yersinia enterocolitica infection in children in Sweden, 2004: a case control study. Epidemiol Infect 2009;137:897–905.

24. Cover TL, Aber RC. Yersinia enterocolitica. N Engl J Med 1989;321:16–24.

25. Natkin J, Beavis KG. Yersinia enterocolitica and Yersinia pseudotuberculosis. Clin Lab Med 1999;19:523–36.

26. El-Maraghi NRH, Mair N. The histopathology of enteric infection with Yersinia pseudotuberculosis. Am J Clin Pathol 1979;71:631–9.

27. Gleason TH, Patterson SD. The pathology of Yersinia enterocolitica ileocolitis. Am J Surg Pathol 1982;6:347–55.

28. Alt B, Glass NR, Sollinger H. Neutropenic enterocolitis in adults. Review of the literature and assessment of surgical intervention. Am J Surg 1985;149:405–8.

29. Williams N, Scott AD. Neutropenic colitis: a continuing surgical challenge. Br J Surg 1997;84:1200–5.

30. Sachak T, Arnold MA, Naini BV, et al. Neutropenic enterocolitis. new insights into a deadly entity. Am J Surg Pathol 2015;39:1635–42.

31. Schmit M, Bethge W, Beck R, et al. CT of gastrointestinal complications associated with hematopoietic stem cell transplantation. AJR Am J Roentgenol 2008;190:712–9.

32. Greenson JK, Stern RA, Carpenter SL, et al. The clinical significance of focal active colitis. Hum Pathol 1997;28:729–33.

33. Shetty S, Anjarwalla SM, Gupta J, et al. Focal active colitis: a prospective study of clinicopathological correlations in 90 patients. Histopathology 2011;59:850–6.

34. Ozdil K, Sahin A, Calhan T, et al. The frequency of microscopic and focal active colitis in patients with irritable bowel syndrome. BMC Gastroenterol 2011;11:96.

35. Volk EE, Shapiro BD, Easley KAS, et al. A cliniocpathologic study of 22 cases of focal active colitis: does it ever represent Crohn's disease? Mod Pathol 1998;11:789–94.

36. Xin W, Brown PL, Greenson JK. The clinical significance of focal active colitis in pediatric patients. Am J Surg Pathol 2003;27:1134–8.

37. Driman DK, Preiksaitis HK. Colorectal inflammation and increased cell proliferation associated with oral sodium phosphate bowel preparation solution. Hum Pathol 1998;29:972–8.

38. Farooq PD, Urrunaga NH, Tang DM, et al. Pseudomembranous colitis. Dis Mon 2015;61:181–206.

39. Bagdasarian N, Rao K, Malani PN. Diagnosis and treatment of Clostridium difficile in adults: a systematic review. JAMA 2015;313:398–408.

40. Ricciardi R, Rothenberger DA, Madoff RD, et al. Increasing prevalence and severity of Clostridium-difficile colitis in hospitalized patients in the United States. Arch Surg 2007;142:624–31.

41. Bouza E. Consequences of Clostridium difficile infection: understanding the healthcare burden. Clin Microbiol Infect 2012;18(Suppl 6):5–12.

42. Leffler DA, Lamont JT. Clostridium difficile Infection. N Engl J Med 2015;372:1539–48.

43. Dupont HL. Diagnosis and management of Clostridium difficile infection. Gastroenterol Hepatol 2013;11:1216–23.

44. Sayedy L, Kothari D, Richards RJ. Toxic megacolon associated Clostridium difficile colitis. World J Gastrointest Endosc 2010;16:293–7.

45. Koss K, Clark MA, Sanders DSA, et al. The outcome of surgery in fulminant Clostridium difficile colitis. Colorectal Dis 2006;8:149–54.

46. Lamontagne F, Labbé AC, Haeck O, et al. Impact of emergency colectomy on survival of patients with fulminant Clostridium difficile colitis during an epidemic caused by a hypervirulent strain. Ann Surg 2007;245:267.

47. Longo WE, Mazuski JE, Virgo KS, et al. Outcome after colectomy for Clostridium difficile colitis. Dis Colon Rectum 2004;47:1620–6.

48. Fishman EK, Kavuru MK, Jones BJ, et al. Pseudomembranous colitis: CT evaluation of 26 cases. Radiology 1981;180:57–60.

49. Boland GW, Lee MJ, Cats AM, et al. Antibiotic induced diarrhea: specificity of abdominal CT for the diagnosis of Clostridium difficile disease. Radiology 1994;191:103–6.

50. Baker ME. Acute infetious and inflammatory enterocolitidies. Radiol Clin North Am 2015;53:1255–71.

51. Fekety R, Shah AB. Diagnosis and treatment of Clostridium difficile Colitis. J Am Med Assoc 1993;269:71–5.

52. Fekety R. Guidelines for the diagnosis and management of Clostridium difficile-associated diarrhea and colitis. Am J Gastroenterol 1997;92:739–50.

53. Cleary RK. Clostridium difficile-associated diarrhea and colitis. Dis Colon Rectum 1998;41:1435–49.

54. Bartlett JG. Clostridium difficile: progress and challenges. Ann N Y Acad Sci 2010;1213:62–9.

55. Kufelnicka AM, Kirn TJ. Effective utilization of evolving methods for the laboratory diagnosis of Clostridium difficile infection. Clin Infect Dis 2011;52:1451–7.

56. Surawicz CM, Brandt LJ, Binion DG, et al. Guidelines for diagnosis, treatment, and prevention of clostridium difficile infections. Am J Gastroenterol 2013;108:478–98.

57. Barbut F, Kajzer C, Planas N, et al. Comparison of three enzyme immunoassays, a cytotoxicity assay, and toxigenic culture for diagnosis of Clostridium difficile-associated diarrhea. J Clin Microbiol 1993;31:963–7.

58. Planche T, Aghaizu A, Holliman R, et al. Diagnosisof Clostridium difficile infection by toxin detection kits: a systematic review. Lancet Infect Dis 2008;8:777–84.

59. Dignan CR, Greenson JK. Can ischemic colitis be differentiated from C difficile colitis in biopsy specimens? Am J Surg Pathol 1997;21:706–10.

60. Ochoa TJ, Cleary TG. Epidemiology and spectrum of disease of Escherichia coli O157. Curr Opin Infect Dis 2003;16:259–63.

61. Karmali MA, Gannon V, Sargeant JM. Verocytotoxin-producing Escherichia coli (VTEC). Vet Microbiol 2010;140:360–70.

62. Nguyen Y, Sperandio V. Enterohemorrhagic E. coli (EHEC) pathogenesis. Front Cell Infect Microbiol 2012;2:90.

63. Pacheco AR, Sperandio V. Shiga toxin in enterohemorrhagic E. coli: regulation and novel anti-virulence strategies. Front Cell Infect Microbiol 2012;2:81.

64. Högenauer C, Langner C, Beubler E, et al. Klebsiella oxytoca as a causative organism of antibiotic-associated hemorrhagic colitis. N Engl J Med 2006;355:2418–26.

65. Cappell MS. Colonic toxicity of administered drugs and chemicals. Am J Gastroenterol 2004;99:1175–90.

66. FitzGerald JF, Hernandez LO. Ischemic colitis. Clin Colon Rectal Surg 2015;28:93–8.

67. Higgins PD, Davis KJ, Laine L. Systematic review: the epidemiology of ischaemic colitis. Aliment Pharmacol Ther 2004;19:729–38.

68. Elder K, Lashner BA, Al Solaiman F. Clinical approach to colonic ischemia. Cleve Clin J Med 2009;76:401–9.

69. Zou X, Cao J, Yao Y, et al. Endoscopic findings and clinicopathologic characteristics of ischemic colitis: a report of 85 cases. Dig Dis Sci 2009;54:2009–15.

70. Glauser PM, Wermuth P, Cathomas G, et al. Ischemic colitis: clinical presentation, localization in relation to risk factors, and long-term results. World J Surg 2011;35:2549–54.

The Many Faces of Medication-Related Injury in the Gastrointestinal Tract

CrossMark

Heewon A. Kwak, MD[a], John Hart, MD[b],*

KEYWORDS

- Gastrointestinal tract • Drug toxicity • Chemotherapy • Immunomodulator • Pathologic features

Key points

- Numerous medications produce clinically significant gastrointestinal toxicity that can be identified by histologic examination

- Gastrointestinal drug toxicity can mimic other, more common inflammatory gastrointestinal disorders; a high index of suspicion is needed to establish a correct diagnosis

- Clinical correlation and careful review of the medication history are especially helpful in recognizing the presence of a drug-induced gastrointestinal injury.

ABSTRACT

Every year many new medications are approved for clinical use, several of which can cause clinically significant gastrointestinal tract toxicity. This article emphasizes the histologic features and differential diagnosis of drug-induced injury to the gastrointestinal mucosa. Ultimately, clinical correlation and cessation of a drug with resolution of symptoms are needed to definitively confirm a drug as a causative factor in mucosal injury. Recognizing histologic features in gastrointestinal biopsies, however, can allow surgical pathologists to play a key role in establishing a diagnosis of drug-induced gastrointestinal toxicity.

OVERVIEW

The Center for Drug Evaluation and Research within the Food and Drug Administration (FDA) regulates over-the-counter and prescription medications. Each year, this organization approves a large number of new drugs and biological agents. Novel drugs that have never been used in humans are classified as "new molecular entities" for purposes of regulatory review; all submitted biological products are included in this category. Many other agents are either the same as, or closely related to, previously approved agents and are intended to compete for use in clinical practice. In 2016, a total of 21 novel drugs received FDA approval for human use.[1] All proposed new medications undergo a rigorous evaluation process designed to not only assess efficacy but also determine a toxicity profile. In 2007 Congress mandated that the FDA provide safety information to the general public and medical professionals relating to medications it has approved for clinical use. For this purpose, the FDA maintains a Web site that is a valuable resource for reports of postmarket drug toxicities.[2] This review is intended to discuss the drugs that most often produce clinically significant gastrointestinal toxicity as well as recently released agents that are emerging as important new sources of mucosal injury.

Disclosure Statement: The authors have nothing to disclose.

[a] Department of Pathology, University of Chicago, 5841 South Maryland Avenue, Chicago, IL, USA;
[b] Department of Pathology, University of Chicago, 5841 South Maryland Avenue, MC 6101, Chicago, IL, USA
* Corresponding author.
E-mail address: John.Hart@uchospitals.edu

Surgical Pathology 10 (2017) 887–908
http://dx.doi.org/10.1016/j.path.2017.07.007

CHEMOTHERAPEUTIC AGENTS

Chemotherapeutic agents increase cell necrosis, autophagy, and/or apoptosis among cells with a high proliferative rate, which unfortunately includes the gastrointestinal epithelium. Once the epithelium is injured, loss of mucosal integrity ensues, resulting in increased permeability and susceptibility to infectious agents. Not surprisingly, a variety of chemotherapeutic agents of several classes can cause gastrointestinal mucosal damage. Platinum adducts (eg, cisplatin, carboplatin, and oxaliplatin), DNA intercalators (eg, doxorubicin), antimetabolites (eg, 5-fluorouracil, capecitabine, 6-mercaptopurine, cytarabine, and gemcitabine) and, to a lesser extent, alkylators (eg, mechlorethamine, melphalan, chlorambucil, and cyclophosphamide) are all capable of producing clinically significant diarrhea due to gastrointestinal mucosal injury.[3] Major risk factors for clinically significant toxicity include patient age (young and elderly), nutritional status, type of malignancy, method of drug delivery, and pretreatment neutropenia.[4]

Chemotherapy-induced gastrointestinal mucosal injury often produces diarrheal symptoms, although some agents may also cause odynophagia, nausea, emesis, anorexia, malabsorption, abdominal pain, and cramping. Common endoscopic findings include mucosal erythema, erosions and ulcers. Severe toxicity is uncommon but can manifest as extensive ulceration with perforation. In this situation, the possibility of individual genetic predisposition to toxicity due to a metabolic defect should be considered. Approximately 20% of patients who develop severe gastrointestinal toxicity after 5-fluorouracil administration prove to have a mutation in *DPYD*. This gene encodes dihydropyrimidine dehydrogenase, which normally promotes drug catabolism; diminished enzymatic activity results in a prolonged serum half-life and toxic drug levels (**Fig. 1**).[5,6]

Chemotherapy-induced injury can occur anywhere in the gastrointestinal tract. One hallmark feature is the presence of scattered withered crypts or glands lined by attenuated epithelial cells that show irregular nuclear spacing and acidophilic cytoplasm, often associated with necrotic epithelial cells in the lumen (**Fig. 2**). This finding is nonspecific and can be seen in other disorders, such as ischemic enterocolitis and graft-versus-host disease (GVHD). Small bowel biopsies may demonstrate villous blunting with increased apoptotic bodies. Some agents can elicit marked cytologic abnormalities that simulate dysplasia, such as cellular enlargement, bizarre and hyperchromatic nuclei, and prominent nucleoli. Affected cells, however, contain ample cytoplasm; typically contain hyperchromatic, smudged nuclei; and show minimal mitotic activity.

Some chemotherapeutic agents produce characteristic mucosal alterations. For example, taxanes inhibit tubulin polymerization into microtubules, leading to mitotic arrest in metaphase and resulting in ring mitotic figures (**Fig. 3**). This phenomenon is commonly identified in the proliferative compartment of the epithelium throughout the gastrointestinal tract.[7,8] Ring mitotic figures are accompanied by increased numbers of normal-appearing mitotic figures as well as scattered apoptotic cellular debris. Glandular crowding, loss of polarity, and nuclear stratification with hyperchromasia are common, and the combination of these features can closely simulate the appearance of dysplasia. These dramatic histologic changes do not necessarily indicate toxicity, however, because they are also seen in asymptomatic individuals who receive these drugs. Mucosal necrosis and bowel perforation reportedly occur, however, in up to 3% of patients with taxane-associated gastrointestinal toxicity.[9] Colchicine is another agent that induces mitotic arrest and produces essentially the same histologic features in mucosal biopsies. Unlike

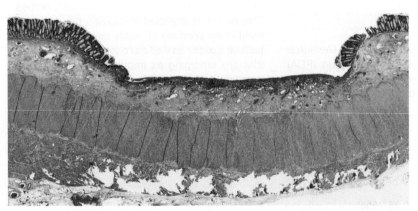

Fig. 1. Severe 5-fluorouracil toxicity produced extensive colonic ulceration in a patient with a *DPYD* mutation [H&E, original magnification ×4].

Fig. 2. Doxorubicin can cause enteric injury characterized by withered crypts, prominent apoptosis, and epithelial cell atypia [H&E, original magnification ×200].

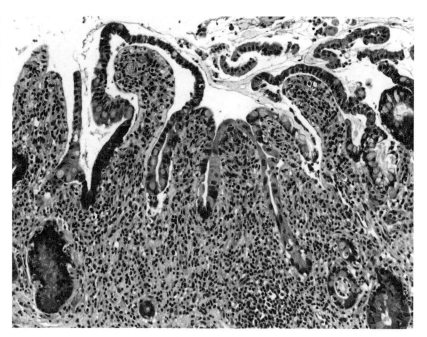

taxanes, however, ring mitotic figures are only seen in patients with symptomatic toxicity, which primarily occurs in those with chronic renal failure and reduced excretion.[10] Colchicine can induce ring mitotic figures in adenomas, carcinomas, and other proliferative lesions, but this feature does not represent drug toxicity.

IMMUNOMODULATORS AND TARGETED AGENTS

Two immunomodulators have been recently FDA approved for use in treatment of human malignancies. Anti–cytotoxic T lymphocyte–associated antigen 4 (CTLA-4) and anti– programmed death 1 (PD-1) medications are approved therapies for several solid tumor types, most commonly melanoma, squamous cell carcinoma, renal cell carcinoma, and non–small cell lung cancer. These agents act by blocking inhibitory receptors on T lymphocytes that tumor cells stimulate to inhibit T-cell activation and antitumoral activity. As a result, they can increase immune-mediated destruction of tumor cells and, in some cases, produce dramatic clinical responses.[11,12] Immune activation, however, can also lead to damage of normal tissues, including the gastrointestinal mucosa, in many cases. All immunomodulators produce similar histologic changes in mucosal biopsies, namely apoptosis in the proliferative compartment of the epithelium accompanied by neutrophilic inflammation and intraepithelial lymphocytosis (**Fig. 4**). When these changes are unassociated with crypt architectural changes, the pattern of injury closely simulates infectious colitis, although most bacterial colitides do not show striking apoptosis in the crypts (**Fig. 5**). Patients who receive immunomodulatory therapy for prolonged periods of time may also develop features of chronic injury with mucosal remodeling, diffuse chronic inflammation, and basal lymphoplasmacytosis, all of which simulate inflammatory bowel disease (**Fig. 6**). Any part of the gastrointestinal tract may be affected; colonic changes are best described, but similar findings occur in the gastric (**Fig. 7**) and small bowel mucosa.[13–15] Rare patients develop ileal or colonic perforation after receiving anti–CTLA-4 therapy.[16]

Idelalisib is an inhibitor of the delta isoform of phosphoinositide 3-kinase that was recently approved for treatment of relapsed chronic lymphocytic leukemia and some forms of non–Hodgkin lymphoma. It has since been shown to cause clinically significant gastrointestinal toxicity in a significant proportion of treated patients. In 2016, the FDA released a warning against use of this drug in combination with other chemotherapeutic agents due to clinically significant toxicity.[17] Histologic features of idelalisab toxicity include prominent intraepithelial lymphocytosis and epithelial cell apoptosis with variable, but often mild, neutrophilic inflammation, similar to features of PD-1 and CTLA-4 inhibitor therapies (**Fig. 8**).[18,19] Given the

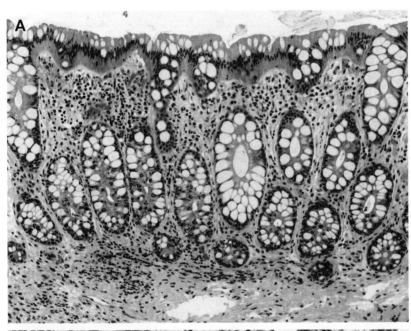

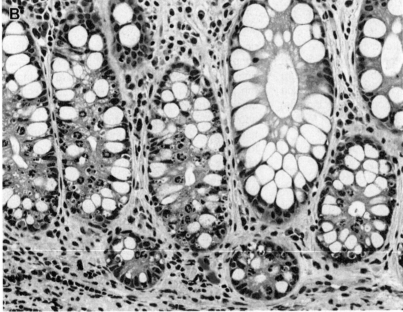

Fig. 3. Taxane-induced colonic mucosal changes include increased mitotic activity and epithelial cell apoptosis without inflammation (*A*) [H&E, original magnification ×200]. Ring mitotic figures that are most evident in the deep crypts (*B*) [H&E, original magnification ×400].

spectrum of histologic changes that can occur in association with all these targeted therapies, it is not surprising that the differential diagnosis includes idiopathic inflammatory bowel disease, bacterial colitis, GVHD, autoimmune enteropathy, and toxicity related to other medications (eg, mycophenolate). Clinical history and knowledge of the medication records are necessary to sort out the specific cause of colitis in an individual patient (**Box 1**).

ANTIBIOTICS

Clinically significant gastrointestinal toxicity occurs at a low rate among users of antibiotic therapy. Some agents indirectly affect the gastrointestinal tract, whereas others are directly toxic. For example, antibacterial agents alter the native intestinal microbiota and can cause diarrheal symptoms. *Clostridium difficile*–associated

Fig. 4. Ipilimumab toxicity manifests with intraepithelial lymphocytosis and prominent apoptosis [H&E, original magnification ×400].

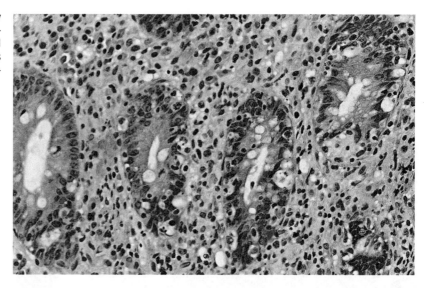

pseudomembranous colitis and *Klebsiella oxytoca*–associated hemorrhagic colitis typically develop after administration of antibiotic therapy, as discussed in Jose Jessurun's article, "The Differential Diagnosis of Acute Colitis: Clues to a Specific Diagnosis," in this issue.[20,21] Penicillin and related agents can induce a hypersensitivity vasculitis that results from immune complex deposition.[22,23] Most patients present with systemic manifestations, such as an erythematous nonpruritic rash, and some may have concomitant renal disease. Gastrointestinal involvement is heralded by acute onset abdominal pain. Endoscopic

biopsy specimens show variably inflamed intestinal mucosa with leukocytoclastic vasculitis characterized by nuclear karyorrhectic debris, mural fibrinoid necrosis, and microthrombi affecting mucosal and submucosal capillaries (**Fig. 9**). In some cases, aggregates of lamina propria neutrophils associated with fibrin deposits may be the only clues to an underlying vasculitis; these features should prompt additional tissue levels and careful correlation with clinical findings when encountered.

Clindamycin, tetracycline, and doxycycline can cause direct caustic injury to mucosae in

Fig. 5. Nivolumab toxicity is associated with active colitis and prominent crypt cell apoptosis. The lamina propria contains a lymphoplasmacytic infiltrate [H&E, original magnification ×200].

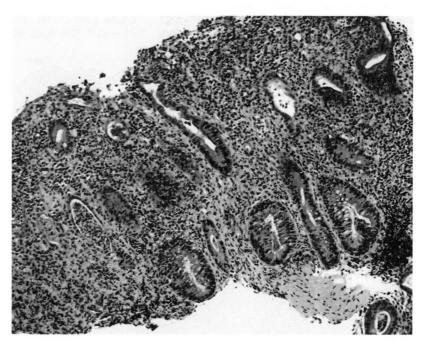

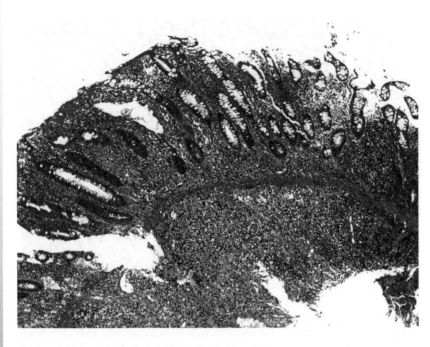

Fig. 6. Ipilimumab toxicity can simulate idiopathic inflammatory bowel disease with dense chronic inflammation in the lamina propria, crypt architectural distortion, and basal lymphoplasmacytosis [H&E, original magnification ×100].

the upper gastrointestinal tract. When dissolved in water (or saliva), these agents have a pH less than 3; prolonged contact of the pill with the mucosa leads to direct acid-related injury. Esophageal injury is most common and usually appears as cratered ulcers in the midesophagus. Gastric ulcers are most common in the body or fundus.[24] Unlike clindamycin and tetracycline, doxycycline produces a type of vascular degeneration that is highly characteristic; capillaries in the superficial lamina propria show smudgy mural necrosis that appears as a dark eosinophilic ringlike structure. Microthrombi may also be seen (**Fig. 10**).[25–27]

BISPHOSPHONATES

The prototypical bisphosphonate, alendronate, prevents osteoclast-mediated bone resorption and is prescribed to treat osteoporosis, Paget disease, and hypercalcemia of malignancy. It is a common cause of pill esophagitis but can also cause gastric and duodenal erosions or ulcers (**Box 2**).[28] The medication is directly injurious on

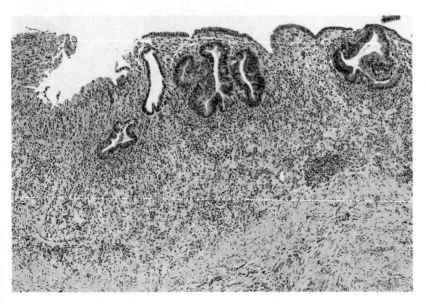

Fig. 7. Nivolumab toxicity is associated with marked epithelial destruction and glandular dropout [H&E, original magnification ×40].

Fig. 8. Idelalisab toxicity in the small bowel results in intraepithelial lymphocytosis and increased epithelial cell apoptosis [H&E, original magnification ×200]. (*Courtesy of* Dr Rhonda Yantiss, Weill Cornell Medicine, New York, NY.)

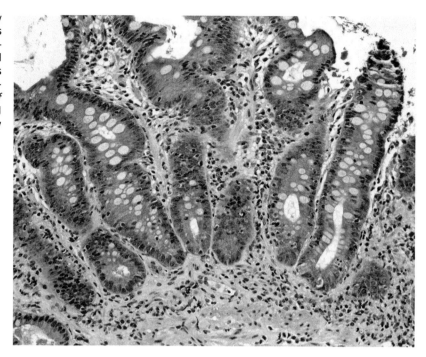

contact with mucosal surfaces and causes a more severe injury with prolonged exposure; recumbent patients of advanced age and those with esophageal dysmotility are at increased risk.[29] Erosions, circumferential ulcers with exudates, edema, and wall thickening are common in the esophagus but may occur in the stomach and duodenum as well.

Biopsies typically show extensive mucosal injury with necrosis of the squamous epithelium and lamina propria with associated inflammation and reactive cytologic atypia in the preserved mucosa.[30] In some cases, the entire squamous lining becomes necrotic and separates from the underlying lamina propria; this finding should not be considered within the spectrum of esophagitis dissecans superficialis. Occasional cases may show colorless or pale yellow, refractile crystalline material, which likely represents a cellulose base found in many drugs.[30]

IRON

Oral iron therapy is directly toxic to the mucosa of the upper gastrointestinal tract, presumably because reactive oxygen species are elaborated on mucosal contact.[31] Iron-associated erosions are encountered in 0.7% of upper endoscopic examinations performed for any reason and are particularly common among older patients.[32,33] Endoscopic findings include erosions, ulcers, erythema, and yellow-brown discoloration of the mucosa.[34,35]

Iron is usually recognizable in hematoxylin-eosin–stained tissue sections; it appears as yellow-brown crystalline material adherent to the

---

Box 1
Drugs that cause prominent epithelial cell apoptosis in the gastrointestinal tract

Mycophenolate
- Closely mimics GVHD (but no skin involvement)
- Prominent eosinophils and lack of endocrine cell clusters are helpful clues

PD-1 and CTLA-4 inhibitors
- Often associated with intraepithelial lymphocytosis
- Some cases of crypt architectural distortion resembling irritable bowel disease

Idelalisib
- Intraepithelial lymphocytosis typically present

Chemotherapeutic agents
- Crypt withering and ulcers often present

Taxanes
- Numerous ring mitoses

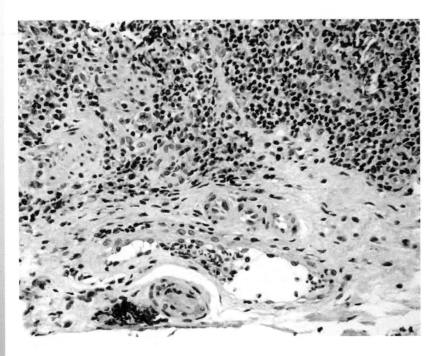

Fig. 9. Antibiotic associated hypersensitivity vasculitis causes subtle abnormalities; occasional capillaries in the colonic mucosa show inflammation and karyorrhectic debris [H&E, original magnification ×400].

surface epithelium or erosions. Encrusted iron may be embedded in the superficial lamina propria (Fig. 11). The background mucosa typically shows features of reactive/chemical gastropathy and erosions are often present. Intracellular iron accumulation is not a feature of iron-induced injury. Rather, this finding usually reflects elevated circulating iron and may be related to either hemolysis or hemochromatosis. Duodenal biopsies can show iron accumulation in the epithelium or macrophages at the villous tips, which has been termed, *pseudomelanosis duodeni*. This finding is unassociated, however, with mucosal injury in most cases and is considered an incidental finding.[32–35]

The differential diagnosis includes other types of crystalline deposits in the mucosa. Barium precipitates are most likely to be confused with iron.

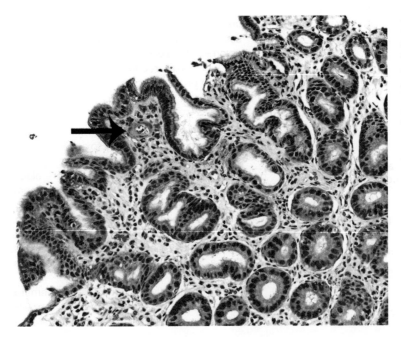

Fig. 10. Doxycycline-induced gastric toxicity often manifests as reactive epithelial changes (chemical gastropathy) associated with amorphous eosinophilic deposits (*arrow*) in vascular walls [H&E, original magnification ×100]. (*Courtesy of* Dr Shu-Yuan Xiao, University of Chicago Medical Center, Chicago, IL.)

They appear as golden crystals, often associated with macrophages in the lamina propria. Osmo-Prep, a tablet form of sodium phosphate, can precipitate as purple-black granular deposits in the superficial gastric mucosa.[36] None of these materials shows Prussian blue staining and, thus, are readily distinguished from iron deposits.

RESINS

Resins are noabsorbable compounds that facilitate ion exchange and excretion of excess ions through the gastrointestinal tract. The only resin definitively shown to cause gastrointestinal injury is sodium polystyrene sulfonate (Kayexalate), which is a cation exchange resin used to treat hyperkalemia in patients with renal failure.[37] Sevelamer is an anion exchange resin used to bind excess phosphate in patients with chronic kidney disease.[38] Cholestyramine, colesevelam, and colestipol are bile acid sequestrants that do not cause gastrointestinal injury but can be histologically confused with other resins.[39]

Kayexalate is formulated with sorbitol, which is a hyperosmotic vehicle that can cause ischemic injury to the gastrointestinal mucosa.[39] Individuals with decreased bowel transit are at increased risk for mucosal injury due to prolonged contact between the medication and the mucosa.[40] Kayexalate can cause injury anywhere in the gastrointestinal tract. Patients may present with bleeding or pain resulting from severe ulcers, tissue necrosis, and even perforation.[41] Crystals may be identified over intact epithelium, but they are generally seen in association with inflamed epithelium, ulcers, ischemic necrosis, or pseudomembranes. Kayexalate crystals are lightly basophilic with narrow rectangular fish scale-like ridges (**Fig. 12**). The crystals are black with acid-fast stain (**Fig. 13**A, B).[42]

On the other hand, the pathologic effects of sevelamer are not well established; it may be seen in biopsies from patients with ulcers or erythema, but most patients have unremarkable endoscopic examinations and are asymptomatic. Crystals are usually encountered in otherwise normal mucosal

Fig. 11. Refractile crystalline iron deposits are associated with an antral erosion [H&E, original magnification ×200].

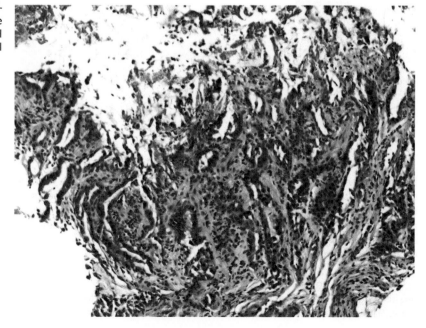

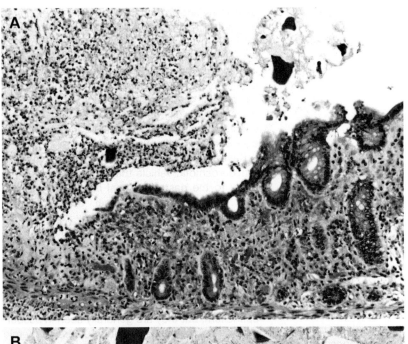

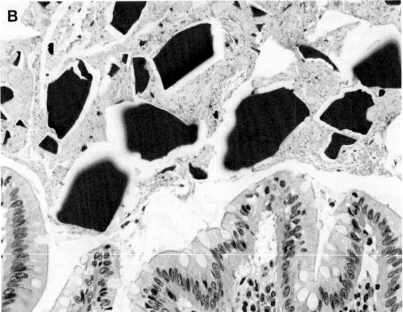

Fig. 12. Kayexalate crystals are present in the inflammatory exudate overlying a colonic ulcer (A) [H&E, original magnification ×200]. The crystals show an internal fish scale pattern (B) [H&E, original magnification ×400].

biopsies, although they may be adherent to polyps, cancers, and ulcers (Fig. 14A). Sevelamer crystals tend to exhibit broad, curved fish scale–like ridges and are 2-toned with a rusty brown to pink central area and yellow periphery (see Fig. 14B). Crystals are magenta with acid-fast stain (see Fig. 13C, D).[38]

Colesevelam, colestipol, and cholestyramine are histologically identical in routinely stained sections. The crystals lack internal fish scale–like ridges and are dark brown, magenta, or orange, in routinely stained sections depending on the tissue thickness and staining conditions (see Fig. 13E, F). They are dull yellow with acid-fast stain.[39]

SARTANS

Olmesartan is an angiotensin II receptor blocker and powerful antihypertensive agent. Olmesartan-

Fig. 13. Several resins can simulate the histologic features of Kayexelate. Kayexelate crystals are jagged and basophilic with an internal structure reminiscent of fish scales (*A*) [H&E, original magnification ×400]. Crystals are black with acid-fast stain (*B*). Sevelamer shows a similar internal structure but also has a 2-toned appearance with pink-to-brown central discoloration and a yellowish periphery [Acid fast bacilli stain, original magnification ×400]. (Photomicrograph *courtesy of* Dr Rhonda Yantiss, Weill Cornell Medicine, New York, NY) (*C*) [H&E, original magnification ×400].

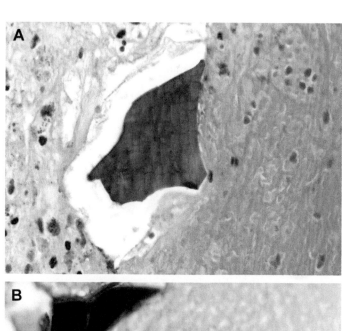

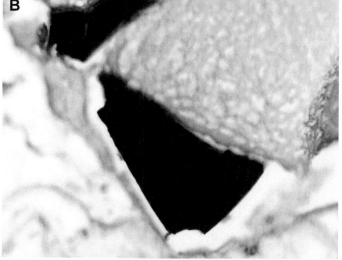

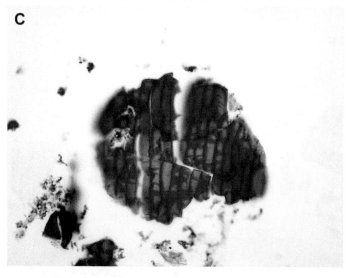

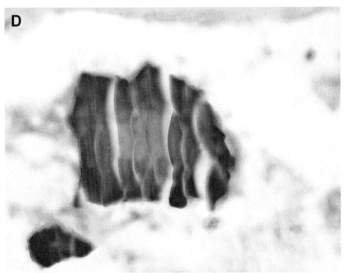

D

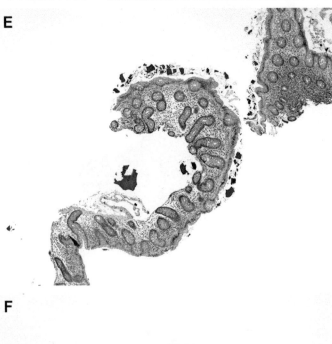

E

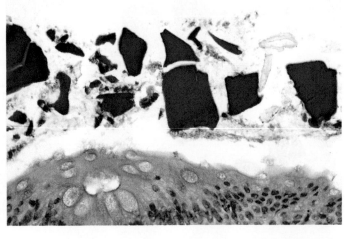

F

Fig. 13. (*continued*). Crystals are magenta with acid-fast stain (*D*) [Acid fast bacilli stain, original magnification ×400]. Cholestyramine can be adherent to ulcers or normal mucosa [H&E, original magnification ×40]. (Photomicrograph *courtesy of* Dr Rhonda Yantiss, Weill Cornell Medicine, New York, NY) (*E*). The resin is brightly eosinophilic and waxy without internal structures [H&E, original magnification x40]. (Photomicrograph *courtesy of* Dr Rhonda Yantiss, Weill Cornell Medicine, New York, NY) (*F*).

Fig. 14. Sevelamer crystals are adherent to the luminal surface of an adenoma [H&E, original magnification ×200]. (Photomicrograph *courtesy of* Dr Rhonda Yantiss, Weill Cornell Medicine, New York, NY) (*A*). They show internal structures reminiscent of Kayexelate, but have a 2-toned pink and yellow appearance [H&E, original magnification ×400]. (Photomicrograph *courtesy of* Dr Rhonda Yantiss, Weill Cornell Medicine, New York, NY) (*B*).

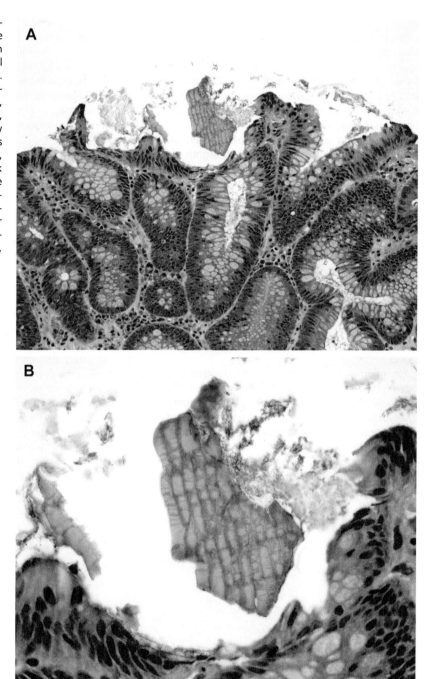

induced injury to the gastrointestinal tract was first reported in 2012 by Rubio-Tapia and colleagues,[43] when 2 patients, previously diagnosed with refractory celiac sprue, noticed improvement of their symptoms during their hospitalizations when the drug was withheld and relapse of symptoms on resuming its use. Numerous additional cases have since been published describing clinical features and histologic findings of olmesartan-related injury in the stomach, small intestine, and colon as well as toxicities caused by other drugs in this class.[44–46] The mechanism of mucosal injury is not clear, but there has been some speculation regarding the importance of HLA-DQ haplotypes and immune dysregulation. Similar to biopsies from patients with celiac disease, overexpression of interleukin-15 has been documented in duodenal biopsies of patients taking olmesartan compared with biopsies obtained after discontinuation of the medication. In addition, in vitro studies have shown disruption of a tight junction protein, ZO-1 (zonula occludens) in olmesartan-treated cells.[47]

Most patients with olmesartan-related gastrointestinal injury are in their seventh to eighth decades of life, reflecting the prevalence of hypertension in this age group. Vigilant clinical suspicion must be maintained because there can be a prolonged interval between initiation of the drug and onset of clinical symptoms. One systemic review reported a range of less than 1 month to 11.5 years between initiation of therapy and symptom onset.[48] Patients with olmesartan-induced gastrointestinal injury commonly present with chronic nonbloody diarrhea and profound weight loss. Upper and lower endoscopy may demonstrate a normal examination, although villous atrophy and ulceration can occur.[43,48,49]

On microscopic examination of duodenal biopsies, the resemblance to celiac disease may be uncanny (**Fig. 15**). Intraepithelial lymphocytes are typically increased and villi are variably blunted; a completely flat mucosa is not uncommon. Some cases show increased subepithelial collagen deposition. A subset of patients has increased intraepithelial lymphocytes and/or subepithelial collagen deposits in biopsies from either the colon (**Fig. 16**) or stomach (**Fig. 17**).[43,45,48] Features that may help exclude celiac disease include the older age of a patient, lack of improvement with a gluten-free diet, and a lack of serologic support for a diagnosis of celiac disease.[43] It can take many months for olmesartan-induced injury to completely resolve.[43,48,50]

NONSTEROIDAL ANTI-INFLAMMATORY DRUGS

Nonsteroidal anti-inflammatory drugs (NSAIDs) are among the most commonly used medications in the United States. They show great efficacy in the treatment of arthritis, musculoskeletal pain, and fever and can be used to prevent thrombotic cardiovascular and cerebrovascular events. NSAIDs do have some undesirable side effects, however, particularly with respect to the gastrointestinal tract. A prospective analysis on adverse drug-related hospital admissions revealed that approximately 5% of hospital admissions were due to adverse drug reactions and 23% of those admissions were related to NSAID use. Aspirin was implicated in 18% of admissions, with gastrointestinal bleeding the most common adverse effect.[51] Age greater than 60 years, prior NSAID-related gastrointestinal events, concurrent corticosteroid use, alcohol, and tobacco are risk factors for NSAID-induced gastrointestinal

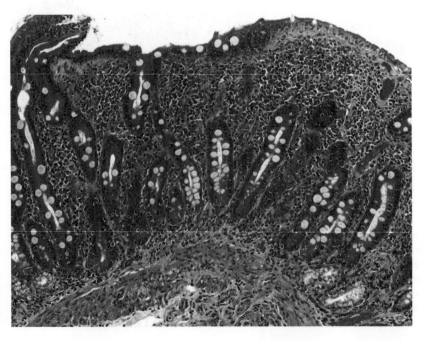

Fig. 15. Olmesartan associated enteropathy can show complete villus blunting, crypt hyperplasia, and intraepithelial lymphocytosis, mimicking celiac disease [H&E, original magnification ×200].

Fig. 16. Olmesartan-associated colonic toxicity produces intraepithelial lymphocytosis and patchy subepithelial collagen deposition [H&E, original magnification ×100].

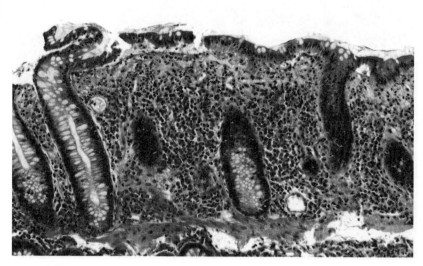

injury.[52,53] Erosions and ulcers are commonly seen within the first 3 months of NSAID use, whereas stricture formation is associated with long-term use.[54] Gastroduodenal erosions and ulcers develop in up to 25% of chronic NSAID users.[52,55]

NSAIDs decrease prostaglandin synthesis through inhibition of the cyclooxygenase (COX) pathway.[1] Although most NSAIDs are nonselective and inhibit both COX-1 and COX-2; selective COX-2 inhibitors reportedly reduce the incidence of gastrointestinal injury.[56] Signs or symptoms related to gastrointestinal toxicity include iron deficiency anemia or melena and abdominal pain, although many patients have no symptoms at all. Endoscopy often demonstrates mucosal erythema, erosions, or ulcers. Abnormalities are most common in the antrum, duodenal bulb, distal ileum, and right colon, but this may be because these portions of the gastrointestinal tract are accessible by routine endoscopy.[57] Capsule video-endoscopy and double-balloon enteroscopy (**Fig. 18**) have shown that NSAID-related injury is common throughout the entire length of the small intestine.[58,59]

Like the nonspecific findings evident by endoscopy, histologic features are banal, and, therefore, clinical correlation with a detailed medication history is necessary for diagnosis. A common pattern of gastric injury is reactive (chemical) gastropathy: foveolar hyperplasia with corkscrewing of the gastric pits and mucin depletion, lamina propria smooth muscle stranding in some cases, and

vascular ectasia. In more severe cases erosions may develop, and deep ulcers requiring surgical intervention can occur (**Fig. 19**). Duodenal involvement is patchy with active inflammation and mucosal architectural distortion that simulates Crohn disease or may manifest with increased intraepithelial lymphocytes that raise the possibility of celiac disease.[60] Pyloric metaplasia can occur near ulcers in the terminal ileum (**Fig. 20**).[61] Thus, one must be cautious when considering a diagnosis of Crohn ileitis in patients with isolated chronic active ileitis. Chronic NSAID use can also lead to diaphragm disease characterized by circular membranes or weblike structures that narrow the lumen.[62] Longer strictures may develop in heavy NSAID users.

NSAIDs are also an important cause of mucosal injury in the colon.[63] NSAID colitis may resemble lymphocytic or collagenous colitis, although the lymphocytosis and collagen deposition are usually patchier and less pronounced than is typical of idiopathic lymphocytic colitis and collagenous colitis. NSAID colitis may show regenerative crypts and lamina propria fibrosis, which overlaps somewhat with ischemic colitis. Eosinophils may be increased, but this is a nonspecific feature (**Fig. 21**). The presence of significant endoscopic mucosal abnormalities is helpful in the distinction between NSAID colitis and either lymphocytic or collagenous colitis, because erosions and mucopus are not typical in the latter conditions. Diarrhea associated with

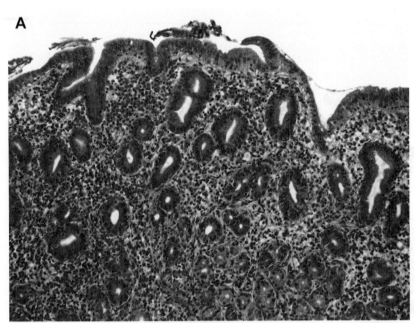

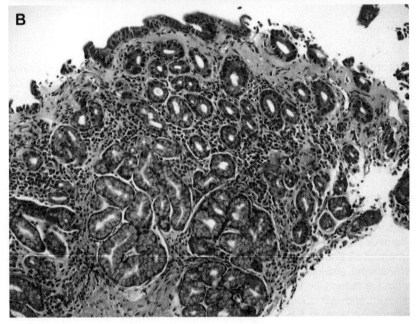

Fig. 17. Olmesartan associated lymphocytic gastritis is associated with prominent intraepithelial lymphocytosis (*A*) [H&E, original magnification ×200]. It should also be considered in the differential diagnosis of collagenous gastritis (*B*) [H&E, original magnification ×200].

NSAID colitis is usually of short duration and may contain blood, in contrast to the chronic watery diarrhea typical of microscopic colitis.

IMMUNOSUPRESSIVE AGENTS

The calcineurin inhibitors and TOR inhibitors rarely produce clinically significant gastrointestinal tract injury. Mycophenolate is an antiproliferative agent, however, used in many solid organ and stem cell transplant patients and is a well-known cause of clinically significant gastrointestinal mucosal toxicity, particularly at high doses and in patients with an elevated serum creatinine. The medication comes in 2 formulations: mycophenolate mofetil, which is absorbed in the stomach, and mycophenolate sodium, which is absorbed in the small intestine. Both drugs curtail proliferation of B lymphocytes and T lymphocytes by inhibiting inosine monophosphate dehydrogenase, an

Fig. 18. Double-balloon enteroscopy demonstrates an ileal web with associated ulcer (*arrow*) in a patient with a long history of heavy NSAID use.

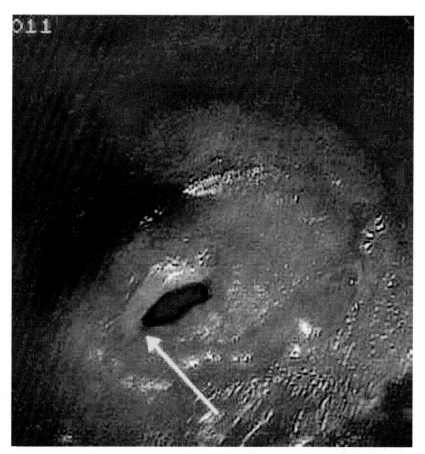

Fig. 19. NSAID-related antral gastritis is characterized by reactive epithelial changes and increased lamina propria eosinophils [H&E, original magnification ×200].

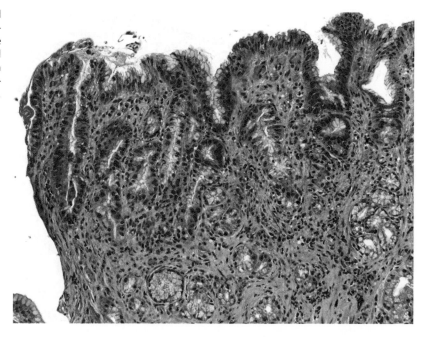

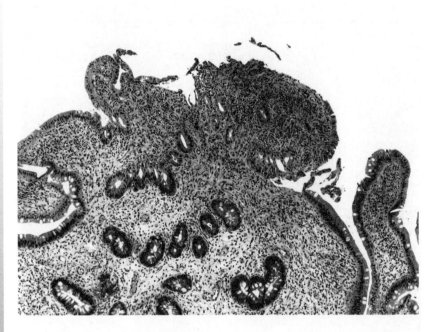

Fig. 20. NSAID-related ileitis can be accompanied by villous architectural distortion and increased eosinophils [H&E, original magnification ×100].

important enzyme in the de novo pathway of purine synthesis. This pathway is also used within intestinal columnar cells, which makes them susceptible to drug-related injury.[64,65] Watery diarrhea is the most common clinical symptom of gastrointestinal toxicity, although nausea, emesis, abdominal pain, malabsorption, and bleeding may also occur. Reported endoscopic findings include erosion, aphthous or confluent ulcers, congestion, and erythema.[64]

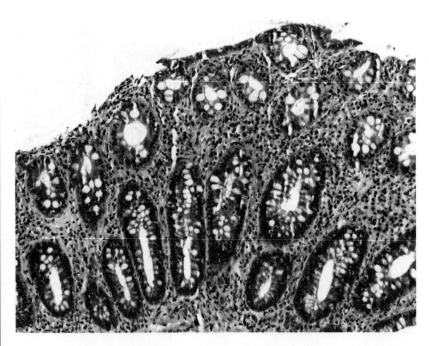

Fig. 21. NSAID-related colitis shows slightly increased intraepithelial lymphocytes, scattered foci of epithelial cell apoptosis, and reactive changes [H&E, original magnification ×200].

Fig. 22. Mycophenolate toxicity is often manifest by prominent apoptosis with crypt dropout [H&E, original magnification ×200].

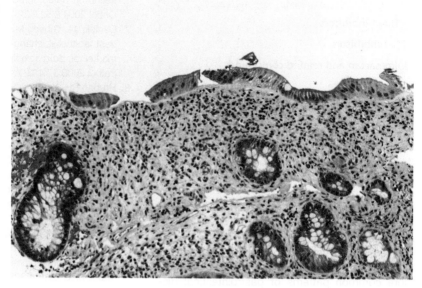

The histologic features of gastrointestinal toxicity are most fully described in colonic biopsies. Crypt cell apoptosis, similar to acute GVHD, is almost always a prominent feature (Fig. 22).[66] Histologic clues favoring mycophenolate-induced colitis over GVHD include increased eosinophils (>15 eosinophils per 10 high-power fields) and the absence of endocrine cell clusters; the latter are characteristic of GVHD.[67] Focal crypt withering and neutrophilic cryptitis are regularly present. Crypt architectural distortion and increased lamina propria mononuclear cell infiltrates can simulate idiopathic inflammatory bowel disease (Fig. 23). It is not clear whether the drug directly causes chronic colitis or results in immune dysregulation that leads to mucosal injury (Box 3). Manifestations

Fig. 23. Mycophenolate toxicity can mimic idiopathic inflammatory bowel disease in the colon; prominent epithelial cell apoptosis is a helpful clue.

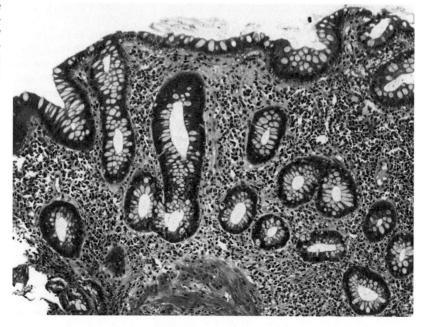

Box 3
Medications that can produce an inflammatory bowel disease –like histologic appearance

CTLA-4 inhibitors

PD-1 inhibitors

Olmesartan and related compounds

Mycophenolate

---

in the upper gastrointestinal tract are similar to those of the colon. Epithelial cell necrosis in the deep glands and crypts is accompanied by patchy, mixed inflammation in the lamina propria.[68,69]

SUMMARY

As this discussion has amply demonstrated, drug-induced gastrointestinal toxicity can take many forms and histologically often closely mimics more common patterns of gastrointestinal disease. The surgical pathologist must always consider the possibility of a drug toxicity, particularly when there is a histologic feature that is atypical or when the available clinical history is incongruent with the biopsy findings. In many cases, a careful review of the medication history is the only way to confirm or exclude the possibility and arrive at the proper diagnosis.

REFERENCES

1. U.S. Food and Drug Administration. Novel Drug Approvals for 2016. 2017. Available at: https://www.fda.gov/drugs/developmentapprovalprocess/druginnovation/ucm483775.htm. Accessed April 19, 2017.
2. U.S. Food and Drug Administration. Postmarket drug safety information for patients and providers. 2016. Available at: https://www.fda.gov/Drugs/DrugSafety/PostmarketDrugSafetyInformationforPatientsandProviders/default.htm. Accessed April 19, 2017.
3. Boussios S, Pentheroudakis G, Katsanos K, et al. Systemic treatment-induced gastrointestinal toxicity: incidence, clinical presentation and management. Ann Gastroenterol 2012;25:106–18.
4. Naidu MU, Ramana GV, Rani PU, et al. Chemotherapy-induced and/or radiation therapy-induced oral mucositis–complicating the treatment of cancer. Neoplasia 2004;6:423–31.
5. Raida M, Schwabe W, Häusler P, et al. Prevalence of a common point mutation in the dihydropyrimidine dehydrogenase (DPD) gene within the 5-splice donor site of intron 14 in patients with severe 5-fluorouracil (5-FU)-related toxicity compared with controls. Clin Cancer Res 2001;2832:2832–9.
6. Lee A, Ezzeldin H, Fourie J, et al. Dihydropyrimidine dehydrogenase deficiency: impact of pharmacogenetics on 5-fluorouracil therapy. Clin Adv Hematol Oncol 2004;8:527–32.
7. Daniels JA, Gibson MK, Xu L, et al. Gastrointestinal tract epithelial changes associated with taxanes: marker of drug toxicity versus effect. Am J Surg Pathol 2008;32:473–7.
8. Hruban RH, Yardley JH, Donehower RC, et al. Taxol toxicity. Epithelial necrosis in the gastrointestinal tract associated with polymerized microtubule accumulation and mitotic arrest. Cancer 1989;63:1944–50.
9. Rose PG, Piver MS. Intestinal perforation secondary to paclitaxel. Gynecol Oncol 1995;57:270–2.
10. Iacobuzio-Donahue CA, Lee EL, Abraham SC, et al. Colchicine toxicity: distinct morphologic findings in gastrointestinal biopsies. Am J Surg Pathol 2001;25:1067–73.
11. Zou W, Wolchok JD, Chen L. PD-L1 (B7-H1) and PD-1 pathway blockade for cancer therapy: mechanisms, response biomarkers, and combinations. Sci Transl Med 2016;8:328rv4.
12. Pardoll DM. The blockade of immune checkpoints in cancer immunotherapy. Nat Rev Cancer 2012;12:252–64.
13. Verschuren EC, van den Eertwegh AJ, Wonders J, et al. Clinical, endoscopic, and histologic characteristics of Ipilimumab-associated colitis. Clin Gastroenterol Hepatol 2016;14:836–42.
14. Chen JH, Pezhouh MK, Lauwers GY, et al. Histopathologic features of colitis due to immunotherapy with Anti-PD-1 antibodies. Am J Surg Pathol 2017;41:643–54.
15. Venditti O, De Lisi D, Caricato M, et al. Ipilimumab and immune-mediated adverse events: a case report of anti-CTLA4 induced ileitis. BMC Cancer 2015;15:87.
16. Dilling P, Walczak J, Pikiel P, et al. Multiple colon perforation as a fatal complication during treatment of metastatic melanoma with ipilimumab - case report. Polski Przeglad Chirurgiczny 2014;86:94–6.
17. U.S. Food and Drug Administration. FDA alerts healthcare professionals about clinical trials with Zydelig (idelalisib) in combination with other cancer medicines. 2016. Available at: https://www.fda.gov/Drugs/DrugSafety/ucm490618.htm. Accessed April 19, 2017.
18. Weidner AS, Panarelli NC, Geyer JT, et al. Idelalisib-associated colitis: histologic findings in 14 patients. Am J Surg Pathol 2015;39:1661–7.
19. Louie CY, DiMaio MA, Matsukuma KE, et al. Idelalisib-associated enterocolitis: clinicopathologic features and distinction from other enterocolitides. Am J Surg Pathol 2015;39:1653–60.
20. Farrell RJ, Lamont JT. Pathogenesis and clinical manifestations of Clostridum difficile diarrhea and colitis. Curr Top Microbiol Immunol 2000;250:109–25.

21. Hogenauer C, Langner C, Beubler E, et al. *Klebsiella oxytoca* as a causative organism of antibiotic-associated hemorrhagic colitis. N Engl J Med 2006;355:2418–26.

22. Hannedouche T, Fillastre JP. Penicillin-induced hypersensitivity vasculitides. J Antimicrob Chemother 1987;20:3–5.

23. Sohagia AB, Gunturu SG, Tong TR, et al. Henoch-schonlein purpura-a case report and review of the literature. Gastroenterol Res Pract 2010;2010:597648.

24. Eng J, Sabanathan S. Drug-induced esophagitis. Am J Gastroenterol 1991;86:1127–33.

25. Kadayifci A, Gulsen MT, Koruk M, et al. Doxycycline-induced pill esophagitis. Dis Esophagus 2004;17:168–71.

26. Xiao SY, Zhao L, Hart J, et al. Gastric mucosal necrosis with vascular degeneration induced by doxycycline. Am J Surg Pathol 2013;37:259–63.

27. Shih AR, Lauwers GY, Mattia A, et al. Vascular injury characterizes doxycycline-induced upper gastrointestinal tract mucosal injury. Am J Surg Pathol 2017;41:374–81.

28. de Groen PC, Lubbe DF, Hirsch LJ, et al. Esophagitis associated with the use of alendronate. N Engl J Med 1996;335:1016–21.

29. Nagano Y, Matsui H, Shimokawa O, et al. Bisphosphonate-induced gastrointestinal mucosal injury is mediated by mitochondrial superoxide production and lipid peroxidation. J Clin Biochem Nutr 2012;51:196–203.

30. Abraham SC, Cruz-Correa M, Lee LA, et al. Alendronate-associated esophageal injury: pathologic and endoscopic features. Mod Pathol 1999;12:1152–7.

31. Mladenka P, Simunek T, Hubl M, et al. The role of reactive oxygen and nitrogen species in cellular iron metabolism. Free Radic Res 2006;40:263–72.

32. Abraham SC, Yardley JH, Wu TT. Erosive injury to the upper gastrointestinal tract in patients receiving iron medication: an underrecognized entity. Am J Surg Pathol 1999;23:1241–7.

33. Kaye P, Abdulla K, Wood J, et al. Iron-induced mucosal pathology of the upper gastrointestinal tract: a common finding in patients on oral iron therapy. Histopathology 2008;53:311–7.

34. Ji H, Yardley JH. Iron medication-associated gastric mucosal injury. Arch Pathol Lab Med 2004;128:821–2.

35. Eckstein RP, Symons P. Iron tablets cause histopathologically distinctive lesions in mucosal biopsies of the stomach and esophagus. Pathology 1996;28:142–5.

36. Matsukuma K, Gui D, Olson KA, et al. OsmoPrep-associated gastritis: a histopathologic mimic of iron pill gastritis and mucosal calcinosis. Am J Surg Pathol 2016;40:1550–6.

37. Harel Z, Harel S, Shah PS, et al. Gastrointestinal adverse events with sodium polystyrene sulfonate (Kayexalate) use: a systematic review. Am J Med 2013;126:264.e9-24.

38. Swanson BJ, Limketkai BN, Liu TC, et al. Sevelamer crystals in the gastrointestinal tract (GIT): a new entity associated with mucosal injury. Am J Surg Pathol 2013;37:1686–93.

39. Arnold MA, Swanson BJ, Crowder CD, et al. Colesevelam and colestipol: novel medication resins in the gastrointestinal tract. Am J Surg Pathol 2014;38:1530–7.

40. Lillemoe KD, Romolo JL, Hamilton SR, et al. Intestinal necrosis due to sodium polystyrene (Kayexalate) in sorbitol enemas: clinical and experimental support for the hypothesis. Surgery 1987;101:267–72.

41. Rashid A, Hamilton SR. Necrosis of the gastrointestinal tract in uremic patients as a result of sodium polystyrene sulfonate (Kayexalate) in sorbitol: an underrecognized condition. Am J Surg Pathol 1997;21:60–9.

42. Abraham SC, Bhagavan BS, Lee LA, et al. Upper gastrointestinal tract injury in patients receiving kayexalate (sodium polystyrene sulfonate) in sorbitol: clinical, endoscopic, and histopathologic findings. Am J Surg Pathol 2001;25:637–44.

43. Rubio-Tapia A, Herman ML, Ludvigsson JF, et al. Severe spruelike enteropathy associated with olmesartan. Mayo Clin Proc 2012;87:732–8.

44. Marthey L, Cadiot G, Seksik P, et al. Olmesartan-associated enteropathy: results of a national survey. Aliment Pharmacol Ther 2014;40:1103–9.

45. Burbure N, Lebwohl B, Arguelles-Grande C, et al. Olmesartan-associated sprue-like enteropathy: a systematic review with emphasis on histopathology. Hum Pathol 2016;50:127–34.

46. Negro A, Rossi GM, Santi R, et al. A case of severe sprue-like enteropathy associated with losartan. J Clin Gastroenterol 2015;49:794.

47. Marietta EV, Nadeau AM, Cartee AK, et al. Immunopathogenesis of olmesartan-associated enteropathy. Aliment Pharmacol Ther 2015;42:1303–14.

48. Ianiro G, Montalto M, Ricci R, et al. Systematic review: sprue-like enteropathy assoiated with olmesartan. Aliment Pharamacol Ther 2014;40:16–23.

49. Khan AS, Peter S, Wilcox CM. Olmesartan-induced enteropathy resembling celiac disease. Endoscopy 2014;46(Suppl 1 UCTN):E97–8.

50. Vane JR, Botting RM. Mechanism of action of nonsteroidal anti-inflammatory drugs. Am J Med 1998;104:2S–8S, [discussion: 21S–2S].

51. Pirmohamed M, James S, Meakin S, et al. Adverse drug reactions as cause of admission to hospital: prospective analysis of 18 820 patients. BMJ 2004;329:15–9.

52. Jaszewski R. Frequency of gastroduodenal lesions in asymptomatic patients on chronic aspirin or nonsteroidal antiinflammatory drug therapy. J Clin Gastroenterol 1990;12:10–3.

53. Carson JL, Strom BL, Morse ML, et al. The relative gastrointestinal toxicity of the nonsteroidal anti-inflammatory drugs. Arch Intern Med 1987;147:1054–9.

54. Allison MC, Howatson AG, Torrance CJ, et al. Gastrointestinal damage associated with the use of nonsteroidal antiinflammatory drugs. N Engl J Med 1992;327:749–54.

55. Laine L. Nonsteroidal anti-inflammatory drug gastropathy. Gastrointest Endosc Clin N Am 1996;6:489–504.

56. Mitchell JA, Akarasereenont P, Thiemermann C, et al. Selectivity of nonsteroidal antiinflammatory drugs as inhibitors of constitutive and inducible cyclooxygenase. Proc Natl Acad Sci U S A 1993;90:11693–7.

57. Gabriel SE, Jaakkimainen L, Bombardier C. Risk for serious gastrointestinal complications related to use of nonsteroidal anti-inflammatory drugs. a meta-analysis. Ann Intern Med 1991;115:787–96.

58. Chutkan R, Toubia N. Effect of nonsteroidal anti-inflammatory drugs on the gastrointestinal tract: diagnosis by wireless capsule endoscopy. Gastrointest Endosc Clin N Am 2004;14:67–85.

59. Matsumoto T, Nakamura S, Esaki M, et al. Endoscopic features of chronic nonspecific multiple ulcers of the small intestine: comparison with nonsteroidal anti-inflammatory drug-induced enteropathy. Dig Dis Sci 2006;51(8):1357–63.

60. Kakar S, Nehra V, Murray JA, et al. Significance of intraepithelial lymphocytosis in small bowel biopsy samples with normal mucosal architecture. Am J Gastroenterol 2003;98:2027–33.

61. Lengeling RW, Mitros FA, Brennan JA, et al. Ulcerative ileitis encountered at ileo-colonoscopy: likely role of non-steroidal agents. Clin Gastroenterol Hepatol 2003;1:160–9.

62. Wang YZ, Sun G, Cai FC, et al. Clinical features, diagnosis, and treatment strategies of gastrointestinal diaphragm disease associated with nonsteroidal anti-inflammatory drugs. Gastroenterol Res Pract 2016;2016:3679741.

63. Bjarnason I, Hayllar J, MacPherson AJ, et al. Side effects of nonsteroidal anti-inflammatory drugs on the small and large intestine in humans. Gastroenterology 1993;104:1832–47.

64. Behrend M. Adverse gastrointestinal effects of mycophenolate mofetil: aetiology, incidence and management. Drug Saf 2001;24:645–63.

65. Allison AC, Eugui EM. Mechanisms of action of mycophenolate mofetil in preventing acute and chronic allograft rejection. Transplantation 2005;80:S181–90.

66. Liapis G, Boletis J, Skalioti C, et al. Histological spectrum of mycophenolate mofetil-related colitis: association with apoptosis. Histopathology 2013;63:649–58.

67. Star KV, Ho VT, Wang HH, et al. Histologic features in colon biopsies can discriminate mycophenolate from GVHD-induced colitis. Am J Surg Pathol 2013;37:1319–28.

68. Nguyen T, Park JY, Scudiere JR, et al. Mycophenolic acid (cellcept and myofortic) induced injury of the upper GI tract. Am J Surg Pathol 2009;33:1355–63.

69. Parfitt JR, Jayakumar S, Driman DK. Mycophenolate mofetil-related gastrointestinal mucosal injury: variable injury patterns, including graft-versus-host disease-like changes. Am J Surg Pathol 2008;32:1367–72.

Mucosal Biopsy After Bone Marrow Transplantation

Maria Westerhoff, MD[a],*, Laura W. Lamps, MD[b]

KEYWORDS

- Hematopoietic stem cell transplant • Graft-versus-host disease
- Diarrhea in immunocompromised patient • Apoptosis • Mycophenolate mofetil toxicity
- Cytomegalovirus • Adenovirus • Neutropenic enterocolitis

Key points

- When faced with a gastrointestinal mucosal biopsy from a bone marrow transplant patient, the 3 main things to consider are graft-versus-host disease (GVHD), infection, and drug toxicity.
- The 2015 National Institutes of Health (NIH) guidelines recommend standardized diagnostic language for GVHD.
- Distinction between acute GVHD and chronic GVHD is no longer based on the interval between diagnosis and transplantation; grading criteria and minimal diagnostic features are not established.
- Apoptotic bodies are characteristic of GVHD, but drug effects and viral infections can also cause this finding.

ABSTRACT

Gastrointestinal mucosal biopsies in the hematopoietic stem cell transplantation setting are challenging because histologic features of graft-versus-host disease (GVHD), which is treated by increasing immunosuppression, overlap with those of other conditions, such as infection, which can get worse with GVHD treatment. More than one condition can occur at the same time. It is important to understand the histologic features of GVHD, drug toxicity, infection, and clinical factors surrounding patients, including timing of biopsy in relation to transplantation, medication history, and laboratory data. Rendering a correct diagnosis and generating a pathology report with standard language that can direct clinical management ensure proper management.

OVERVIEW

Graft-versus-host disease (GVHD) is an important complication of hematopoietic stem cell transplantation (HSCT), particularly in the context of allogeneic bone marrow transplantation. It results from donor immune cells that recognize the recipient host as foreign and mediate an immune-mediated attack on host cells. Gastrointestinal involvement occurs in up to 50% of GVHD patients; it is the second most common site involved after skin.[1,2] Optimal endoscopic biopsy protocols evaluating for GVHD have not been determined.[3,4] Sampling of the entire gastrointestinal tract has the highest yield for diagnosing GVHD and ruling out potential mimics. Flexible sigmoidoscopy with rectal biopsy may be considered when patients are unable to tolerate full upper and lower endoscopy.[5]

Disclosure Statement: Dr M. Westerhoff has nothing to disclose. Dr L.W. Lamps receives royalties from Elsevier for editing and authoring work.
[a] Anatomic Pathology, University of Washington Medical Center, 1959 Northeast Pacific Street, BB 220, Seattle, WA 98195, USA; [b] Department of Pathology, University of Michigan, 5231F, 1301 Catherine Street, Ann Arbor, MI 48109-5602, USA
* Corresponding author.
E-mail address: mariawesterhoff@gmail.com

surgpath.theclinics.com

GRAFT-VERSUS-HOST DISEASE

CLINICAL FEATURES

Although GVHD classification has been historically based on the interval between HSCT and onset of symptoms, the 2005 National Institutes of Health (NIH) consensus guidelines recommended use of clinical manifestations and test results to classify GVHD rather than an arbitrary time cut-off.[6] Acute GVHD usually occurs within 100 days of transplantation but may persist, recur, or develop beyond that time period and can only be diagnosed in the absence of chronic GVHD. Chronic GVHD may occur with or without features of acute GVHD. Its diagnosis requires at least 1 diagnostic clinical sign or at least 1 distinctive clinical feature with biopsy confirmation. The only clinical features sufficient for diagnosing chronic gastrointestinal GVHD without further investigation are esophageal webs or strictures in the upper esophagus to midesophagus. Biopsies are performed to confirm GVHD when these diagnostic clinical manifestations are not present or other disorders are clinically considered.[7]

PATHOGENESIS OF GRAFT-VERSUS-HOST DISEASE

GVHD has an initiating and an efferent stage. The pretransplant conditioning regimen damages host cells and triggers the initial phase. Antigen-presenting cells are recruited to damaged tissue, where they present host antigens to donor lymphocytes. The donor T cells attack the host, in particular the stem cells in the gut, and delay healing after injury.[8] Loss of mucosal integrity leads to translocation of microbial products into the circulation, promoting cytokine elaboration and propagating tissue injury.

Although GVHD occurs in allogeneic HSCT, a similar syndrome can also occur in autologous HSCT. Autologous HSCT is commonly performed in patients with plasma cell myeloma and involves reinfusion of a patient's own hematopoietic progenitors after chemotherapy.[9–12] Women, in particular those with a history of breast cancer, are more likely to develop GVHD-like syndrome after autologous HSCT.[9] Presumably, loss of self-tolerance results from disruption in these patients. The female preponderance may be parity related; hematopoietic microchimerism may develop from fetal cells persisting in maternal circulation, and GVHD-like syndrome results from the allogeneic fetal immune cells included in the autologous transplantation.[9,13] The histologic features of GVHD in autologous HSCT are identical to those occurring in the allogeneic transplant setting.

MORPHOLOGIC FEATURES OF GRAFT-VERSUS-HOST DISEASE

GVHD causes apoptosis of epithelial cells in the regenerative zones of the gastrointestinal mucosae where stem cells reside: basal epithelium of the esophagus, neck regions of gastric glands, and basolateral aspects of enterocolonic crypts (Box 1).[14] Apoptotic cells may have an exploding appearance, contain shrunken cells with

---

Box 1
Key features of graft-versus-host disease in the modern era

Clinical features

- Interval between transplant and symptoms no longer used to distinguish acute from chronic GVHD

- Esophageal webs and stenoses in upper third to middle third of esophagus are the only diagnostic features of chronic GVHD

- Nausea, vomiting, and anorexia are common in acute and chronic GVHD; require biopsy

Pathologic features

- Apoptotic bodies in stem cell compartment of gastrointestinal epithelium are seen in acute and chronic GVHD

- Chronic GVHD also shows crypt architectural distortion, pyloric metaplasia, or Paneth cell metaplasia

- Severe GVHD showing ulcers and widespread crypt dropout

- Histologic features of gastrointestinal GVHD overlapping with those of other important differential diagnoses

eosinophilic cytoplasm and condensed nuclei, or appear as karyorrhectic debris surrounded by a clear halo (Figs. 1–4). Severe GVHD may result in complete crypt or gland destruction with erosions. Endocrine cells are often spared, possibly because they are nonproliferative differentiated cells.[15] Inflammation, in particular neutrophilic inflammation, is typically sparse.

The diagnosis of GVHD may be challenging, and minimal histologic criteria for a diagnosis are lacking.[7] Some investigators require at least 1 apoptotic body per biopsy fragment to consider GVHD.[13,14] This criterion clearly depends on the sizes of tissue fragments, number of examined levels, and elimination of confounding factors that may also cause apoptosis. Other investigators require a total number of apoptotic bodies at least equal to the number of biopsy pieces or scattered apoptotic bodies in multiple crypts.[16]

Mucosal biopsies from the gastrointestinal tract are crucial to establishing a diagnosis that directs appropriate therapy for a patient. In 1 study, approximately 10% of patients referred to an institution for treatment of presumptive GVHD without biopsy confirmation were found to have an alternative explanation for their symptoms.[17] The timing of gastrointestinal biopsy can influence the severity of GVHD findings, as can the effects of immunosuppressive therapy; minimal GVHD can be partially masked by immunosuppressive therapy.[7] Endoscopic examination performed shortly after HSCT shows poorer correlation between endoscopy and histology. One study analyzed 112 patients who underwent endoscopic biopsies within the first 100 days of HSCT and found no association between the degree of endoscopic mucosal injury and the presence of GVHD at any site in the gastrointestinal tract.[4] In another series, 23% of patients had a normal first endoscopic examination despite histologically confirmed acute GVHD, but only 3% of patients had normal endoscopic findings when GVHD was histologically diagnosed on a second endoscopy.[18] Biopsies of the upper and lower gastrointestinal tract should be obtained to optimally evaluate for GVHD, even in the setting of an entirely normal macroscopic evaluation. The 2015 NIH consensus guidelines recommend a minimum of 8 to 20 serial tissue sections be examined.[7]

GRADING OF GRAFT-VERSUS-HOST DISEASE

GVHD was traditionally graded using a 4-tiered system (Figs. 5–8):

Grade I: individual cell apoptosis, rare apoptotic, exploding cells in basolateral regions of crypts and negligible lymphocytic infiltrate

Grade II: individual crypt involvement by apoptosis, crypts lined by apoptotic cells, crypts containing luminal apoptotic debris, and variable lymphocytes, neutrophils, and eosinophils

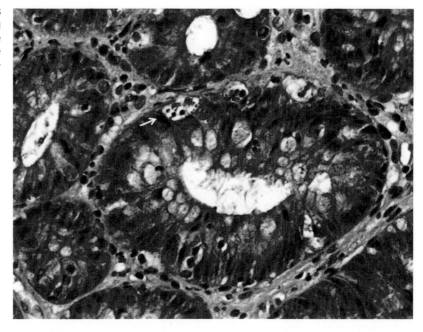

Fig. 1. Apoptotic cells can have an exploding appearance, where nuclei seem to have exploded into karyorrhectic debris (*arrow*).

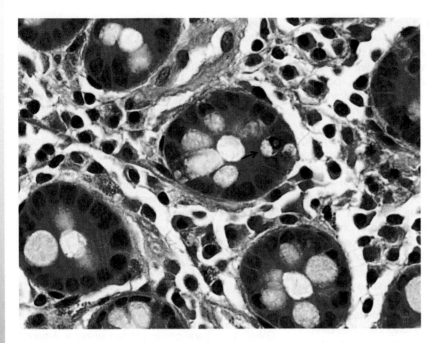

Fig. 2. An apoptotic body (*arrow*) showing a pyknotic nucleus.

Grade III: contiguous crypt destruction resulting in stretches of mucosa devoid of epithelium

Grade IV: denuded mucosa with loss of the surface epithelium and crypts

Grading GVHD in routine practice is controversial because histologic grade does not necessarily correlate with treatment regimens or clinical course.[19] The 2015 NIH guidelines[7] recognize the lack of consensus regarding GVHD grading in gastrointestinal biopsies but also acknowledge that detection of a high-grade (III–IV) lesion is relevant to treatment decisions.[16] Severe GVHD (grade IV) is an independent factor correlating

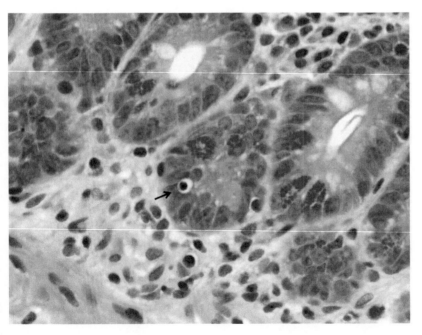

Fig. 3. An apoptotic cell (*arrow*) appearing as a pyknotic nucleus surrounded by a halo.

Fig. 4. Another morphologic appearance of an apoptotic cell (*arrow*), showing a shrunken cell with eosinophilic cytoplasm and karyorrhectic debris.

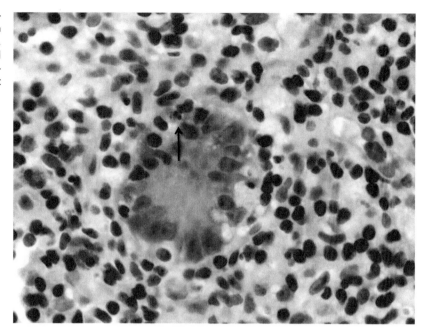

with lack of treatment response and worse overall survival.[20] If an institution elects to use a grading system, the site of highest histologic grade should be noted.[7]

PATHOLOGIC FEATURES OF CHRONIC GRAFT-VERSUS-HOST DISEASE

Esophageal webs, strictures, and stenoses are the only macroscopic findings diagnostic of chronic gastrointestinal GVHD. Multiple microscopic features suggest disease chronicity, including crypt architectural distortion, Paneth cells distal to the hepatic flexure or pyloric metaplasia in the small bowel, lamina propria and submucosal fibrosis, and lymphoplasmacytic inflammation.[7,21,22] These findings are not specific for chronic GVHD and overlap with features of idiopathic inflammatory bowel disease (**Fig. 9**). Thus, care should be taken to not

Fig. 5. Grade 1 of the 4-tiered traditional GVHD grading system shows individual cell apoptotic bodies (*arrow*) without substantial inflammation.

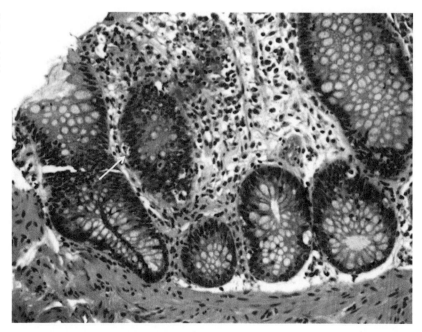

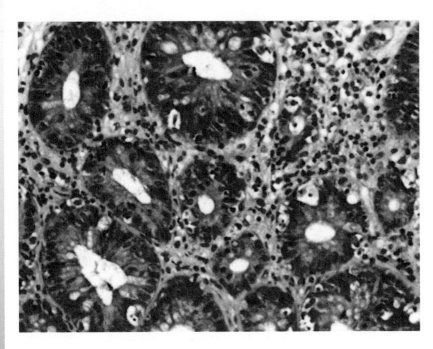

Fig. 6. Grade 2 GVHD is exemplified here as crypts lined by apoptotic cells.

overdiagnose Crohn disease or ulcerative colitis after HSCT and concomitant immunosuppression.[22,23]

REPORTING GRAFT-VERSUS-HOST DISEASE

The NIH guidelines provide 3 categories for reporting GVHD: not GVHD, possible GVHD, and likely GVHD (**Table 1**).[7] The not GVHD category is rendered when there is no histologic evidence of GVHD. The possible GVHD category is used when some features of GVHD are present, but alternate diagnoses are possible, such as viral infection or an adverse drug reaction. The likely GVHD category encompasses both unequivocal GVHD and features consistent with GVHD. It can

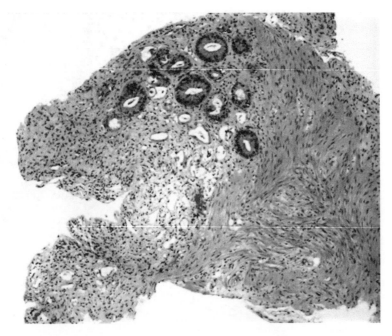

Fig. 7. Grade 3/4 GVHD shows multiple contiguous crypts that are damaged and widespread loss of crypts.

Fig. 8. A high-power magnification of Fig. 7, highlighting the damaged crypts, characterized by attenuated crypt epithelium and apoptoses (*arrow*). This would qualify as a high-grade GVHD (grade 3/4) in the traditional grading system.

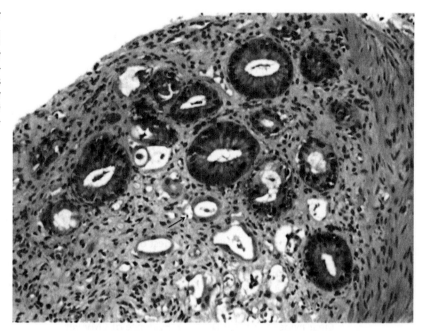

be used when findings are minimal, but no alternative conditions explain them, or when biopsies are taken long enough after chemotherapy or radiotherapy so that the apoptotic crypt epithelial cells seen are not likely to be due to prior treatment. This category can also be used when patients have serologic evidence of cytomegalovirus (CMV) but no histologic or immunohistochemical evidence of inclusions associated with apoptotic bodies on biopsy.[7]

DIFFERENTIAL DIAGNOSIS OF GASTROINTESTINAL GRAFT-VERSUS-HOST DISEASE

Evaluating gastrointestinal mucosal biopsies in the HSCT setting is challenging because many clinically relevant etiologies cause similar findings (**Box 2**). Chemotherapeutic agents, mycophenolate mofetil (MMF), nonsteroidal anti-inflammatory drugs (NSAIDs), proton pump

Fig. 9. This colon shows chronic GVHD: there is marked crypt architectural distortion simulating inflammatory bowel disease. The inset shows crypt cell apoptotic bodies (*arrows*).

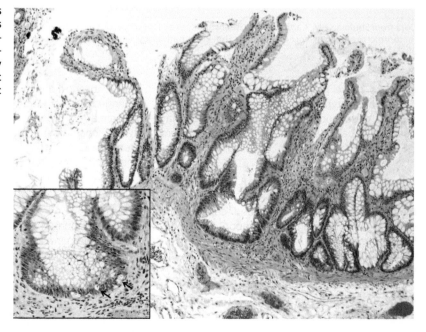

Table 1
How to sign out a pathologic diagnosis of graft-versus-host disease

Category	Definition	Examples	Comments
Recommendation for Final Diagnosis Categories			
Not GVHD Possible GVHD	No evidence for GVHD Evidence of GVHD but other possible explanations	• Obvious CMV enteritis with inclusions near the apoptotic changes • Focal colonic ulcers with marked apoptotic cryptitis and destruction of crypts associated with use of MMF • Coinfection with known active viral hepatitis • Clinical features that suggest or favor a drug reaction	Indicate possible alternate diagnoses and reasons for suspicion
Likely GVHD	Clear evidence of GVHD without a competing cause of injury OR Clear evidence of GVHD with mitigating factors OR GVHD most likely diagnosis but relevant clinical information is limited OR GVHD is validated by sequential biopsy or by absence of competing diagnosis	• Abundant epithelial apoptosis without clinical or histologic evidence of drug injury or infection • Evidence of CMV yet abundant apoptotic epithelial changes that are not associated with CMV infected cells by immunostaining • Single or rare apoptotic epithelial changes without other features of active GVHD and no alternative explanations • Limited sample or minimal or focal findings • Proximity to recent chemotherapy or radiotherapy	Included old categories of "consistent with" and "unequivocal" GVHD

Data from Shulman HM, Cardona DM, Greenson JK, et al. NIH consensus development project on criteria for clinical trials in chronic graft-versus-host disease: II. The 2014 pathology working group report. Biol Blood Marrow Transplant 2015;21(4):589–603.

inhibitors, bowel preparations, and viral infections can all cause crypt cell apoptosis. Cord colitis is a recently described infectious disorder that may develop in patients who receive umbilical cord HSCT.

CHEMOTHERAPY-INDUCED INJURY

Methotrexate, 5- fluorouracil, and capecitabine often cause diarrhea and feature apoptotic epithelial cells, crypt loss and atrophy, and severe regenerative epithelial cell atypia (**Figs. 10–13**).[24–26] Chemotherapy-related changes generally resolve within 3 weeks of treatment cessation, although long-term therapy can lead to progressive mucosal damage and crypt architectural distortion in the absence of significant inflammation. These changes overlap with those of chronic GVHD and ischemia.[27,28] Hence, establishing the timing between chemotherapy and biopsy is important, because GVHD and chemotherapy effect within the first 21 days after HSCT is indistinguishable.[13]

MYCOPHENOLATE MOFETIL (CELLCEPT)

MMF-related injury shows histologic similarities to GVHD. This immunosuppressive agent is used after solid organ transplants and HSCT to prevent graft rejection as well as GVHD prophylaxis.[30,31] The drug inhibits a key enzyme in the de novo purine synthesis pathway, inosine 5'- monophosphate dehydrogenase, thereby reducing B-lymphocyte and

---

Box 2
Pitfalls to graft-versus-host disease diagnosis

Timing of biopsy

- Earlier biopsy in disease course may show more discordance between endoscopic appearance and histologic changes

- Within first 21 days after transplant, apoptotic bodies in gastrointestinal biopsy may be related to pretransplant myeloablative chemotherapy, indistinguishable from GVHD

Sampling

- Endoscopic undersampling may lead to missed diagnosis of GVHD

- A minimum of 8–20 serial tissue sections should examined to look for apoptoses

Other diseases with overlapping features

- Drug effect

  o PPIs cause apoptotic bodies in comparable amounts to GVHD in the antrum; hence, examine fundus for GVHD

  o MMF can cause apoptotic bodies, crypt dropout, architectural disarray, and features mimicking ischemia

  o Other: chemotherapy, NSAIDs, bowel preparation

- Infections

  o CMV can cause apoptotic bodies; viral cytopathic effect preferentially affects endothelium: enlarged cells with nuclear and cytoplasmic viral inclusions

  o Adenovirus can cause apoptotic bodies; viral cytopathic effect that preferentially affects epithelium: cells are not enlarged and contain smudgy nuclear inclusions; employ immunohistochemical staining because inclusions can be easily missed

---

T-lymphocyte proliferation.[32] The precise mechanisms of gastrointestinal toxicity are not completely known, although the drug may directly affect enterocytes by stunting regenerative capacity.[33] MMF may indirectly affect enterocytes by altering lymphocyte proliferation, thereby promoting susceptibility to infection, or autoimmune reactions.[34,35]

Both MMF and GVHD feature crypt cell apoptosis and chronic mucosal damage with significant crypt architectural disarray (**Figs. 14–17**).[34,36,37] Crypt abnormalities can be so pronounced that they mimic

Fig. 10. Crypt atrophy and dropout is evident in this bowel biopsy from a patient with chemotherapy-induced injury. The histologic findings overlap with those of chronic GVHD. It is important to establish when the biopsy is taken, as chemotherapy-related changes and GVHD are histologically indistinguishable within the first 21 days after HSCT. Chemotherapy-related changes generally resolve within 3 weeks of stopping treatment.

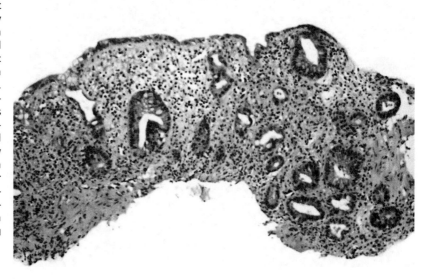

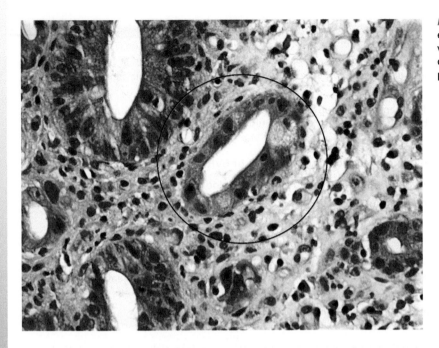

Fig. 11. Chemotherapy effect: this high-power view of a colon biopsy demonstrates an atrophic crypt (*circled*).

chronic idiopathic inflammatory bowel disease.[38,39] Less frequently, MMF-related injury produces atrophic, dilated crypts lined by attenuated epithelium simulating ischemia.[36–39]

MMF can produce histologic changes at every level of the tubular gastrointestinal tract. Esophageal findings include active esophagitis with erosions and/or ulcers and reactive epithelial changes.[35,37] Reported gastric findings include increased apoptotic debris in glandular epithelium, *Helicobacter*-negative chronic active gastritis and erosions, ballooned parietal cells with cytoplasmic clearing, and reactive gastropathy.[35,37] Duodenal biopsies can contain apoptotic debris and show celiac disease–like features with intraepithelial lymphocytosis and villous blunting, foveolar

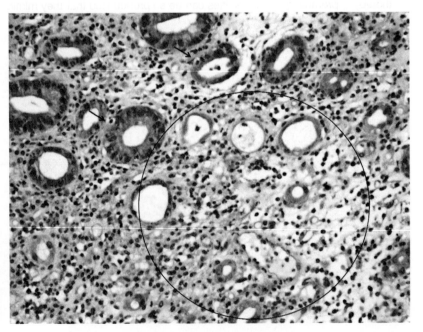

Fig. 12. Chemotherapy effect: this colon biopsy shows damaged crypts with attenuated cytoplasm (*circled*) and apoptotic bodies (*arrow*). The findings can be indistinguishable from GVHD.

Fig. 13. Severe regenerative epithelial atypia can be seen in chemotherapy effect, even simulating neoplasia.

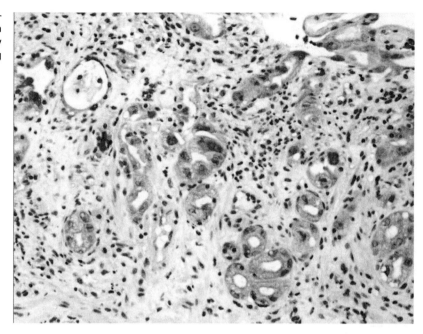

metaplasia, and active inflammation.[35] Reported ileal findings include GVHD-like features, granulomatous enteritis, and active enteritis.[37]

Because features of GVHD, MMF toxicity, and viral infection can overlap histologically, and all occur in the bone marrow transplant setting, several studies have examined whether there are histologic features that can reliably distinguish between them. Star and colleagues[40] evaluated HSCT patients who developed diarrhea while taking MMF and compared their gastrointestinal biopsy samples to those of solid organ transplant patients with MMF-related colitis as well as to those of GVHD. They found that greater than 15 eosinophils/10 high-power fields, lack of endocrine cell aggregates, and lack of apoptotic microabscesses (ie, >3 apoptotic epithelial cells in a crypt) were more strongly associated with MMF-

Fig. 14. MMF injury may induce crypt dropout with inflammation, as seen in this figure. An area of crypt dropout is circled.

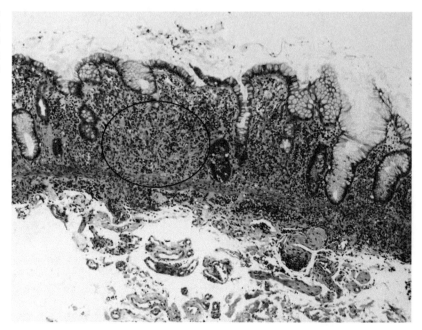

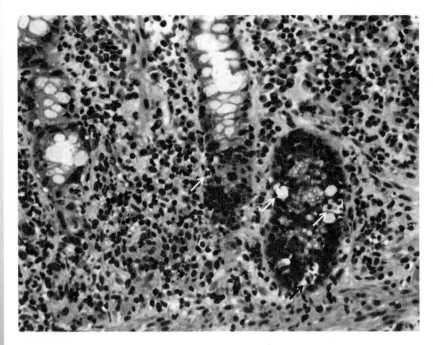

Fig. 15. In this colon biopsy showing MMF-related injury, numerous apoptotic bodies (*arrows*) are present in intestinal crypts.

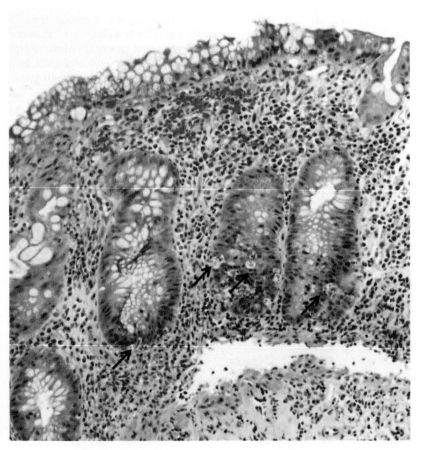

Fig. 16. This photo is of a colon biopsy showing MMF effect; apoptotic bodies are indicated by arrows. The findings are similar to that seen in GVHD and, therefore, require correlation with medication history and clinical findings.

Fig. 17. This follow-up colon sample was obtained from the same patient affected by MMF-toxicity, whose biopsies were featured in **Figs. 14–16.** These biopsies obtained after MMF cessation show improvement of histologic features, including reduction of inflammation and apoptotic bodies.

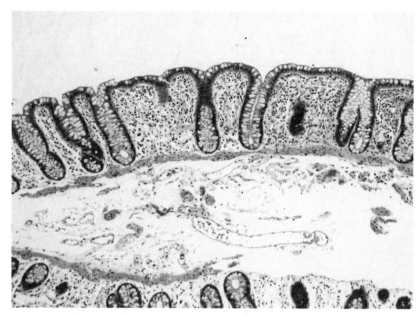

related colitis than GVHD. Other investigators, however, have reported eosinophils to be more typical of GVHD, particularly in the upper gastrointestinal tract, where density of eosinophils reportedly correlates with severity of GVHD.[13,16,41] Ultimately, the histologic features of MMF-related injury substantially overlap with those of GVHD; distinction between these entities requires careful correlation with clinical findings.

PROTON PUMP INHIBITOR EFFECT

Proton pump inhibitors are used for controlling gastroesophageal reflux disease. Their use is associated with increased numbers of apoptotic epithelial cells in gastric antral biopsies, similar to that seen in GVHD.[42] Because gastric fundic mucosa does not have this similar increase in apoptosis, sampling of the fundus is more useful for diagnosing GVHD of the stomach (**Fig. 18**).[43]

BOWEL PREPARATION

Bowel preparations are performed to improve endoscopic visualization; this often involves oral cleansing with polyethylene glycol or sodium phosphate solutions. These preparatory agents can mildly increase crypt cell apoptosis in the range of 12 apoptotic bodies per 100 crypts.[44] In addition, focal active colitis (ie, foci of crypts with infiltrating neutrophils, normal crypt architecture, and no basal plasma cells), accompanied by mucosal hemorrhage, can also be seen with these agents.

NONSTEROIDAL ANTI-INFLAMMATORY DRUGS

NSAIDs can cause several inflammatory changes in the gastrointestinal tract, including apoptosis, active or ischemic enterocolitis, ulcers, erosions, intraepithelial lymphocytosis, chemical gastropathy, and fibrotic strictures or diaphragms in the small intestine.[45] These drugs reduce inflammation by inhibiting cyclooxygenase, a key enzyme in prostaglandin synthesis, and induction of the inflammatory cascade. The exact mechanism by which NSAIDs induce apoptosis is unclear, but it may be related to increased arachidonic acid levels; arachidonic acid increases ceramide production and alters cell membrane permeability with subsequent cytochrome c release, leading to apoptosis.[46]

CORD COLITIS

Umbilical cord blood is an alternative to HSCT that allows for significant mismatch between donor and recipient HLA, thereby increasing access to transplantation.[29] Both related and unrelated cord blood transplants are successfully performed for a variety of hematologic disorders and metabolic storage diseases in pediatric patients. Unrelated HLA-mismatched cord blood transplants result in delayed engraftment and less GVHD, but similar relapse rates, overall survival, and leukemia-free survival compared with matched unrelated donor bone marrow or peripheral blood stem cell transplants.[29,47,48] Cord colitis was

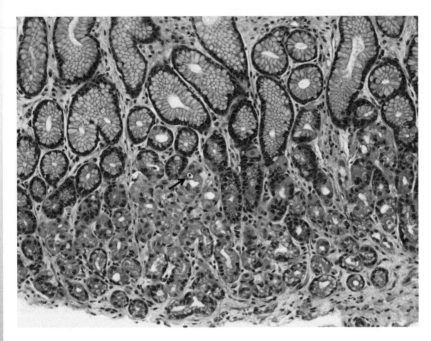

Fig. 18. Mild GVHD in the gastric fundus is characterized by occasional apoptotic epithelial cells (*arrow*). Acid-suppressive therapy can also cause apoptosis, but this is usually limited to the antrum. Hence, it is important to evaluate the fundus if GVHD is of clinical concern, especially if the patient is also taking proton pump inhibitor therapy.

originally described as an antibiotic-responsive, culture-negative diarrhea, although data from DNA sequencing suggest the disorder is due to a bacterium, *Bradyrhizobium enterica*.[49] Although cord colitis can feature occasional apoptotic bodies, it was initially reported to differ from GVHD because of granulomatous inflammation affecting the gastrointestinal tract. In addition, cord colitis can have active colitis with Paneth cell metaplasia and crypt distortion, mimicking Crohn disease. The 2015 NIH guidelines state that cord colitis syndrome is not sufficiently distinct from colonic GVHD to allow separation of these entities based on histology alone. Large studies, including controls who received cord blood and non–cord blood HSCT have shown that neither granulomas nor histologic features of chronicity are specific to cord blood recipients.[7] Granulomas, crypt distortion, and Paneth cell metaplasia may also be encountered in GVHD and CMV colitis.[50] Regardless of controversy, it is important to be aware of cord colitis syndrome because it seems to be a treatable infection that can affect cord blood recipients and shows histologic features that may be seen in GVHD and other infections that can occur in the HSCT population.[51]

INFECTION

The immunocompromised state of HSCT patients renders them susceptible to a variety of infections. GVHD treatment is based on increasing immunosuppression, which exacerbates most infectious conditions; hence, it is important to recognize infectious agents and distinguish them from GVHD. Detection of organisms can be facilitated by immunohistochemistry and multiple tissue levels as well as laboratory and clinical evaluation.

CYTOMEGALOVIRUS

CMV infection is one of the most common infections afflicting immunocompromised patients and is a well-known cause of epithelial cell apoptosis.[52] Viral cytopathic effect involves endothelial and stromal cells more often than epithelial cells and is characterized by enlarged cells that may contain cytoplasmic and nuclear inclusions. Glassy, basophilic nuclear inclusions are surrounded by a clear halo and thickened nuclear membrane. Cytoplasmic inclusions are granular and eosinophilic (**Figs. 19–21**). Apoptosis results from direct cytopathic effect as well as tissue ischemia from endothelial involvement.[53] CMV infection and GVHD can coexist. The 2015 NIH guidelines state that a diagnosis of "likely GVHD" can be rendered in the context of a CMV infection, if abundant apoptotic crypt cells are remote from CMV inclusions. Possible GVHD is the recommended diagnosis if apoptotic bodies are only present in close proximity to CMV-infected cells, implying that CMV may be a source of the apoptotic changes.[7] Immunohistochemistry for CMV and correlation with blood polymerase chain reaction

Fig. 19. A CMV-infected endothelial cell (*circled*) features a prominent nuclear inclusion associated with apoptosis (*arrow*) in the crypt epithelium. Hence, CMV infection is another cause for apoptotic bodies and must be considered in the differential diagnosis for GVHD.

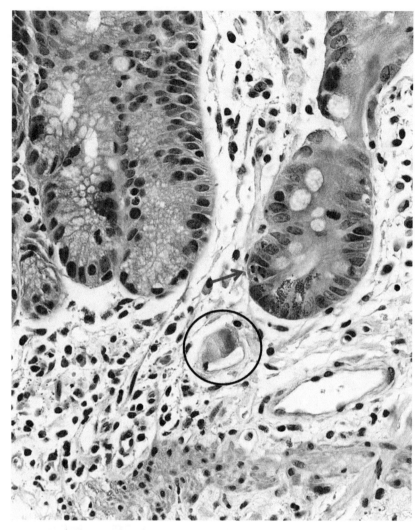

(PCR) testing are helpful tools, although there is not complete concordance between CMV in biopsies and a positive serum PCR assay.[54,55] Many HSCT patients receive prophylactic ganciclovir to decrease the incidence of CMV disease.

ADENOVIRUS

Adenovirus is an important cause of post-transplant diarrhea. The virus almost exclusively infects epithelial cells, producing basophilic, smudged intranuclear inclusions without nuclear enlargement (**Fig. 22**). Adenovirus infection causes gastrointestinal epithelial cell apoptosis with or without active inflammation.[56–58] Although the viral cytopathic effect is usually present in hematoxylin-eosin–stained sections, infected cells can be easily overlooked; thus, immunohistochemistry should be considered when infection is suspected.[59] Preemptive treatment of adenovirus is not standard of care, although affected patients have reduced overall survival and increased hospitalizations compared with HSCT patients without adenovirus. Some investigators suggest weekly adenovirus blood PCR studies until day 100 post-transplant may reduce virus-associated morbidity.[60]

STRONGYLOIDES STERCORALIS

Strongyloides stercoralis is an intestinal nematode capable of causing disseminated, fulminant, and even fatal infections in some immunocompromised patients, in particular those receiving corticosteroids.[61,62] Humans are transcutaneously infected through contact with contaminated soil; filariform larvae migrate to the small intestine, where the female larvae reside and lay eggs. Rhabditiform larvae hatch and are excreted into the stool or molt into filariform larvae within the

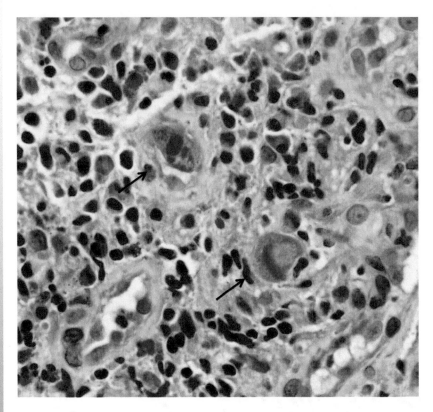

Fig. 20. CMV viral cytopathic effect is featured in this photo. There are enlarged cells with eosinophilic cytoplasmic and basophilic nuclear inclusions (*arrows*).

host; the latter allows the parasite to reinfect the host indefinitely. Hyperinfection, or accelerated autoinfection, is characterized by increased larval migration into the lungs and systemic circulation. Glucocorticoid therapy transforms chronic, subclinical strongyloidiasis into hyperinfection. The stomach, small bowel, and large bowel can all be affected; biopsies show larval and adult forms as well as eggs (30–36 μm by 50–58 μm). Organisms infiltrating the lamina propria are

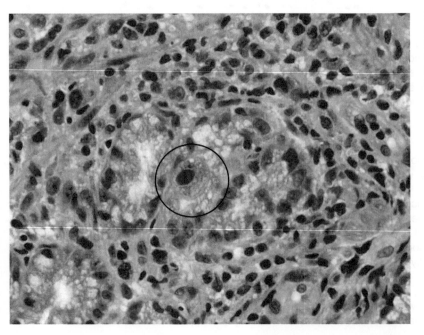

Fig. 21. A glandular epithelial cell infected by CMV (*circled*). The cell is enlarged and contains a glassy, basophilic nuclear inclusions.

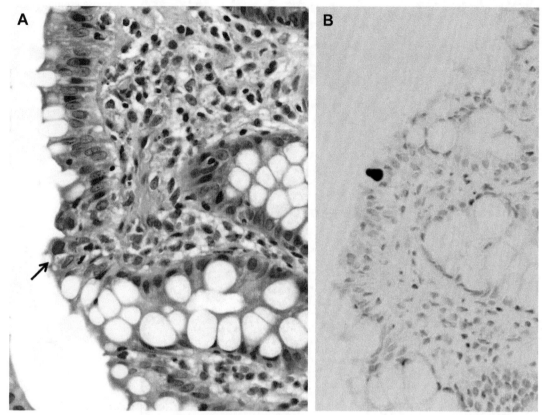

Fig. 22. Adenovirus infection. Intranuclear adenovirus inclusions (*arrow*) are basophilic with a smudged appearance (*A*). Immunohistochemistry highlights the infected cell (*B*).

accompanied by eosinophilic infiltrates, the density of which correlates with parasite burden. Nodules of eosinophils should prompt tissue levels to look for organisms, particularly in immunocompromised patients. Larval forms have cross-sectional diameters of 12 μm to 18 μm, and adult female larvae have diameters of 30 μm to 45 μm with visible internal organs and sharply pointed tails (**Figs. 23–25**).[61] Chronic infection can cause crypt architectural distortion that mimics inflammatory bowel disease.[63] Serologic studies facilitate the diagnosis, but stool examinations are often negative, even in the face of significant infection.[64,65]

IDIOPATHIC ESOPHAGEAL ULCERS

Idiopathic esophageal (and sometimes gastric) ulcers were initially described in patients with AIDS but can occur after HSCT and solid organ transplants.[58,66–68] These lesions are often large with heaped-up edges and mucosal bridges that traverse the ulcer bed. They can bleed or perforate. The pathogenesis remains unclear; CMV, *Candida albicans*, and herpes simplex virus infections

should be excluded prior to rendering a diagnosis because treatment requires immunosuppressive therapy.

NEUTROPENIC ENTEROCOLITIS

Neutropenic enterocolitis (typhlitis) is a life-threatening condition typically encountered in the setting of chemotherapy-induced neutropenia.[69] The chemotherapeutic agents particularly associated with neutropenic enterocolitis are cytosine arabinoside, cisplatin, vincristine, adriamycin, 5-fluorouracil, and mercaptopurine.[45] The mucosal damage from chemotherapy results in tissue invasion by luminal bacteria or other microorganisms, which can lead to perforation and sepsis. This disease is highly fatal and requires aggressive management, such as surgical resection and antibiotics.[70] Clinical features include neutropenia, bowel wall thickening on imaging studies, abdominal pain, signs of an acute abdomen, and fever, although similar findings can be seen in patients with GVHD, MMF-related injury, ischemia, and relapsed leukemia.[71] Almost all cases involve the cecum and right

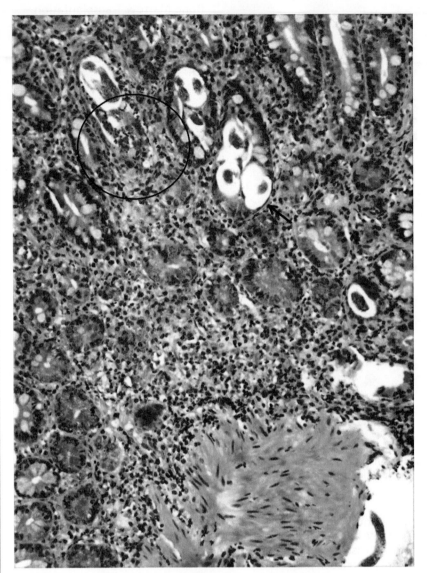

Fig. 23. Strongyloidiasis (*arrow*) is accompanied by dense eosinophilic infiltrates (*circled*).

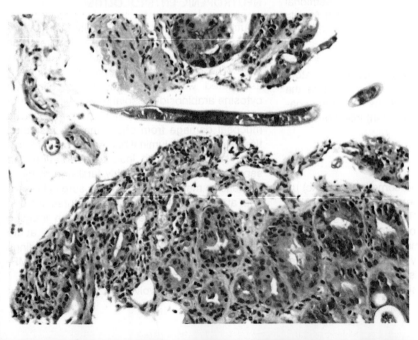

Fig. 24. An adult *Strongyloides* worm. A sharply pointed tail and visible internal organs are present.

Fig. 25. An adult *Strongyloides* worm has a sharply pointed tail (*arrow*) and visible internal organs.

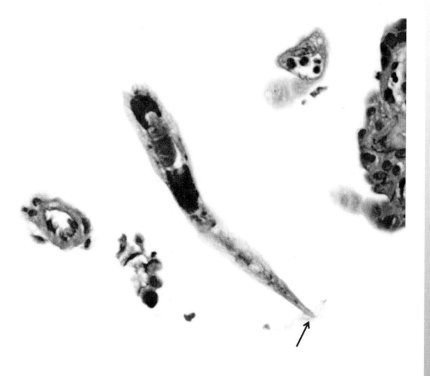

colon and show ulcers, mural edema, severe epithelial injury, and hemorrhage unaccompanied by neutrophilic infiltrates; apoptosis is not a prominent feature. Invasive bacteria and/or fungi are common, including *Clostridium septicum,* vancomycin-resistant *Enterococcus*, and *Klebsiella.*

SUMMARY

Gastrointestinal mucosal biopsies from HSCT patients pose several diagnostic challenges because features of GVHD overlap with those of other disorders. Distinction between GVVHD and its mimics is important; the former is treated by increasing immunosuppression, which can exacerbate infections and lead to life-threatening illness. Knowledge of the clinical scenario, timing of the biopsy, medication regimens, and laboratory data are important when evaluating biopsies from these complicated patients.

REFERENCES

1. Przepiorka D, Smith TL, Folloder J, et al. Risk factors for acute graft-versus-host disease after allogeneic blood stem cell transplantation. Blood 1999;94(4): 1465–70.

2. Wild D, Sung AD, Cardona D, et al. The diagnostic yield of site and symptom-based biopsies for acute gastrointestinal graft-versus-host disease: a 5-year retrospective review. Dig Dis Sci 2016;61(3):806–13.

3. Snover DC, Weisdorf SA, Vercellotti GM, et al. A histopathologic study of gastric and small intestinal graft-versus-host disease following allogeneic bone marrow transplantation. Hum Pathol 1985; 16(4):387–92.

4. Ross WA, Ghosh S, Dekovich AA, et al. Endoscopic biopsy diagnosis of acute gastrointestinal graft-versus-host disease: Rectosigmoid biopsies are more sensitive than upper gastrointestinal biopsies. Am J Gastroenterol 2008;103(4):982–9.

5. Aslanian H, Chander B, Robert M, et al. Prospective evaluation of acute graft-versus-host disease. Dig Dis Sci 2012;57(3):720–5.

6. Filipovich AH, Weisdorf D, Pavletic S, et al. National Institutes of Health consensus development project on criteria for clinical trials in chronic graft-versus-host disease: I. Diagnosis and staging working group report. Biol Blood Marrow Transplant 2005; 11(12):945–56.

7. Shulman HM, Cardona DM, Greenson JK, et al. NIH consensus development project on criteria for clinical trials in chronic graft-versus-host disease: II. The 2014 pathology working group report. Biol Blood Marrow Transplant 2015;21(4): 589–603.

8. Takashima S, Kadowaki M, Aoyama K, et al. The wnt agonist R-spondin1 regulates systemic graft-versus-host disease by protecting intestinal stem cells. J Exp Med 2011;208(2):285–94.

9. Holmberg L, Kikuchi K, Gooley TA, et al. Gastrointestinal graft-versus-host disease in recipients of autologous hematopoietic stem cells: Incidence, risk factors, and outcome. Biol Blood Marrow Transplant 2006;12(2):226–34.

10. Drobyski WR, Hari P, Keever-Taylor C, et al. Severe autologous GVHD after hematopoietic progenitor cell transplantation for multiple myeloma. Bone Marrow Transplant 2009;43(2):169–77.

11. Krishna SG, Barlogie B, Lamps LW, et al. Recurrent spontaneous gastrointestinal graft-versus-host disease in autologous hematopoietic stem cell transplantation. Clin Lymphoma Myeloma Leuk 2010; 10(1):E17–21.

12. Cogbill CH, Drobyski WR, Komorowski RA. Gastrointestinal pathology of autologous graft-versus-host disease following hematopoietic stem cell transplantation: A clinicopathological study of 17 cases. Mod Pathol 2011;24(1):117–25.

13. Washington K, Jagasia M. Pathology of graft-versus-host disease in the gastrointestinal tract. Hum Pathol 2009;40(7):909–17.

14. Meisel JL, Bergman D, Graney D, et al. Human rectal mucosa: Proctoscopic and morphological changes caused by laxatives. Gastroenterology 1977;72(6):1274–9.

15. Lampert IA, Thorpe P, van Noorden S, et al. Selective sparing of enterochromaffin cells in graft versus host disease affecting the colonic mucosa. Histopathology 1985;9(8):875–86.

16. Shulman HM, Kleiner D, Lee SJ, et al. Histopathologic diagnosis of chronic graft-versus-host disease: National institutes of health consensus development project on criteria for clinical trials in chronic graft-versus-host disease: II. Pathology working group report. Biol Blood Marrow Transplant 2006;12(1): 31–47.

17. Jacobsohn DA, Montross S, Anders V, et al. Clinical importance of confirming or excluding the diagnosis of chronic graft-versus-host disease. Bone Marrow Transplant 2001;28(11):1047–51.

18. Martinez C, Rosales M, Calvo X, et al. Serial intestinal endoscopic examinations of patients with persistent diarrhea after allo-SCT. Bone Marrow Transplant 2012;47(5):694–9.

19. Martin P, Nash R, Sanders J, et al. Reproducibility in retrospective grading of acute graft-versus-host disease after allogeneic marrow transplantation. Bone Marrow Transplant 1998;21(3):273–9.

20. Ferrara JL, Harris AC, Greenson JK, et al. Regenerating islet-derived 3-alpha is a biomarker of gastrointestinal graft-versus-host disease. Blood 2011; 118(25):6702–8.

21. Akpek G, Chinratanalab W, Lee LA, et al. Gastrointestinal involvement in chronic graft-versus-host disease: A clinicopathologic study. Biol Blood Marrow Transplant 2003;9(1):46–51.

22. Nepal S, Navaneethan U, Bennett AE, et al. De novo inflammatory bowel disease and its mimics after organ transplantation. Inflamm Bowel Dis 2013;19(7): 1518–27.

23. Baron FA, Hermanne JP, Dowlati A, et al. Bronchiolitis obliterans organizing pneumonia and ulcerative colitis after allogeneic bone marrow transplantation. Bone Marrow Transplant 1998;21(9):951–4.

24. Jewell LD, Fields AL, Murray CJ, et al. Erosive gastroduodenitis with marked epithelial atypia after hepatic arterial infusion chemotherapy. Am J Gastroenterol 1985;80(6):421–4.

25. Soldini D, Gaspert A, Montani M, et al. Apoptotic enteropathy caused by antimetabolites and TNF-alpha antagonists. J Clin Pathol 2014;67(7):582–6.

26. Lee FD. Importance of apoptosis in the histopathology of drug related lesions in the large intestine. J Clin Pathol 1993;46(2):118–22.

27. Sparano JA, Dutcher JP, Kaleya R, et al. Colonic ischemia complicating immunotherapy with interleukin-2 and interferon-alpha. Cancer 1991; 68(7):1538–44.

28. Beck PL, Wong JF, Li Y, et al. Chemotherapy- and radiotherapy-induced intestinal damage is regulated by intestinal trefoil factor. Gastroenterology 2004;126(3):796–808.

29. Ballen KK, Gluckman E, Broxmeyer HE. Umbilical cord blood transplantation: The first 25 years and beyond. Blood 2013;122(4):491–8.

30. Maris MB, Niederwieser D, Sandmaier BM, et al. HLA-matched unrelated donor hematopoietic cell transplantation after nonmyeloablative conditioning for patients with hematologic malignancies. Blood 2003;102(6):2021–30.

31. Minagawa K, Yamamori M, Katayama Y, et al. Mycophenolate mofetil: Fully utilizing its benefits for GvHD prophylaxis. Int J Hematol 2012;96(1):10–25.

32. Sievers TM, Rossi SJ, Ghobrial RM, et al. Mycophenolate mofetil. Pharmacotherapy 1997;17(6): 1178–97.

33. Gil-Vernet S, Amado A, Ortega F, et al. Gastrointestinal complications in renal transplant recipients: MITOS study. Transplant Proc 2007;39(7):2190–3.

34. Papadimitriou JC, Cangro CB, Lustberg A, et al. Histologic features of mycophenolate mofetil-related colitis: A graft-versus-host disease-like pattern. Int J Surg Pathol 2003;11(4):295–302.

35. Nguyen T, Park JY, Scudiere JR, et al. Mycophenolic acid (cellcept and myfortic) induced injury of the upper GI tract. Am J Surg Pathol 2009;33(9): 1355–63.

36. Selbst MK, Ahrens WA, Robert ME, et al. Spectrum of histologic changes in colonic biopsies in patients

treated with mycophenolate mofetil. Mod Pathol 2009;22(6):737–43.

37. Parfitt JR, Jayakumar S, Driman DK. Mycophenolate mofetil-related gastrointestinal mucosal injury: Variable injury patterns, including graft-versus-host disease-like changes. Am J Surg Pathol 2008;32(9): 1367–72.

38. Lee S, de Boer WB, Subramaniam K, et al. Pointers and pitfalls of mycophenolate-associated colitis. J Clin Pathol 2013;66(1):8–11.

39. Liapis G, Boletis J, Skalioti C, et al. Histological spectrum of mycophenolate mofetil-related colitis: Association with apoptosis. Histopathology 2013; 63(5):649–58.

40. Star KV, Ho VT, Wang HH, et al. Histologic features in colon biopsies can discriminate mycophenolate from GVHD-induced colitis. Am J Surg Pathol 2013;37(9):1319–28.

41. Daneshpouy M, Socie G, Lemann M, et al. Activated eosinophils in upper gastrointestinal tract of patients with graft-versus-host disease. Blood 2002;99(8): 3033–40.

42. Katz PO, Gerson LB, Vela MF. Guidelines for the diagnosis and management of gastroesophageal reflux disease. Am J Gastroenterol 2013;108(3): 308–28, [quiz: 329].

43. Welch DC, Wirth PS, Goldenring JR, et al. Gastric graft-versus-host disease revisited: Does proton pump inhibitor therapy affect endoscopic gastric biopsy interpretation? Am J Surg Pathol 2006;30(4): 444–9.

44. Driman DK, Preiksaitis HG. Colorectal inflammation and increased cell proliferation associated with oral sodium phosphate bowel preparation solution. Hum Pathol 1998;29(9):972–8.

45. Parfitt JR, Driman DK. Pathological effects of drugs on the gastrointestinal tract: a review. Hum Pathol 2007;38(4):527–36.

46. Jana NR. NSAIDs and apoptosis. Cell Mol Life Sci 2008;65(9):1295–301.

47. Rocha V, Labopin M, Sanz G, et al. Transplants of umbilical-cord blood or bone marrow from unrelated donors in adults with acute leukemia. N Engl J Med 2004;351(22):2276–85.

48. Rocha V, Cornish J, Sievers EL, et al. Comparison of outcomes of unrelated bone marrow and umbilical cord blood transplants in children with acute leukemia. Blood 2001;97(10):2962–71.

49. Bhatt AS, Freeman SS, Herrera AF, et al. Sequence-based discovery of bradyrhizobium enterica in cord colitis syndrome. N Engl J Med 2013;369(6):517–28.

50. Shimoji S, Kato K, Eriguchi Y, et al. Evaluating the association between histological manifestations of cord colitis syndrome with GVHD. Bone Marrow Transplant 2013;48(9):1249–52.

51. Milano F, Shulman HM, Guthrie KA, et al. Late-onset colitis after cord blood transplantation is consistent with graft-versus-host disease: Results of a blinded histopathological review. Biol Blood Marrow Transplant 2014;20(7):1008–13.

52. Washington K, Bentley RC, Green A, et al. Gastric graft-versus-host disease: A blinded histologic study. Am J Surg Pathol 1997;21(9):1037–46.

53. Tzankov A, Stifter G, Tschorner I, et al. Detection of apoptoses in gastro-intestinal graft-versus-host disease and cytomegalovirus colitis by a commercially available antibody against caspase-3. Pathol Res Pract 2003;199(5):337–40.

54. Brainard JA, Greenson JK, Vesy CJ, et al. Detection of cytomegalovirus in liver transplant biopsies. A comparison of light microscopy, immunohistochemistry, duplex PCR and nested PCR. Transplantation 1994;57(12):1753–7.

55. Muir SW, Murray J, Farquharson MA, et al. Detection of cytomegalovirus in upper gastrointestinal biopsies from heart transplant recipients: Comparison of light microscopy, immunocytochemistry, in situ hybridisation, and nested PCR. J Clin Pathol 1998; 51(11):807–11.

56. Adeyi OA, Randhawa PA, Nalesnik MA, et al. Post-transplant adenoviral enteropathy in patients with small bowel transplantation. Arch Pathol Lab Med 2008;132(4):703–5.

57. Kaufman SS, Magid MS, Tschernia A, et al. Discrimination between acute rejection and adenoviral enteritis in intestinal transplant recipients. Transplant Proc 2002;34(3):943–5.

58. Lipson DA, Berlin JA, Palevsky HI, et al. Giant gastric ulcers and risk factors for gastroduodenal mucosal disease in orthotopic lung transplant patients. Dig Dis Sci 1998;43(6):1177–85.

59. Solomon IH, Hornick JL, Laga AC. Immunohistochemistry is rarely justified for the diagnosis of viral infections. Am J Clin Pathol 2016;147(1):96–104.

60. Rustia E, Violago L, Jin Z, et al. Risk factors and utility of a risk-based algorithm for monitoring cytomegalovirus, epstein-barr virus, and adenovirus infections in pediatric recipients after allogeneic hematopoietic cell transplantation. Biol Blood Marrow Transplant 2016;22(9):1646–53.

61. Rivasi F, Pampiglione S, Boldorini R, et al. Histopathology of gastric and duodenal strongyloides stercoralis locations in fifteen immunocompromised subjects. Arch Pathol Lab Med 2006;130(12): 1792–8.

62. Keiser PB, Nutman TB. Strongyloides stercoralis in the immunocompromised population. Clin Microbiol Rev 2004;17(1):208–17.

63. Weight SC, Barrie WW. Colonic strongyloides stercoralis infection masquerading as ulcerative colitis. J R Coll Surg Edinb 1997;42(3):202–3.

64. Siddiqui AA, Berk SL. Diagnosis of strongyloides stercoralis infection. Clin Infect Dis 2001;33(7): 1040–7.

65. Rodriguez EA, Abraham T, Williams FK. Severe strongyloidiasis with negative serology after corticosteroid treatment. Am J Case Rep 2015;16: 95–8.

66. Bach MC, Valenti AJ, Howell DA, et al. Odynophagia from aphthous ulcers of the pharynx and esophagus in the acquired immunodeficiency syndrome (AIDS). Ann Intern Med 1988;109(4):338–9.

67. Farrell JJ, Cosimi AB, Chung RT. Idiopathic giant esophageal ulcers in a renal transplant patient responsive to steroid therapy. Transplantation 2000;70(1):230–2.

68. Dang S, Atiq M, Krishna S, et al. Idiopathic esophageal ulcers after autologous hemopoetic stem cell transplant: Possible role of IgA levels. Ann Hematol 2008;87(12):1031–2.

69. Bavaro MF. Neutropenic enterocolitis. Curr Gastroenterol Rep 2002;4(4):297–301.

70. Machado NO. Neutropenic enterocolitis: A continuing medical and surgical challenge. N Am J Med Sci 2010;2(7):293–300.

71. Sachak T, Arnold MA, Naini BV, et al. Neutropenic enterocolitis: new insights into a deadly entity. Am J Surg Pathol 2015;39(12):1635–42.

Emerging Concepts in Gastric Neoplasia

Heritable Gastric Cancers and Polyposis Disorders

Rachel S. van der Post, MD[a],*,
Fátima Carneiro, MD, PhD[b,c,d,e]

KEYWORDS

- Hereditary gastric cancer • Signet ring cell • Stomach • E-cadherin • CDH1 • CTNNA1 • GAPPS
- Gastric polyposis

Key points

- Hereditary diffuse gastric cancer results from germline mutations in *CDH1* (40% of families) and *CTNNA1* (few families reported).
- Small intramucosal foci of signet ring cell carcinoma, in situ signet ring cell carcinoma, and pagetoid lesions can be observed in *CDH1* mutation carriers.
- Gastric adenocarcinoma and proximal polyposis displays fundic gland polyposis, dysplasia, and intestinal-type or mixed-type adenocarcinoma.
- Fundic gland polyposis occurs in familial adenomatous polyposis (FAP), attenuated FAP, and MUTYH-associated polyposis syndromes.
- Gastric polyps in juvenile, Peutz-Jeghers, and Cowden polyposis cannot be reliably distinguished from each other or sporadic hyperplastic polyps.

ABSTRACT

Hereditary gastric cancer is a relatively rare disease with specific clinical and histopathologic characteristics. Hereditary gastric cancer of the diffuse type is predominantly caused by germline mutations in *CDH1*. The inherited cause of familial intestinal gastric cancer is unknown. Gastric adenocarcinoma and proximal polyposis of the stomach is a hereditary cancer syndrome caused by germline mutations in promoter 1B of *APC*. Other well-defined cancer syndromes, such as Lynch, Li-Fraumeni, and hereditary breast or ovarian cancer syndromes, are associated with increased risk of gastric cancer. This article reviews important histopathologic features and emerging concepts regarding gastric carcinogenesis in these syndromes.

OVERVIEW

Most (>80%) gastric carcinomas are sporadic; familial aggregation occurs in 10% to 20% of patients and fewer than 3% of cases can be attributed to known inherited causes.[1] Gastric

---

Disclosure Statement: The authors have nothing to disclose.
[a] Department of Pathology, Radboud University Medical Centre, Postbox 9101, Nijmegen 6500 HB, The Netherlands; [b] Department of Pathology, Centro Hospitalar de São João, Porto, Portugal; [c] Department of Pathology, Faculty of Medicine of the University of Porto (FMUP), Alameda Professor Hernâni Monteiro, Porto 4200-319, Portugal; [d] Institute of Molecular Pathology and Immunology of the University of Porto (Ipatimup), Rua Júlio Amaral de Carvalho, 45, Porto 4200-135, Portugal; [e] Institute for Research Innovation in Health (i3S), Rua Júlio Amaral de Carvalho, 45, Porto 4200-135, Portugal
* Corresponding author.
E-mail address: Chella.vanderpost@radboudumc.nl

carcinomas diagnosed at advanced stage have a poor prognosis; every effort should be made to prevent or detect it at early stages when potentially curable.

Familial gastric carcinoma can be classified as hereditary diffuse gastric cancer, familial intestinal gastric cancer, and familial gastric cancer when the histologic subtype is unknown.[2] Advanced gastric cancers are often classified as "poorly differentiated adenocarcinoma" at the time of biopsy, although an attempt should be made to categorized them according to the World Health Organization or Laurén schemes. The latter classifies tumors as intestinal and diffuse types; tumors that cannot be placed in one of these categories are considered indeterminate and mixed type.[3]

The purpose of this review was to describe the histologic and clinical characteristics of several gastric cancer syndromes, including other primary malignancies and types of gastrointestinal polyps. This article focuses on important histopathologic features and emerging concepts in (1) hereditary diffuse gastric cancer, (2) familial intestinal gastric cancer, (3) gastric adenocarcinoma and proximal polyposis of the stomach and similar polyposis syndromes, as well as (4) other hereditary cancer syndromes, as enumerated in **Tables 1** and **2**.

HEREDITARY DIFFUSE GASTRIC CANCER

CDH1 GERMLINE MUTATION

Identification of *CDH1* germline mutations in the Maori population defined a newly recognized autosomal dominant cancer-susceptibility syndrome termed "hereditary diffuse gastric cancer."[4] Following this discovery, many families around the world with clustering of gastric cancer have been tested to identify novel *CDH1* germline mutations. *CDH1* encodes E-cadherin, a transmembrane calcium-dependent protein with important roles in cell-cell adhesion at the *adherens* junctions.[5,6]

Germline *CDH1* alterations can affect the entire coding sequence and include small frameshifts, splice-site, nonsense, and missense mutations, as well as large rearrangements.[7] Most truncating mutations are pathogenic and several missense mutations have a deleterious effect on E-cadherin function.[8] Individuals with germline *CDH1* mutations have a single functional *CDH1* allele. Inactivation of the wild-type allele by a somatic second-hit molecular mechanism (ie, promoter hypermethylation, loss of heterozygosity) leads to biallelic inactivation and development of diffuse gastric cancer.[9–12] Biallelic *CDH1* inactivation leads to loss of E-cadherin function and abnormal

immunohistochemical staining for E-cadherin compared with complete membranous staining in normal epithelium.[11–14] Aberrant E-cadherin staining patterns include absence of immunoreactivity, weak membranous staining, "dotlike" staining, and cytoplasmic staining.[15]

Individuals with a pathogenic germline *CDH1* mutation are at 60% to 70% increased risk for diffuse gastric cancer and women are at risk for lobular breast cancer (40%).[1,16] There is no evidence that individuals with *CDH1* mutations are at significantly increased risk for other cancer types. Testing for germline *CDH1* mutations is recommended in families that fulfill 1 of the following 3 criteria[1]:

1. Two or more documented cases of gastric cancer at any age in first-degree or second-degree relatives, with at least 1 confirmed diffuse gastric cancer.
2. Personal history of diffuse gastric cancer before the age of 40 years.
3. Personal or family history (first-degree or second-degree relatives) of diffuse gastric cancer and lobular breast cancer, 1 diagnosed before the age of 50 years.

Genetic testing also can be considered in patients with bilateral lobular breast cancer before the age of 50 years, families with multiple cases of lobular breast cancer, families with clustering of diffuse gastric cancer and cleft lip/cleft palate, and any patient diagnosed with in situ or pagetoid spread of signet ring cells in the gastric mucosa.[1]

Prophylactic total gastrectomy is advised for individuals with a proven pathogenic germline *CDH1* mutation.[1] These resection specimens generally show no specific gross abnormalities, but multiple invasive intramucosal cancers (pT1a) are almost always detected when the entire stomach is processed for histology (**Fig. 1A**).[13,17,18] In most cases, these tiny (<0.1–10 mm) foci are restricted to the superficial mucosa. They are composed of relatively small signet ring cells at the neck-zone level that enlarge toward the mucosal surface.[14] Foci are found throughout the stomach and even in gastric metaplasia beyond the pylorus.[1]

Two typical precursor lesions of intraepithelial signet ring cell carcinoma include signet ring cell carcinoma in situ (Tis) and pagetoid spread of signet ring cell carcinoma. The former is defined as a disorganized proliferation of signet ring cells that replaces normal glandular epithelial cells, but is confined by the basement membrane. Pagetoid spread of signet ring cells appears as a linear proliferation of signet ring cells between normal epithelial cells and the

Table 1
Characteristics of hereditary diffuse gastric cancer and familial intestinal gastric cancer

Syndrome	Gene Mutation	Mode of Inheritance	Gastric Cancer Lifetime Risk	Histology	Associated Malignancies	Important Histologic Clues	Important Clinical Clues
Hereditary diffuse gastric cancer associated with *CDH1* germline mutation	*CDH1*	Autosomal dominant	70%–80%	Diffuse	Lobular breast cancer	Mucosal foci Abnormal E-cadherin immunostaining	Familial clustering, lobular breast cancer, young age of diagnosis, cleft lip/palate
Hereditary diffuse gastric cancer associated with *CTNNA1* germline mutation	*CTNNA1*	Autosomal dominant	Unknown	Diffuse	None	Abnormal a-E-catenin immunostaining	Familial clustering and/or young age of diagnosis
Familial intestinal gastric cancer	None	Autosomal dominant	Unknown	Intestinal	None	Unknown	Familial clustering of without polyposis

Table 2
Characteristics of gastric polyposis syndromes

Syndrome	Gene Mutation	Mode of Inheritance	Associated Gastric Polyps	Estimates of Gastric Cancer Lifetime Risk	Histology Gastric Cancer	Important Histologic Clues	Locations of Associated Other Malignancies	Important Clinical Clues
Gastric adenocarcinoma with proximal polyposis	Point mutations in Exon 1B of APC	Autosomal dominant	Fundic gland polyps, few hyperplastic polyps and adenomas	Increased	Intestinal and mixed	Fundic gland polyposis with antral sparing	None	Gastric polyposis without colorectal polyposis and without use of acid-suppression therapy
Attenuated familial adenomatous polyposis	APC	Autosomal dominant	Predominantly fundic gland polyps, foveolar adenomas, and pyloric gland adenomas	Not increased	Intestinal	Fundic gland polyps	Colorectum, thyroid, duodenum, adrenal gland, small bowel, brain	Colorectal and duodenal polyposis
MUTYH-associated polyposis	MUTYH (MYH)	Autosomal recessive	Predominantly fundic gland polyps, adenomas	Not increased	Intestinal	Fundic gland polyps	Colorectum, thyroid, duodenum	Colorectal and duodenal polyposis

Syndrome	Gene	Inheritance	Polyps	Risk	Gastric cancer		Extra-gastric malignancies	Clinical features
Peutz-Jeghers syndrome	LKB1 (STK11)	Autosomal dominant	Hamartomatous polyps	29%	Intestinal	Colonic Peutz-Jeghers polyps	Colorectum, small bowel, pancreas, lung, breast, gynecologic tract	Gastrointestinal polyposis, perioral pigmentation, diversity of malignancies
Juvenile polyposis syndrome	SMAD4 (DPC4/MADH4) or BMPR1A	Autosomal dominant	Hamartomatous (juvenile) polyps	10%–30%	Intestinal and diffuse	SMAD4 immunostain, colonic juvenile polyps	Colorectum, duodenum, pancreas	Juvenile polyps throughout the gastrointestinal tract
PTEN hamartoma tumor syndrome	PTEN	Autosomal dominant	Hamartomatous polyps, ganglioneuromas	Increased	Intestinal and diffuse	Multiple polyps, mucocutaneous lesions	Breast, thyroid, endometrium, colorectum, kidney, skin (melanoma)	Macrocephaly, mucocutaneous lesions, gastrointestinal polyps (hamartomas, adenomas, ganglioneuromas, lipomas), diffuse esophageal glycogenic acanthosis

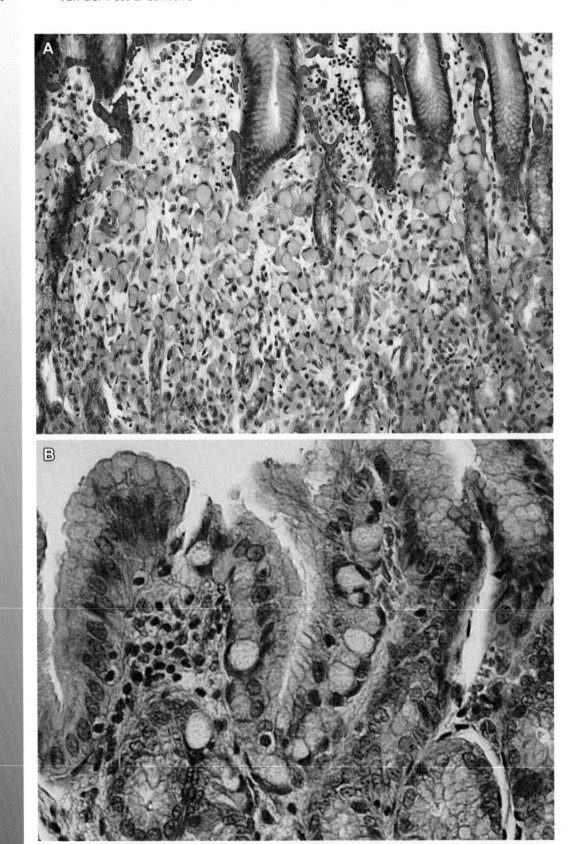

Fig. 1. (*A*) Typical *CDH1*-associated intramucosal signet ring cell carcinoma [H&E, original magnification ×100]. (*B*) Pagetoid spread of signet ring cells [H&E, original magnification ×250].

basement membrane (see **Fig.** 1B). Confirmation of these precursors by an experienced histopathologist is recommended because benign signet cell–like changes may mimic these lesions.[1] Most resection specimens contain few, or no precursor lesions despite the presence of numerous foci of intramucosal signet ring cell carcinomas.

It is not clear how long early lesions of hereditary diffuse gastric cancer can remain indolent and predicting progression of disease is challenging. Inactivation of the second *CDH1* allele is an early event, but other driver alterations that may play a role in the pathogenesis of diffuse gastric cancer have not been clarified. Early hereditary diffuse gastric cancers have an "indolent" phenotype and contain uniform signet ring cells with low Ki-67 labeling and normal p53 immunoexpression. Advanced hereditary diffuse gastric cancers display an "aggressive" phenotype with a mixture of pleomorphic cells, increased Ki-67 staining, and aberrant p53 expression.[15]

Advanced gastric carcinomas associated with a pathogenic *CDH1* germline mutation, often show gastric wall thickening due to diffuse infiltration by cancer cells. Although hereditary diffuse gastric carcinomas are histologically indistinguishable from sporadic diffuse gastric cancers, the presence of in situ lesions, pagetoid spread, or multifocal intramucosal signet ring cells in otherwise normal mucosa, are important clues.

CTNNA1 GERMLINE MUTATION

Approximately 60% to 70% of families that fulfill the current testing criteria for hereditary diffuse gastric cancer lack germline *CDH1* mutations.[16,19,20] Three families with clustering of diffuse gastric cancer have been recently reported to carry germline *CTNNA1* mutations.[16,21] *CTNNA1* encodes α-E-catenin, which is involved in intercellular cell adhesion and forms a complex with β-catenin to bind the cytoplasmic domain of E-cadherin to the cytoskeleton.[22–24] Diffuse gastric cancers identified in *CTNNA1* mutation carriers can show loss of immunohistochemical staining for α-E-catenin with preservation of E-cadherin. The clinical features of these kindreds are similar to those of families with *CDH1*-mutations and include intramucosal signet ring cell carcinomas, but available data are not sufficient to make a statement regarding disease penetrance.[21]

OTHER MUTATIONS DESCRIBED IN HEREDITARY DIFFUSE GASTRIC CANCER

Hansford and colleagues[16] reported results from targeted sequencing of 55 cancer-associated genes in 144 families with hereditary diffuse gastric cancer who lacked detectable germline *CDH1* mutations. They identified 2 families with germline *CTNNA1* mutations, as well as truncating germline mutations in *BRCA2*, *PRSS1*, *ATM*, *PALB2*, *SDHB*, *STK11*, and *MSR1*.[16] These results do not suggest a new type of hereditary diffuse gastric cancer, but reflect clustering of diffuse gastric cancer that is sometimes seen in the context of familial cancer syndromes. Other germline mutations affecting *MAP3K6* and *MYD88* have been described, but their significance is not known.[25,26] It is possible that some families have abnormalities at the *CDH1 locus* or changes affecting proteins that interact with E-cadherin pathway that have not yet been identified. Next-generation sequencing and similar methods may identify other genes responsible for hereditary diffuse gastric cancer in the future.

FAMILIAL INTESTINAL GASTRIC CANCER

Patients with familial intestinal gastric cancer are at increased risk for intestinal-type gastric carcinoma. Definitional criteria for this disorder depend on the incidence of gastric carcinoma in the population. In 1999, the International Gastric Cancer Linkage Consortium proposed diagnostic criteria analogous to the Amsterdam criteria in high-incidence countries (eg, Portugal, Japan).[2] Diagnostic criteria for countries with low incidence include at least 2 first-degree or second-degree relatives affected by intestinal-type gastric cancer, with 1 diagnosed before the age of 50 years; or 3 or more relatives with intestinal-type gastric cancer diagnosed at any age.[2] The diagnosis should be considered when there is a history of intestinal-type gastric cancer in families without polyposis. Familial intestinal gastric cancers show no histologic features that distinguish them from sporadic intestinal-type gastric cancers. One family with clustering of intestinal-type gastric cancer and heterozygous mutations in the immunity gene *IL12RB1* was reported, but additional research is required to determine whether such mutations increase gastric cancer risk.[27] No other inherited mutations have been reported in patients with familial intestinal gastric cancer. *Helicobacter pylori* eradication seems to be the most important strategy for preventing gastric cancer in first-degree relatives of patients with gastric cancer.[28]

GASTRIC POLYPOSIS AND GASTRIC CANCER PREDISPOSITION

BACKGROUND

Most gastric polyps are sporadic, consist mostly of epithelial elements, and they are related to high rates of *H pylori* infection. Gastric polyps that develop in patients with a polyposis syndrome are often multiple and can be divided into the following:

- Fundic gland polyps seen in gastric adenocarcinoma and proximal polyposis of the stomach, complete and attenuated familial adenomatous polyposis, and MUTYH-associated polyposis syndromes.
- Hamartomatous polyps seen in Peutz-Jeghers syndrome, juvenile polyposis syndrome, and Cowden (phosphatase and tensin homolog [PTEN] hamartoma tumor) syndrome.

Other syndromes in which gastric polyps are sometimes reported include neurofibromatosis type 1, McCune-Albright syndrome, and Cronkhite-Canada syndrome, the latter of which is likely a nonheritable immune-mediated disorder. There is no definite increased gastric cancer risk among patients with neurofibromatosis type 1, McCune-Albright syndrome, or Cronkhite-Canada syndrome.[29]

FUNDIC GLAND POLYPOSIS SYNDROMES

GAPPS (Gastric Adenocarcinoma and Proximal Polyposis of the Stomach)-Related Gastric Polyposis and Cancer

In 2012, gastric adenocarcinoma and proximal polyposis of the stomach was recognized as a heritable form of gastric cancer. Affected kindreds exhibit a specific clinicopathologic phenotype with 10 to hundreds of fundic gland polyps involving oxyntic mucosa, occasional hyperplastic and adenomatous polyps, and an increased risk for intestinal-type or mixed-type gastric adenocarcinoma.[30] The gastric antrum and pylorus are typically spared, and the small intestine and colon are unaffected.[31]

Li and colleagues[32] recently described point mutations in the *Adenomatous Polyposis Coli* (*APC*) gene promoter 1B that cosegregated with disease in 6 families afflicted by gastric adenocarcinoma and proximal polyposis of the stomach. These point mutations specifically affect the promoter 1B of *APC* and lead to an increased risk of gastric polyps and adenocarcinoma, but affected families do not have the full familial adenomatous polyposis phenotype and have a low risk for colonic polyposis and colorectal cancer.[32] To date, 9 families with gastric adenocarcinoma and proximal polyposis of the stomach are reported worldwide; the youngest patient presented with generalized gastric adenocarcinoma at the age of 26 years.[30,32-34]

Familial Adenomatous Polyposis and Gastric Fundic Gland Polyposis

Fundic gland polyps are the most common polyp type in Western countries, comprising almost 80% of all gastric polyps.[35] They characteristically contain cystically dilated oxyntic glands lined by parietal and chief cells. Fundic gland polyposis is a frequent gastric manifestation of familial adenomatous polyposis, which is an autosomal dominant syndrome caused by a pathogenic mutation in *APC* leading to hundreds to thousands of colorectal polyps and adenocarcinoma. Patients with attenuated forms of disease have fewer colorectal polyps (<100), but similar upper endoscopic manifestations compared with familial adenomatous polyposis. Gastric findings include predominantly fundic gland polyps (**Fig. 2**), as well as fewer foveolar-type adenomas and pyloric gland adenomas that may show high-grade dysplasia in rare cases.[36] In Western countries, gastric cancer is extremely rare and lifetime risk does not seem to be increased compared with the healthy population.[37-40] Patients with familial adenomatous polyposis usually undergo upper gastroendoscopy primarily for surveillance of duodenal and ampullary adenomas and cancer.[41]

MUTYH-Associated Polyposis and Gastric Fundic Gland Polyposis

MUTYH-associated polyposis is an autosomal recessive syndrome caused by mutations in the *MUTYH* gene. Approximately 10% to 30% of patients develop a limited number of gastric polyps, mostly fundic gland polyps and adenomas.[42,43] A recent study reported a ninefold higher incidence of gastric cancer in monoallelic *MUTYH* mutation carriers.[44] Patients with MUTYH-associated polyposis regularly undergo upper gastroendoscopy for surveillance of duodenal polyps and cancer.[39,42]

GASTRIC HAMARTOMATOUS POLYPOSIS

Hamartomatous gastric polyps occur in the context of Peutz-Jeghers syndrome, juvenile polyposis syndrome, Cowden (PTEN hamartoma tumor) syndrome, and McCune-Albright syndrome. Many of these lesions lack specific histologic features that allow their separation from each other and sporadic hyperplastic polyps.[29,45]

Peutz-Jeghers Syndrome

Peutz-Jeghers syndrome is caused by a germline mutation in *LKB1* (*STK11*). Gastric polyps show a less developed arborizing pattern of smooth muscle compared with hamartomatous polyps in the

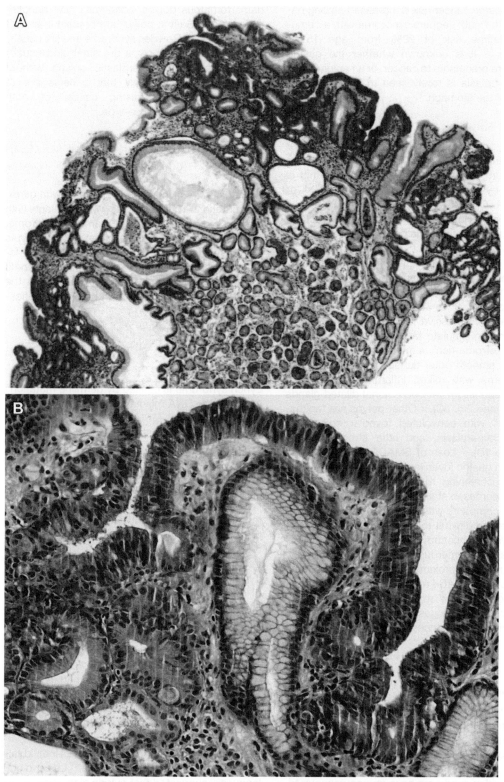

Fig. 2. (*A*) Fundic gland polyp with low-grade dysplasia associated with familial adenomatous polyposis [H&E, original magnification ×100]. (*B*) Magnification of dysplastic area of (*A*) [H&E, original magnification ×250].

colon. Gastric cancer risk is increased among patients with Peutz-Jeghers syndrome with a cumulative lifetime risk of 29% from age 15 to 64 years.[46] It is unknown whether the gastric polyps are precursors to cancer, or an epiphenomenon; dysplasia is rarely seen in Peutz-Jeghers polyps of the stomach.[39]

Juvenile Polyposis

Juvenile polyposis syndrome is a rare disorder characterized by multiple juvenile polyps in the colorectum, small intestine, and stomach that is caused by a germline mutation in SMAD4 or BMPR1A. Clinical criteria for a diagnosis include (1) 5 or more juvenile polyps in the colorectum, (2) any number of juvenile polyps in other parts of the gastrointestinal tract, or (3) any number of juvenile polyps in a patient with a family history of juvenile polyps.[41] Juvenile gastric polyps usually range up to 2 to 3 cm in greatest dimension, but approach 9 to 10 cm in some patients (Fig. 3A, B).[47] Massive juvenile polyposis of the stomach can simulate Ménétrier disease. Polyps may be "stroma-rich" with elongated filiform projections, smooth outer surfaces, prominent stromal edema with mixed inflammation, and flat surface epithelium with occasional dilated glands or cysts (see Fig. 3C).[47] Other polyps are "epithelium-rich" with convoluted foveolar epithelium, surface hyperplasia, and little stromal edema (see Fig. 3D).[47] Loss of SMAD4 immunostaining occurs in gastric juvenile polyps and can be used as a prescreening method; lesional epithelium shows decreased staining intensity or absence of staining compared with normal epithelium, but results may be difficult to interpret.[39,47,48] Foveolar-type dysplasia occurs in approximately 32% of patients with numerous gastric polyps.[47] Gastric cancer risk is approximately 10% to 30% among patients with SMAD4 mutations.[41,47] Complete or partial gastrectomy may be considered for patients with massive gastric polyposis, high-grade dysplasia, and/or cancer.[41]

Phosphatase and Tensin Homolog Hamartoma Tumor Syndrome (Including Cowden Syndrome)

PTEN hamartoma tumor syndrome comprises a heterogeneous group of disorders, including Cowden (most cases), Bannayan-Riley-Ruvalcaba, and Proteus syndrome, all of which result from various germline mutations in PTEN. Patients with Cowden syndrome have mucocutaneous tricholemommas and papillomas, thyroid lesions, fibrocystic disease and breast cancer, and a spectrum of gastrointestinal polyps including hamartomatous polyps, adenomas, and ganglio-neuromas.[49] Gastric polyps are present in almost all patients with Cowden syndrome and are usually numerous. Gastric polyps are small and usually simulate sporadic hyperplastic polyps without dysplasia.[50,51] It is likely that patients are at increased risk for gastric cancer of both intestinal-type and diffuse-type.[52,53]

OTHER HEREDITARY CANCER SYNDROMES IN WHICH GASTRIC CANCER RISK IS INCREASED

Gastric cancer is increased in patients with germline mutations in BRCA1/2, as well as patients with Lynch syndrome and Li-Fraumeni syndrome. Although families sometimes meet the phenotypic criteria for hereditary diffuse gastric cancer or familial intestinal gastric cancer, patients benefit most from surveillance strategies based on the mutated gene, rather than morphologic classification of the tumor.

LYNCH SYNDROME AND GASTRIC CANCER RISK

Lynch syndrome is caused by germline mutations in one of the DNA mismatch repair genes: MLH1, PMS2, MSH2, or MSH6. Mutations in EPCAM, which is directly upstream to MSH2, can also lead to silencing of MSH2 from transcription. Lynch syndrome is associated with colorectal and endometrial cancer. The frequency of gastric cancer ranges from 0.2% to 3.0% depending on patient population, gender, and the gene that is mutated.[41,54] The cumulative gastric cancer risk is 2% to 6% by the age of 70 years in most Western countries.[41,54,55] There seems to be no clustering of gastric cancer in most families with Lynch syndrome. In view of the relatively low risk of gastric cancer and lack of established benefit, surveillance is not recommended among patients with gastric cancer in Europe.[56] On the other hand, American guidelines state that gastroscopy can be considered in individuals with Lynch syndrome at age 30 to 35 years with testing for, and eradication of, H pylori. Recommendations and evidence for ongoing regular surveillance are lacking, but gastric screening may be considered in affected patients.[41] A Finnish study did not find a difference in rates of polyps, H pylori infection, atrophy, or intestinal metaplasia between individuals with, and without, Lynch syndrome.[57] Lee and colleagues[58] suggested that pyloric gland adenomas may be a precursor to gastric cancer in Lynch syndrome, but others have not substantiated these results. Approximately 75% of individuals with

Fig. 3. (*A*) Macroscopic image of gastrectomy specimen of a patient with a germline *SMAD4* mutation and massive gastric polyposis. (*B*) Overview image of juvenile polypoid projections [H&E, original magnification ×10].

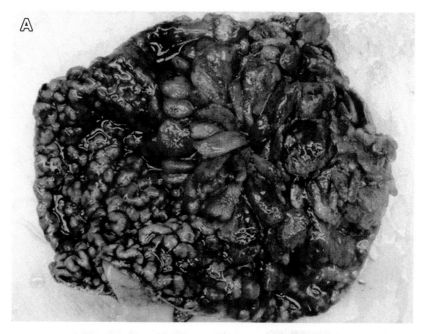

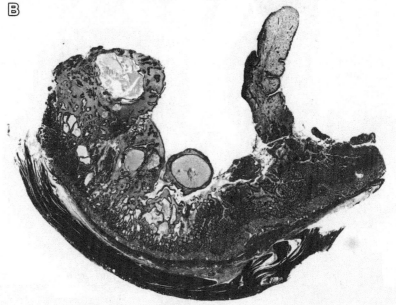

Lynch syndrome show an intestinal phenotype and most show microsatellite instability.[55,59,60]

LI-FRAUMENI SYNDROME AND GASTRIC CANCER RISK

Li-Fraumeni syndrome is caused by a *TP53* germline mutation and characterized by an increased cancer risk for a wide spectrum of tumors starting at young age, including sarcomas, brain tumors, leukemia, and carcinomas of breast, lung, and stomach. Individuals with Li-Fraumeni syndrome have a cumulative risk of gastric cancer of approximately 5%; both intestinal-type and diffuse-type have been reported.[61–63]

HEREDITARY BREAST AND OVARIAN CANCER AND GASTRIC CANCER RISK

Hereditary breast or ovarian cancer syndrome is caused by *BRCA1* or *BRCA2* germline mutations. It is one of the most well-defined and most common hereditary syndromes. A meta-analysis of more than 30 studies reported a relative risk of

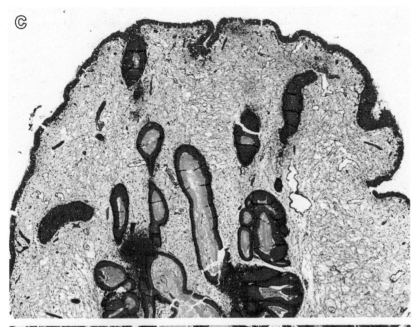

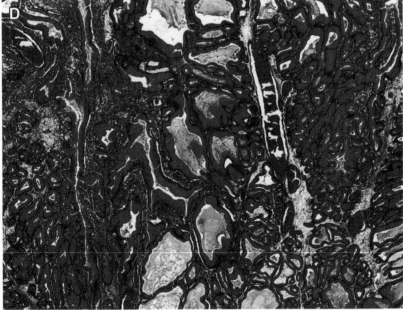

Fig. 3. (continued). (C) Stroma-rich juvenile polyp [H&E, original magnification ×100]. *(D)* Epithelium-rich juvenile polyp [H&E, original magnification ×100].

gastric cancer of approximately 1.7.[64] Details about histopathological characteristics are not reported.

SUMMARY

Important clues to the possibility of a heritable gastric cancer include elements of the patient history, such as other primary malignancies, known gastrointestinal polyps, and a family history of

cancer. Hereditary diffuse gastric cancer results from *CDH1*-germline mutations. Carriers often have small mucosal foci of signet ring cell carcinoma, in situ and pagetoid spread of signet ring cells, and are at high risk for diffuse-type gastric cancer. Some families with a pathogenic mutation in *CTNNA1* have been described; a search of other gene mutations in hereditary diffuse gastric cancer families is ongoing. No definite inherited mutations have been described for familial intestinal gastric cancer. It is important to exclude and treat *H pylori* in family members of patients who present with intestinal gastric cancer at young age (<40 years) or in families that show clustering of intestinal-type gastric cancer. Gastric polyposis can be divided into fundic gland polyposis and hamartomatous polyposis. Gastric adenocarcinoma and proximal polyposis syndrome are characterized by fundic gland polyposis with dysplasia and intestinal-type or mixed-type adenocarcinoma. Fundic gland polyposis also can be seen in patients with familial adenomatous polyposis and *MUTYH*-associated polyposis. Juvenile, Peutz-Jeghers, and PTEN hamartoma syndrome–related polyps cannot be reliably differentiated from each other or from sporadic hyperplastic polyps, so these possibilities should be considered only in the appropriate clinical context. Other hereditary cancer syndromes with increased gastric cancer risk include *BRCA1/2* germline mutations, Lynch syndrome, and Li-Fraumeni syndrome. Important clinicopathological clues include the personal or familial clustering of malignancies, but no distinctive histologic characteristics of gastric carcinomas in these syndromes have been reported.

REFERENCES

1. van der Post RS, Vogelaar IP, Carneiro F, et al. Hereditary diffuse gastric cancer: updated clinical guidelines with an emphasis on germline CDH1 mutation carriers. J Med Genet 2015;52(6):361–74.
2. Caldas C, Carneiro F, Lynch HT, et al. Familial gastric cancer: overview and guidelines for management. J Med Genet 1999;36(12):873–80.
3. Lauren P. The two histological main types of gastric carcinoma: diffuse and so-called intestinal-type carcinoma. An attempt at a histo-clinical classification. Acta Pathol Microbiol Scand 1965;64:31–49.
4. Guilford P, Hopkins J, Harraway J, et al. E-cadherin germline mutations in familial gastric cancer. Nature 1998;392(6674):402–5.
5. Berx G, Becker KF, Hofler H, et al. Mutations of the human E-cadherin (CDH1) gene. Hum Mutat 1998;12(4):226–37.
6. van Roy F, Berx G. The cell-cell adhesion molecule E-cadherin. Cell Mol Life Sci 2008;65(23):3756–88.
7. Oliveira C, Seruca R, Carneiro F. Hereditary gastric cancer. Best Pract Res Clin Gastroenterol 2009;23(2):147–57.
8. Oliveira C, Pinheiro H, Figueiredo J, et al. Familial gastric cancer: genetic susceptibility, pathology, and implications for management. Lancet Oncol 2015;16(2):e60–70.
9. Grady WM, Willis J, Guilford PJ, et al. Methylation of the CDH1 promoter as the second genetic hit in hereditary diffuse gastric cancer. Nat Genet 2000;26(1):16–7.
10. Oliveira C, Ferreira P, Nabais S, et al. E-Cadherin (CDH1) and p53 rather than SMAD4 and Caspase-10 germline mutations contribute to genetic predisposition in Portuguese gastric cancer patients. Eur J Cancer 2004;40(12):1897–903.
11. Barber M, Murrell A, Ito Y, et al. Mechanisms and sequelae of E-cadherin silencing in hereditary diffuse gastric cancer. J Pathol 2008;216(3):295–306.
12. Oliveira C, Sousa S, Pinheiro H, et al. Quantification of epigenetic and genetic 2nd hits in CDH1 during hereditary diffuse gastric cancer syndrome progression. Gastroenterology 2009;136(7):2137–48.
13. Carneiro F, Huntsman DG, Smyrk TC, et al. Model of the early development of diffuse gastric cancer in E-cadherin mutation carriers and its implications for patient screening. J Pathol 2004;203(2):681–7.
14. Huntsman DG, Carneiro F, Lewis FR, et al. Early gastric cancer in young, asymptomatic carriers of germ-line E-cadherin mutations. N Engl J Med 2001;344(25):1904–9.
15. van der Post RS, Gullo I, Oliveira C, et al. Histopathological, molecular, and genetic profile of hereditary diffuse gastric cancer: current knowledge and challenges for the future. Adv Exp Med Biol 2016;908:371–91.
16. Hansford S, Kaurah P, Li-Chang H, et al. Hereditary diffuse gastric cancer syndrome: CDH1 mutations and beyond. JAMA Oncol 2015;1(1):23–32.
17. Rogers WM, Dobo E, Norton JA, et al. Risk-reducing total gastrectomy for germline mutations in E-cadherin (CDH1): pathologic findings with clinical implications. Am J Surg Pathol 2008;32(6):799–809.
18. Charlton A, Blair V, Shaw D, et al. Hereditary diffuse gastric cancer: predominance of multiple foci of signet ring cell carcinoma in distal stomach and transitional zone. Gut 2004;53(6):814–20.
19. Benusiglio PR, Malka D, Rouleau E, et al. CDH1 germline mutations and the hereditary diffuse gastric and lobular breast cancer syndrome: a multicentre study. J Med Genet 2013;50(7):486–9.
20. van der Post RS, Vogelaar IP, Manders P, et al. Accuracy of hereditary diffuse gastric cancer testing criteria and outcomes in patients with a germline mutation in CDH1. Gastroenterology 2015;149(4):897–906.e19.
21. Majewski IJ, Kluijt I, Cats A, et al. An alpha-E-catenin (CTNNA1) mutation in hereditary diffuse gastric cancer. J Pathol 2013;229(4):621–9.
22. Rimm DL, Koslov ER, Kebriaei P, et al. Alpha 1(E)-catenin is an actin-binding and -bundling protein mediating the attachment of F-actin to the membrane adhesion complex. Proc Natl Acad Sci U S A 1995;92(19):8813–7.

23. Koslov ER, Maupin P, Pradhan D, et al. Alpha-catenin can form asymmetric homodimeric complexes and/or heterodimeric complexes with beta-catenin. J Biol Chem 1997;272(43):27301–6.

24. Vasioukhin V, Bauer C, Degenstein L, et al. Hyperproliferation and defects in epithelial polarity upon conditional ablation of alpha-catenin in skin. Cell 2001;104(4):605–17.

25. Gaston D, Hansford S, Oliveira C, et al. Germline mutations in MAP3K6 are associated with familial gastric cancer. PLoS Genet 2014;10(10):e1004669.

26. Vogelaar IP, Ligtenberg MJ, van der Post RS, et al. Recurrent candidiasis and early-onset gastric cancer in a patient with a genetically defined partial MYD88 defect. Fam Cancer 2016;15(2):289–96.

27. Vogelaar IP, van der Post RS, van de Vosse E, et al. Gastric cancer in three relatives of a patient with a biallelic IL12RB1 mutation. Fam Cancer 2015; 14(1):89–94.

28. Choi YJ, Kim N. Gastric cancer and family history. Korean J Intern Med 2016;31(6):1042–53.

29. Brosens LA, Giardiello FM, Offerhaus GJ, et al. Syndromic gastric polyps: at the crossroads of genetic and environmental cancer predisposition. Adv Exp Med Biol 2016;908:347–69.

30. Worthley DL, Phillips KD, Wayte N, et al. Gastric adenocarcinoma and proximal polyposis of the stomach (GAPPS): a new autosomal dominant syndrome. Gut 2012;61(5):774–9.

31. Declich P, Arrigoni GS, Omazzi B, et al. Sporadic fundic gland polyps and proximal polyposis associated with gastric adenocarcinoma share a common antral G cell hyperplasia. Gut 2013;62(7):1088–9.

32. Li J, Woods SL, Healey S, et al. Point mutations in exon 1B of APC reveal gastric adenocarcinoma and proximal polyposis of the stomach as a familial adenomatous polyposis variant. Am J Hum Genet 2016;98(5):830–42.

33. Repak R, Kohoutova D, Podhola M, et al. The first European family with gastric adenocarcinoma and proximal polyposis of the stomach: case report and review of the literature. Gastrointest Endosc 2016;84(4):718–25.

34. Yanaru-Fujisawa R, Nakamura S, Moriyama T, et al. Familial fundic gland polyposis with gastric cancer. Gut 2012;61(7):1103–4.

35. Carmack SW, Genta RM, Schuler CM, et al. The current spectrum of gastric polyps: a 1-year national study of over 120,000 patients. Am J Gastroenterol 2009;104(6):1524–32.

36. Wood LD, Salaria SN, Cruise MW, et al. Upper GI tract lesions in familial adenomatous polyposis (FAP): enrichment of pyloric gland adenomas and other gastric and duodenal neoplasms. Am J Surg Pathol 2014;38(3):389–93.

37. Arnason T, Liang WY, Alfaro E, et al. Morphology and natural history of familial adenomatous polyposis-associated dysplastic fundic gland polyps. Histopathology 2014;65(3):353–62.

38. Garrean S, Hering J, Saied A, et al. Gastric adenocarcinoma arising from fundic gland polyps in a patient with familial adenomatous polyposis syndrome. Am Surg 2008;74(1):79–83.

39. Brosens LA, Wood LD, Offerhaus GJ, et al. Pathology and genetics of syndromic gastric polyps. Int J Surg Pathol 2016;24(3):185–99.

40. Offerhaus GJ, Giardiello FM, Krush AJ, et al. The risk of upper gastrointestinal cancer in familial adenomatous polyposis. Gastroenterology 1992;102(6): 1980–2.

41. Syngal S, Brand RE, Church JM, et al. ACG clinical guideline: genetic testing and management of hereditary gastrointestinal cancer syndromes. Am J Gastroenterol 2015;110(2):223–62, [quiz: 263].

42. Nielsen M, Morreau H, Vasen HF, et al. MUTYH-associated polyposis (MAP). Crit Rev Oncol Hematol 2011;79(1):1–16.

43. Vogt S, Jones N, Christian D, et al. Expanded extracolonic tumor spectrum in MUTYH-associated polyposis. Gastroenterology 2009;137(6):1976–85.e1-10.

44. Win AK, Reece JC, Dowty JG, et al. Risk of extracolonic cancers for people with biallelic and monoallelic mutations in MUTYH. Int J Cancer 2016; 139(7):1557–63.

45. Lam-Himlin D, Park JY, Cornish TC, et al. Morphologic characterization of syndromic gastric polyps. Am J Surg Pathol 2010;34(11):1656–62.

46. Giardiello FM, Brensinger JD, Tersmette AC, et al. Very high risk of cancer in familial Peutz-Jeghers syndrome. Gastroenterology 2000;119(6):1447–53.

47. Gonzalez RS, Adsay V, Graham RP, et al. Massive gastric juvenile-type polyposis: a clinicopathological analysis of 22 cases. Histopathology 2017;70(6): 918–28.

48. Langeveld D, van Hattem WA, de Leng WW, et al. SMAD4 immunohistochemistry reflects genetic status in juvenile polyposis syndrome. Clin Cancer Res 2010;16(16):4126–34.

49. Pilarski R, Burt R, Kohlman W, et al. Cowden syndrome and the PTEN hamartoma tumor syndrome: systematic review and revised diagnostic criteria. J Natl Cancer Inst 2013;105(21):1607–16.

50. Coriat R, Mozer M, Caux F, et al. Endoscopic findings in Cowden syndrome. Endoscopy 2011;43(8): 723–6.

51. Levi Z, Baris HN, Kedar I, et al. Upper and lower gastrointestinal findings in PTEN mutation-positive Cowden syndrome patients participating in an active surveillance program. Clin Transl Gastroenterol 2011;2:e5.

52. Al-Thihli K, Palma L, Marcus V, et al. A case of Cowden's syndrome presenting with gastric carcinomas and gastrointestinal polyposis. Nat Clin Pract Gastroenterol Hepatol 2009;6(3):184–9.

53. Hamby LS, Lee EY, Schwartz RW. Parathyroid adenoma and gastric carcinoma as manifestations of Cowden's disease. Surgery 1995;118(1):115–7.

54. Koornstra JJ, Mourits MJ, Sijmons RH, et al. Management of extracolonic tumours in patients with Lynch syndrome. Lancet Oncol 2009;10(4):400–8.

55. Capelle LG, Van Grieken NC, Lingsma HF, et al. Risk and epidemiological time trends of gastric cancer in Lynch syndrome carriers in the Netherlands. Gastroenterology 2010;138(2):487–92.

56. Vasen HF, Blanco I, Aktan-Collan K, et al. Revised guidelines for the clinical management of Lynch syndrome (HNPCC): recommendations by a group of European experts. Gut 2013;62(6):812–23.

57. Renkonen-Sinisalo L, Sipponen P, Aarnio M, et al. No support for endoscopic surveillance for gastric cancer in hereditary non-polyposis colorectal cancer. Scand J Gastroenterol 2002;37(5):574–7.

58. Lee SE, Kang SY, Cho J, et al. Pyloric gland adenoma in Lynch syndrome. Am J Surg Pathol 2014; 38(6):784–92.

59. Gylling A, Abdel-Rahman WM, Juhola M, et al. Is gastric cancer part of the tumour spectrum of hereditary non-polyposis colorectal cancer? A molecular genetic study. Gut 2007;56(7):926–33.

60. Aarnio M, Salovaara R, Aaltonen LA, et al. Features of gastric cancer in hereditary non-polyposis colorectal cancer syndrome. Int J Cancer 1997;74(5):551–5.

61. Corso G, Pedrazzani C, Marrelli D, et al. Familial gastric cancer and Li-Fraumeni syndrome. Eur J Cancer Care 2010;19(3):377–81.

62. Masciari S, Dewanwala A, Stoffel EM, et al. Gastric cancer in individuals with Li-Fraumeni syndrome. Genet Med 2011;13(7):651–7.

63. Ruijs MW, Verhoef S, Rookus MA, et al. TP53 germline mutation testing in 180 families suspected of Li-Fraumeni syndrome: mutation detection rate and relative frequency of cancers in different familial phenotypes. J Med Genet 2010;47(6):421–8.

64. Friedenson B. BRCA1 and BRCA2 pathways and the risk of cancers other than breast or ovarian. MedGenMed 2005;7(2):60.

Problematic Colorectal Polyps

Is It Cancer and What Do I Need to Do About It?

Maurice B. Loughrey, MD, MRCP, FRCPath[a],
Neil A. Shepherd, DM, FRCPath[b],*

KEYWORDS

- Colorectum • Polyp • Adenoma • Epithelial misplacement • Pseudo-invasion • Adenocarcinoma
- Polypectomy

Key points

- Benign submucosal misplacement of epithelium can closely mimic adenocarcinoma, especially within large adenomatous polyps arising in the sigmoid colon.

- Such diagnostically difficult adenomatous polyps are selected into bowel cancer screening programs because larger polyps are more likely to bleed; detection of occult blood is a widely used screening method.

- Distinction relies mainly on careful routine morphologic evaluation of key discriminatory features, often assisted by examining multiple levels of the relevant block(s).

- Adenocarcinomas arising within colorectal polypectomy specimens require systematic assessment of features that may indicate the risk of residual disease and inform management decision-making regarding the need for further endoscopic or surgical intervention.

ABSTRACT

Two issues commonly arise for pathologists reporting adenomatous polyps of the colorectum. Particularly problematic within large sigmoid colonic adenomas is the distinction between benign misplacement of epithelium into the submucosa and invasive malignancy. This distinction requires careful morphologic evaluation of key discriminatory features, assisted only rarely by the application of selected adjunctive immunohistochemistry. Following a diagnosis of adenocarcinoma within a polypectomy or other local excision specimen, systematic assessment is required of features that may indicate the risk of residual local and/or nodal neoplastic disease and inform management decision-making regarding the need for further endoscopic or surgical intervention.

OVERVIEW

Adenomatous polyps of the colorectum form a substantial component of the routine gastrointestinal workload in most surgical pathology laboratories. Reporting of such polyps is usually straightforward, requiring a diagnosis of adenoma subtype and grade of dysplasia and, for intact polypectomies, an assessment of size and margin

---

Disclosure: The authors have no conflicts of interest to disclose.
[a] Department of Histopathology, Royal Victoria Hospital, Grosvenor Road, Belfast, Northern Ireland BT12 6BA, UK; [b] Gloucestershire Cellular Pathology Laboratory, Cheltenham General Hospital, Sandford Road, Cheltenham, Gloucestershire GL53 7AN, UK
* Corresponding author.
E-mail address: neil.a.shepherd@nhs.net

status with respect to involvement by dysplasia. Some adenomas, however, particularly larger adenomas located within the sigmoid colon, may cause difficulty in two respects. Firstly, the distinction between true invasive malignancy and misplacement of adenomatous epithelium within the submucosa (so-called epithelial misplacement or "pseudo-invasion") has been long recognized and may be extremely problematic in some cases.[1–3] Secondly, if a diagnosis of early-stage colorectal adenocarcinoma is made within a polypectomy or other local excision specimen, this raises the question of what further treatment is required, if any.[4–7]

These two conundra require careful and systematic consideration of relevant morphologic features in conjunction with endoscopy, assisted in some cases by the application of selected additional immunohistochemical markers. These two common and problematic issues form the basis of this review article.

EPITHELIAL MISPLACEMENT VERSUS ADENOCARCINOMA

The phenomenon of epithelial misplacement is most frequently encountered in large adenomatous polyps located within the sigmoid colon, to such an extent that a diagnosis of epithelial misplacement should be made only in polyps arising at other sites after careful consideration of a diagnosis of adenocarcinoma. Epithelial misplacement is typically a result of repeated traumatic injury to the polyp. In the sigmoid colon, this is a consequence of the narrow bowel lumen, often in association with hypertrophy of the muscularis propria, as a result of diverticular disease, and the solid fecal state in this distal location. After all, these polyps are commonest in the older Western population and this is the very population with high rates of sigmoid colonic diverticular disease. Further, peristaltic activity is prominent here and any intraluminal lesion will be subjected to marked propulsive forces, providing a further reason for traumatic forces to the larger polyp. It is likely that mucosal prolapse is also contributory in many cases. Traumatic injury can result in luminal bleeding, generating a positive fecal occult blood test and accounting for the high prevalence of this phenomenon in bowel cancer screening pathology.[8]

To minimize the risk of missing a focal microscopic finding of diagnostic importance, all adenomas routinely should be processed in their entirety for histologic examination, with careful orientation to allow visualization of the polypectomy base resection margin. Polyps with equivocal features should be examined through multiple levels (at least six), which may reveal evidence of the true diagnosis. The most useful morphologic features used to distinguish epithelial misplacement (Fig. 1) from adenocarcinoma are listed in Table 1. In most cases, systematic evaluation of these features, through levels if necessary, will allow a definitive diagnosis.

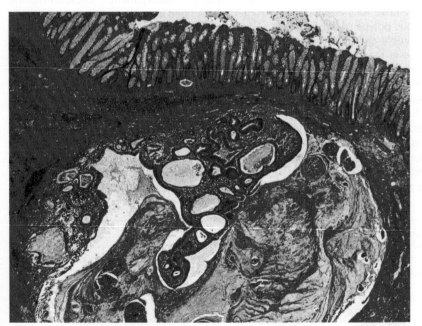

Fig. 1. Classic epithelial misplacement in a sigmoid colonic adenomatous polyp. Although this is beneathsurface non-adenomatous epithelium, the misplaced epithelium appears adenomatous, is accompanied by lamina propria, and forms mucin cysts. The classic changes help to ease the interpretation, as epithelial misplacement of the more concerning features seen in the two more isolated glandular structures seen in the upper left of the field [H&E, original magnification ×50].

Table 1
A comparison of the histopathologic features valuable in differentiating epithelial misplacement from invasive adenocarcinoma

	Epithelial Misplacement (EM)	Adenocarcinoma
Epithelial "differentiation"	Usually similar to that of the surface adenomatous component	Variable and usually different to the surface adenomatous component
Lamina propria accompaniment	Characteristic but may be lacking when there is secondary inflammation and epithelial destruction	Usually absent. Can be present in rare, very well differentiated carcinoma
Accompaniment by nonadenomatous epithelium	Characteristically seen when EM is due to previous intervention	Absent
Hemosiderin deposition	Characteristic and indicative of previous necrosis and/or hemorrhage	Usually absent
Mucosal prolapse changes	Often present	Usually absent
Mucus cysts	Characteristic. They likely represent EM that has become "detached" from the more superficial components	Only present, usually, in mucinous tumors
Continuity with surface adenomatous component	Characteristic but often only appreciated in multiple levels and/or three-dimensional (3D) reconstruction studies	Usually absent but some cases do show continuity, even in 3D reconstruction studies
Involvement of muscularis propria (MP)	Usually absent. Very rarely, especially after previous intervention, involvement of the MP can be seen in EM	Present if at least pT2
Budding	Usually absent but a similar phenomenon can be seen as a result of epithelial destruction and/or inflammation	Often present
Desmoplastic reaction to glands	Usually absent but fibromuscular stromal proliferation can accompany EM	Usually present
Lymphatic and/or vascular invasion	Absent	Diagnostic of cancer

From Loughrey MB, Shepherd NA. The pathology of bowel cancer screening. Histopathology 2015;66:70; with permission.

Pitfalls

! Infiltrating adenocarcinoma may coexist with epithelial misplacement in adenomatous polyps but this phenomenon is rare.

! Gland rupture in the setting of epithelial misplacement may result in apparent single-cell infiltration or "tumor budding."

! Previous endoscopic intervention, in particular partial polypectomy, can generate a desmoplastic stromal response closely mimicking adenocarcinoma, most prominent toward the mucosal surface (a clue to benignity).

! Although lymphatic or venous invasion is considered diagnostic of adenocarcinoma, very occasionally there may be "vascular intrusion" of adenomatous glands into submucosal vessels.

! Endometriosis may form a polypoid mucosal lesion in the colorectum and can mimic adenocarcinoma.

A low-power view, to assess lobular or haphazard glandular architecture, is most useful, along with evaluation of the periglandular stroma to assess if this represents lamina propria or desmoplastic reaction. Benign adenomas with an element of mucosal prolapse may have accompanying prominent muscular stroma, and distinction of this from a desmoplastic stromal reaction is diagnostically important.[8] Hemosiderin deposition is strongly suggestive of epithelial misplacement, indicating concurrent traumatic vascular injury. No one feature, however, is pathognomonic in isolation (see Table 1).

Poorly recognized, in the literature at least, is the ability of these adenomatous polyps to show mimicry of vascular invasion, so-called vascular intrusion. So, adenomatous epithelium can be forced into blood vessels, either at the time of endoscopic intervention or in the laboratory. Fig. 2 is a good example of this phenomenon. Here it is clear that the intravascular epithelium has been subject to artifactual distortion, especially when one compares it with the adjacent adenomatous epithelium that has not been so affected. Furthermore, the vessel is an arteriole with atheroma demonstrable and invasion into such a structure would seem, at best, unlikely (see Fig. 2). We also recognize an artifact of orientation of adenomatous polyps mimicking venous invasion. In this situation, neoplastic glandular epithelium can be seen, often deeply, surrounded by a ring of muscularis, resembling venous invasion in the submucosa (Fig. 3).

Deeper levels will in fact demonstrate that the muscle is not venous in origin but is derived from the muscularis mucosae and that a complex interweaving of that muscle layer, and the adenomatous epithelium, causes mimicry of venous invasion (see Fig. 3). Further, epithelium can be forced into lymphatic spaces and pathologists are exhorted to confirm true lymphovascular invasion and not be misled by these artifacts.

The differential diagnosis is particularly problematic when glands demonstrating high-grade dysplasia are misplaced and/or when submucosal misplacement is accompanied by gland rupture, mucin extravasation, and secondary inflammatory change. This may result in apparent single-cell infiltration, mimicking tumor budding, and a stromal reaction closely mimicking adenocarcinoma.[9,10] Similarly, prior endoscopic intervention, in particular partial or attempted polypectomy, can generate a desmoplastic stromal response closely mimicking adenocarcinoma.[11] Importantly, this is most prominent toward the mucosal surface and is associated with significant regenerative-type cytologic changes, features less prominent within deeper glands (so-called "reverse maturation"). This represents an important clue to benignity in this setting. Also helpful in this regard is the finding of foci of nondysplastic glandular epithelium located within submucosa, accompanying misplaced adenomatous epithelium, strongly suggesting all of the submucosal epithelium represents misplacement rather than adenocarcinoma (Fig. 4). This finding is most often

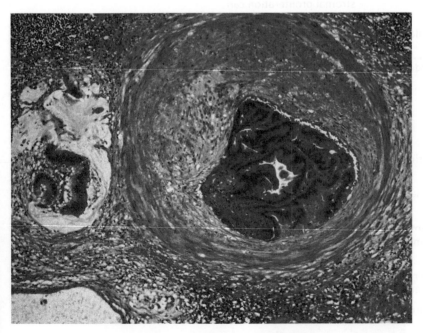

Fig. 2. Vascular intrusion of adenomatous epithelium. Here, within an arteriole (note the atheroma), there is intruded adenomatous epithelium showing marked artifactual change, contrasting with adjacent adenomatous epithelium (*left*), which has not been subject to such artifact [H&E, original magnification ×50].

Fig. 3. In (*A*), in the deep submucosa, is a circumscribed area, surrounded by muscle, containing neoplastic epithelium. It would be easy to interpret this as venous invasion in the submucosa. Note the worried pathologist's green pen marks!! Deeper levels (*B*) show that the area is actually in continuity with the overlying adenomatous epithelium and simply represents a very convoluted muscularis mucosae [H&E, original magnification ×50].

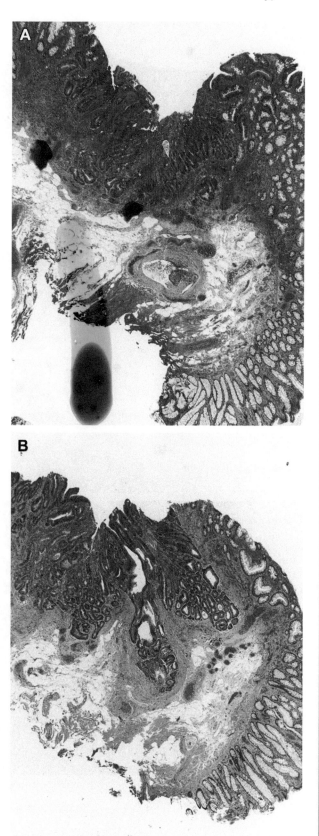

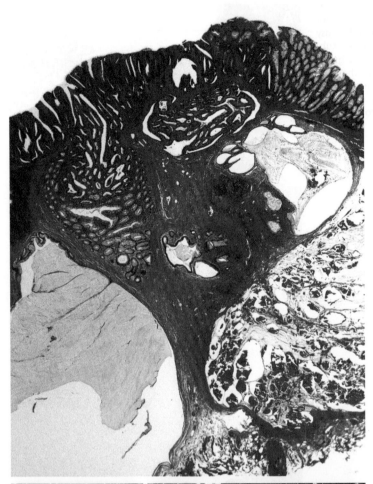

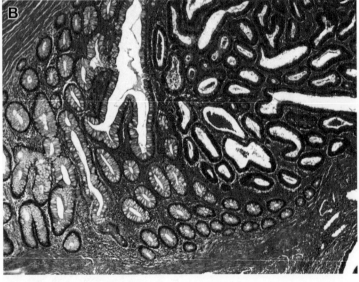

Fig. 4. (A) All the features of epithelial misplacement, with mucus cysts prominent below, but there is also accompaniment of the misplaced adenomatous epithelium by nonadenomatous epithelium, better seen at higher power in (B). The latter is a characteristic feature of previous intervention, whether endoscopic or surgical [H&E, original magnification A ×50, B ×100].

encountered following previous endoscopic intervention.[11]

When convincing features of epithelial misplacement are found in one part of an adenoma, it provides supportive evidence that other, less definitive, features are also due to epithelial misplacement rather than adenocarcinoma. However, rarely epithelial misplacement and adenocarcinoma can coexist, further emphasizing the diagnostic difficulties (Fig. 5). Given overlapping features, some cases may be frankly impossible to confidently diagnose. The difficulties are compounded by the recent description of "adenoma-like adenocarcinoma."[12] These lesions show features that very closely resemble epithelial misplacement and the main distinguishing feature, not evident in biopsies, is the presence of neoplastic epithelium within the muscularis propria or beyond in "adenoma-like adenocarcinoma."

Epithelial misplacement is usually the result of necrosis of a superficial part of an adenomatous polyp and one can understand why the epithelium is then misplaced into the submucosa. One characteristic phenomenon in this situation is the inversion of adenomatous epithelium such that the tubulovillous adenomatous surface is inverted and ends up facing the diathermy excision margin.[8] This is often associated with prominent muscle proliferation suggesting that mucosal prolapse is also a factor in the generation of the epithelial misplacement. It also should be recognized that colorectal lymphoglandular complexes have a natural micro-anatomical defect of the muscularis mucosae and misplacement into the submucosal component of the lymphoglandular complex is not uncommon. Perhaps thankfully, this is more commonly seen in right-sided colonic adenomatous polyps (and also in serrated polyps, especially in the right colon) and is less common in sigmoid colonic adenomatous polyps (Fig. 6).

At this point, it is appropriate to emphasize that this diagnostic difficulty, namely epithelial misplacement versus adenocarcinoma, is very particularly seen in population-based bowel cancer screening programs.[2,8] The latter most commonly use the detection of fecal occult blood and these larger polyps are more prone to bleeding. Nevertheless, that does not entirely explain the extraordinary problems that have occurred in the UK screening programs (and also in other European population screening programs, such as in the Republic of Ireland, the Netherlands and Slovenia). In the United Kingdom, this problem and the issues over misdiagnosis of polyp cancer and overtreatment thereof have necessitated the establishment of an "Expert Board," to help ensure accurate interpretation and appropriate management of such cases.[13]

The diagnostic issues are such that the UK Expert Board is composed of three "expert" gastrointestinal pathologists, as those pathologists do not necessarily agree and a consensus diagnosis is required to drive patient management. In fact, that experience of the Board has shown that general pathologists heavily overcall epithelial misplacement as cancer. Fifty percent of all Expert Board cases, where there is a diagnostic agreement among the three Board pathologists, are downgraded from malignant to benign by that consensus diagnosis.[13] Further, in 3% of cases, the Expert Board has made the dual diagnosis of both epithelial misplacement and adenocarcinoma in the same polyp (see Fig. 2). Thus, although this phenomenon should be regarded as rare and should not be overdiagnosed, it is clear that the dual diagnosis does occur, further underpinning the diagnostic difficulties in many of these cases.

As there have been such difficulties in the interpretation of routine hematoxylin-eosin–stained sections, there have been some attempts to develop adjunctive methods, especially immunohistochemistry.[14–17] p53 and Ki-67 may be of some value in selected situations but are less useful when the submucosal glands in question demonstrate high-grade dysplasia, as both biomarkers are likely to be strongly positive whether these glands represent epithelial misplacement or adenocarcinoma.[11] Of other available immunohistochemical markers, we find desmin (or other smooth muscle stains, such as smoothelin) useful on occasion, in demonstrating the preservation of the muscularis mucosae, often with thickening and distortion, in adenomas with epithelial misplacement (Fig. 7) and destruction of the muscularis mucosae in adenocarcinoma (Fig. 8). Like other immunohistochemical aids in this setting, however, the findings of desmin immunohistochemistry may be equivocal and thereby unhelpful, especially in the presence of heavy inflammation.

Given the experience of these very difficult cases of large adenomatous polyps of the sigmoid colon, we have been looking for alternative adjunctive tests to enable epithelial misplacement to be differentiated from adenocarcinoma.[2] Spectroscopic methods, especially infrared spectroscopy, hold some promise, but computerized three-dimensional reconstruction methodology has proved disappointing.[2] Although continuity between the surface adenomatous lesion and that in the submucosa is readily demonstrable in multiple levels in these polyps, tantalizingly it would appear that early polyp cancers also demonstrate considerable

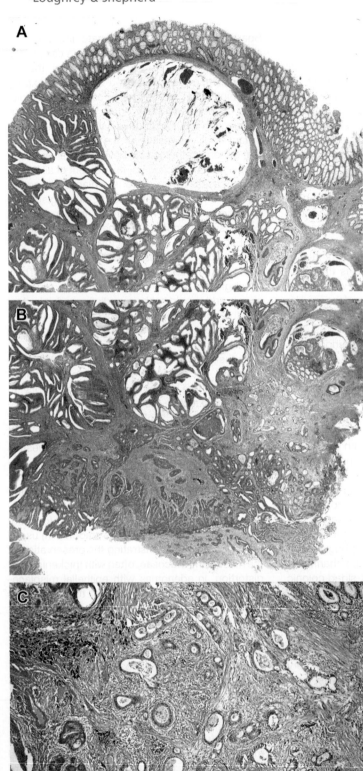

Fig. 5. The dual diagnosis of both epithelial misplacement and adenocarcinoma in the same polyp. (*A*) Classic changes of epithelial misplacement in the head of the polyp. (*B*) The deeper aspect of the polyp. In the upper part of the field there is epithelial misplacement but below there are very different features. High power of one area shows isolated neoplastic tubules (*C*), indicative of invasive adenocarcinoma, even if there is adjacent hemosiderin pigmentation. Some of the neoplastic glands show a cribriform morphology [H&E, original magnification (*A, B*) ×50, *C* ×200].

Fig. 6. Adenomatous involvement of a lymphoglandular complex. This feature is less commonly seen in sigmoid colonic adenomatous polyps and is a more common feature of right-sided polyps, both adenomatous and serrated [H&E, original magnification ×100].

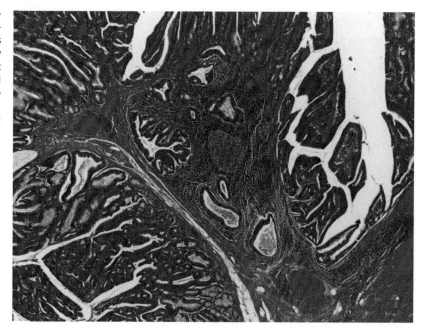

continuity and thus this time-consuming and expensive methodology does not appear to have a role in this diagnostic arena.[2]

A final consideration is that glands located within submucosa, or deeper within the bowel wall, may, on occasion, represent endometriosis and this represents another potential mimic of adenocarcinoma (**Fig. 9**).[18,19] Benign endometriotic glands may be interpreted as "atypical," and this is a particular diagnostic pitfall in diagnostic biopsies sampled from a polypoid lesion, especially when, as is so often the case, the clinical, endoscopic, and radiological features are all suggestive of malignancy, less so when interpreting a polypectomy specimen, in which more of the characteristics surrounding endometriotic stroma should be present. Once this differential diagnosis is considered, it is easily confirmed or refuted by immunohistochemistry for estrogen receptor or

CD10. In general, we find the former marker more useful, as it demonstrates nuclear staining for both epithelial and stromal components of the endometriosis (see **Fig. 9**).

MANAGEMENT OF MALIGNANT COLORECTAL POLYPS

Malignant colorectal polyps usually represent stage pT1 colorectal adenocarcinomas and such "polyp cancers" are broadly considered to have a risk of regional lymph node metastatic disease of approximately 10%. When locally resected, the pathology specimen generated includes no lymph nodes but the morphologic features of the cancer within the local excision specimen offer some insight into refining the risk of lymph node involvement by metastatic disease, informing the

Fig. 7. A composite illustration of epithelial misplacement on hematoxylin-eosin (H&E) (*A*) and desmin immunohistochemistry (*B*). The latter shows smooth muscle proliferation between the misplaced epithelium, presumably the result of mucosal prolapse, but no evidence of destruction of the muscularis mucosae [H&E, original magnification ×50].

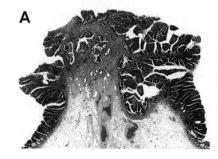
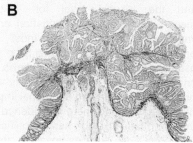

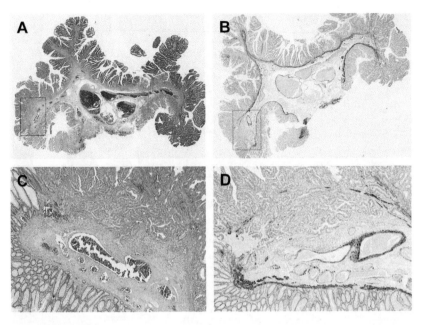

Fig. 8. A composite illustration of adenocarcinoma arising in an adenomatous polyp, on H&E (*A, C*) and desmin immunohistochemistry (*B, D*). C and D represent high power views of the box insets in A and B. The destruction of the muscularis mucosae and infiltration by adenocarcinoma beyond its confines is better appreciated in the desmin immunohistochemistry preparation [H&E, original magnification (*A, B*) ×20, (*C, D*) ×100].

management decision that needs to balance the risk of residual disease against the morbidity and mortality potential of the required surgical procedure for that patient. This has been the subject of numerous original research publications over many decades, and several recent systematic reviews, but the evidence base is limited, in that most reports describe single-center retrospective observational series involving relatively few cases.[4,20]

There is a general consensus that, for cancers detected within polypectomy specimens, polypectomy is considered sufficient treatment (therapeutic polypectomy) in the absence of any adverse histologic features within the cancer (**Box 1**). Features traditionally considered adverse in this regard include poor differentiation, lymphovascular invasion, and advanced depth of tumor invasion, the latter represented by the Haggitt level for pedunculated specimens and the Kikuchi level for sessile specimens.[6,7,21–23] Poor differentiation and lymphovascular invasion are the most established predictive features for regional lymph node metastatic disease. Systematic reviews and meta-analyses have recently highlighted tumor budding (**Fig. 10**) as an additional important predictive feature and there is evidence to suggest that lymphatic invasion has a significantly stronger value than venous invasion in predicting regional lymph node metastatic disease and these features should be assessed separately, using additional immunohistochemical stains if

necessary.[4,20] Evidence based on a standardized and reproducible method of tumor budding assessment is awaited with interest.[6,10,24–26]

Given concerns around applying Haggitt and Kikuchi systems of substaging in routine practice, some publications have favored a shift to more quantitative measures of substaging, specifically in the form of measuring depth or width of tumor invasion.[6,7,27] Measurement of depth of invasion (typically from the muscularis mucosae) is fraught with difficulties resulting from the vagaries of tumor shape, with exophytic, polypoid tumors typically including a significant noninvasive component, the transition point to invasive neoplasia often ill-defined, and more endophytic, often ulcerated, lesions usually lacking any identifiable structures to reliably measure from. The muscularis mucosae is almost invariably destroyed by any invasive neoplasm, so measurement of invasive depth from this structure is always a crude estimate.[27] These issues apply to a much lesser extent to measurement of width of invasion and this feature may be the best measure of tumor size and more reliable than tumor depth as a predictor of lymph node metastatic disease. An appropriate cutoff level for management purposes is still to be determined, but 4 mm has been suggested by several larger studies.[6,7] Importantly, this assessment of width also may be possible in piecemeal polypectomy specimens, even if tumor is present in multiple fragments, should width exceed the agreed cutoff level for management in any one fragment.

Fig. 9. A high-power view of the colonic mucosa (*A*) in polypoid endometriosis, when endometrial glands and stroma are present within that mucosa. The contrast of the very benign-looking colonic epithelium with the endometrial glands (below) may trap the unwary into thinking that the endometrial glands are neoplastic, be that dysplasia or frank malignancy. (*B*) demonstrates estrogen receptor immunohistochemistry whereby both the endometrial epithelium and its stroma show strong nuclear staining, contrasting with the negative superficial colonic epithelium above [H&E, original magnification ×100].

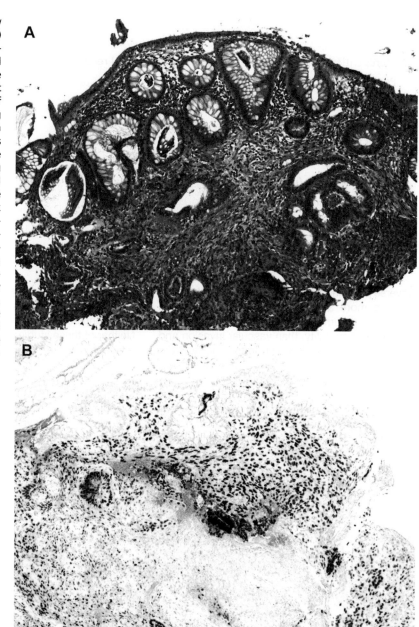

Assessment of margin involvement within polypectomy specimens is controversial and requires very careful consideration. Many older studies tended not to provide a detailed definition of such margin involvement, making interpretation of any comparison between studies difficult.[7] As a consequence, there is confusion over what constitutes the actual margin and what degree of clearance is regarded as acceptable in polyp cancers that extend close to this margin. Current guidelines generally consider a margin clearance of less than 1 mm as needing consideration of further therapy but do not provide any detail on margin assessment.[28–31]

The controversies about margin involvement are further exemplified by the fact that many studies combine all pT1 cancers and the margin is often difficult to assess in sessile tumors. Perhaps the pooled data analysis by Hassan and colleagues[5] in 2005 gives the most useful data on margin involvement in pedunculated polyps. This article shows that margin involvement is the commonest

---

Box 1
Important pathologic features of malignant colorectal polyps

Features critical to management (and may trigger surgical resection):

  Poor differentiation

  Lymphovascular invasion

  Margin involvement

Features that may influence management:

  Distinguishing venous invasion from lymphatic invasion

  Width of invasion (in millimeters)

  Depth of invasion (in millimeters)

  Tumor budding

  Haggitt/Kikuchi level

---

adverse pathologic parameter and critically that it predicts more adverse results, namely residual disease, recurrent disease, hematogenous spread, and mortality, than vascular invasion and poor differentiation. However, in that study, it did not appear to be a predictor of lymph node involvement by tumor. The latter means that one might not be able to justify surgical resection after the removal of a polyp cancer that demonstrates only margin involvement, as the excision of potentially involved regional lymph nodes is the most likely prognostically advantageous result of such a resection.

Two of the largest available relevant studies define margin positivity, as tumor cells present at the resection margin and also offer some guidance on handling artifacts related to diathermy, commonplace in such polypectomy specimens.[6,7] Neither of these studies report any cases in which residual tumor was identified at the polypectomy site within the subsequent surgical resection specimen, when tumor within the original polypectomy specimen was clear (even by less than 1 mm) of the diathermied resection margin. These two studies provide evidence for a conservative approach to margin assessment in polypectomy specimens, reporting such a margin as positive only if tumor cells are present at the resection margin or within the zone of diathermy artifact to such an extent that completeness of excision

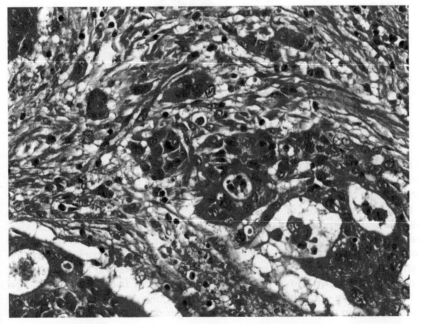

Fig. 10. Tumor budding in a polyp cancer. This was the only adverse prognostic parameter in a small colonic polyp cancer. Resection was undertaken and one mesocolic lymph node was positive for metastatic cancer.

cannot be confidently assessed. Furthermore, in the absence of other adverse histologic features, margin involvement as defined should not necessarily trigger surgical intervention, and follow-up by endoscopy and local reexcision of any residual endoscopic disease may be more appropriate, similar to recommended management of margin involvement by adenoma.

In general, endoscopic piecemeal resection of polyps should be avoided, if possible, as this compromises pathologic assessment of pathologic features of potential utility in deciding subsequent management, in particular assessment of completeness of excision. Piecemeal resection is, however, inevitable for a significant proportion of larger polyps. Margin involvement is unassessable in almost all such specimens. Reexamination of the polypectomy site at follow-up endoscopy is generally advised, in the absence of adverse features indicating consideration of surgical intervention.

The importance of optimal handling of polypectomy specimens within the laboratory cannot be overemphasized to allow adequate histologic assessment. The intact polypectomy should be adequately fixed in formalin, before dissection and submission of the entire polyp for histologic examination. Identification of the base margin and appropriate orientation of this is important, if possible. Smaller polyps may be bisected, but larger polyps (>10 mm) should be dissected to keep the central portion containing the stalk or base intact and this block or blocks identified and processed separately from those containing the peripheral fragments and examined through multiple levels. It may be helpful to paint the base margin of larger, sessile or semipedunculated, polyps but this is considered unnecessary for stalked polyps.

So, in summary, the further management of patients with polyp cancers remains a vexatious subject despite the considerable literature on the subject. The parameters that determine whether or not major surgery is indicated, after polyp cancer endoscopic resection, remain uncertain and we believe that, in the future, we will rely more on parameters such as width and depth of carcinoma, with some evidence from studies that we have been involved in that these measurements are associated with good levels of interobserver agreement, and tumor budding, rather than more traditional parameters, some of which, like Haggitt grouping, are associated, in the United Kingdom at least, with poor levels of interobserver agreement. Suffice to say that the management of individual patients with polyp cancers should be discussed in a multidisciplinary team meeting/tumor board with all relevant clinicians, including physicians, endoscopists, pathologists, surgeons, radiologists, oncologists and specialist nurses present. Further, the establishment of national bowel cancer screening programs, in which polyp cancers make up approximately one-quarter of all cancer cases, with their comprehensive databases, will give us clear answers to these management conundra once survival data are available in these programs.

REFERENCES

1. Muto T, Bussey HJ, Morson BC. The evolution of cancer of the colon and rectum. Cancer 1975;36: 2251–70.
2. Shepherd NA, Griggs RK. Bowel cancer screening-generated diagnostic conundrum of the century: pseudoinvasion in sigmoid colonic polyps. Mod Pathol 2015;28(suppl 1):S88–94.
3. Pascal RR, Hertzler G, Hunter S, et al. Pseudoinvasion with high-grade dysplasia in a colonic adenoma. Distinction from adenocarcinoma. Am J Surg Pathol 1990;14:694–7.
4. Bosch SL, Teerenstra S, de Wilt JH, et al. Predicting lymph node metastasis in pT1 colorectal cancer: a systematic review of risk factors providing rationale for therapy decisions. Endoscopy 2013;45:827–34.
5. Hassan C, Zullo A, Risio M, et al. Histologic risk factors and clinical outcome in colorectal malignant polyp: a pooled-data analysis. Dis Colon Rectum 2005;48:1588–96.
6. Brown IS, Bettington ML, Bettington A, et al. Adverse histological features in malignant colorectal polyps: a contemporary series of 239 cases. J Clin Pathol 2016;69:292–9.
7. Ueno H, Mochizuki H, Hashiguchi Y, et al. Risk factors for an adverse outcome in early invasive colorectal carcinoma. Gastroenterology 2004;127: 385–94.
8. Loughrey MB, Shepherd NA. The pathology of bowel cancer screening. Histopathology 2015;66: 66–77.
9. Lugli A, Karamitopoulou E, Zlobec I. Tumour budding: a promising parameter in colorectal cancer. Br J Cancer 2012;106:1713–7.
10. Wang LM, Kevans D, Mulcahy H, et al. Tumor budding is a strong and reproducible prognostic marker in T3N0 colorectal cancer. Am J Surg Pathol 2009;33:134–41.
11. Panarelli NC, Somarathna T, Samowitz WS, et al. Diagnostic challenges caused by endoscopic biopsy of colonic polyps: a systematic evaluation of epithelial misplacement with review of problematic polyps from the Bowel Cancer Screening Program, United Kingdom. Am J Surg Pathol 2016;40: 1075–83.

12. Gonzalez RS, Cates JM, Washington MK, et al. Adenoma-like adenocarcinoma: a subtype of colorectal carcinoma with good prognosis, deceptive appearance on biopsy and frequent KRAS mutation. Histopathology 2016;68:183–90.

13. Griggs RK, Novelli MR, Sanders DS, et al. Challenging diagnostic issues in adenomatous polyps with epithelial misplacement in bowel cancer screening: 5 years' experience of the Bowel Cancer Screening Programme Expert Board. Histopathology 2017;70:466–72.

14. Hansen TP, Fenger C, Kronborg O. The expression of p53, Ki-67 and urokinase plasminogen activator receptor in colorectal adenomas with true invasion and pseudoinvasion. APMIS 1999; 107:689–94.

15. Yantiss RK, Bosenberg MW, Antonioli DA, et al. Utility of MMP-1, p53, E-cadherin, and collagen IV immunohistochemical stains in the differential diagnosis of adenomas with misplaced epithelium versus adenomas with invasive adenocarcinoma. Am J Surg Pathol 2002;26:206–15.

16. Yantiss RK, Goldman H, Odze RD. Hyperplastic polyp with epithelial misplacement (inverted hyperplastic polyp): a clinicopathologic and immunohistochemical study of 19 cases. Mod Pathol 2001;14: 869–75.

17. Mueller J, Mueller E, Arras E, et al. Stromelysin-3 expression in early (pT1) carcinomas and pseudoinvasive lesions of the colorectum. Virchows Arch 1997;430:213–9.

18. Yantiss RK, Clement PB, Young RH. Endometriosis of the intestinal tract: a study of 44 cases of a disease that may cause diverse challenges in clinical and pathologic evaluation. Am J Surg Pathol 2001; 25:445–54.

19. Kelly P, McCluggage WG, Gardiner KR, et al. Intestinal endometriosis morphologically mimicking colonic adenocarcinoma. Histopathology 2008;52: 510–4.

20. Beaton C, Stephenson BM, Williams GL. Risk of lymph node metastasis in malignant colorectal polyps. Colorectal Dis 2014;16:67.

21. Kikuchi R, Takano M, Takagi K, et al. Management of early invasive colorectal cancer. Risk of recurrence and clinical guidelines. Dis Colon Rectum 1995;38: 1286–95.

22. Haggitt RC, Glotzbach RE, Soffer EE, et al. Prognostic factors in colorectal carcinomas arising in adenomas: implications for lesions removed by endoscopic polypectomy. Gastroenterology 1985; 89:328–36.

23. Cooper HS, Deppisch LM, Kahn EI, et al. Pathology of the malignant colorectal polyp. Hum Pathol 1998; 29:15–26.

24. Egashira Y, Yoshida T, Hirata I, et al. Analysis of pathological risk factors for lymph node metastasis of submucosal invasive colon cancer. Mod Pathol 2004;17:503–11.

25. Graham RP, Vierkant RA, Tillmans LS, et al. Tumor budding in colorectal carcinoma: confirmation of prognostic significance and histologic cutoff in a population-based cohort. Am J Surg Pathol 2015; 39:1340–6.

26. Ishikawa Y, Akishima-Fukasawa Y, Ito K, et al. Histopathologic determinants of regional lymph node metastasis in early colorectal cancer. Cancer 2008; 112:924–33.

27. Watanabe T, Itabashi M, Shimada Y, et al. Japanese Society for Cancer of the Colon and Rectum (JSCCR) guidelines 2014 for treatment of colorectal cancer. Int J Clin Oncol 2015;20:207–39.

28. Loughrey MB, Quirke P, Shepherd NA. Standards and datasets for reporting cancers: dataset for colorectal cancer histopathology reports. 3rd edition. London: Royal College of Pathologists; 2014. Available at: https://www.rcpath.org/resourceLibrary/dataset-for-colorectal-cancer-histopathology-reports-3rd-edition-.html. Accessed August 15, 2017.

29. Quirke P, Risio M, Lambert R, et al. Quality assurance in pathology in colorectal cancer screening and diagnosis—European recommendations. Virchows Arch 2011;458:1–19.

30. Williams JG, Pullan RD, Hill J, et al. Management of the malignant colorectal polyp: ACPGBI position statement. Colorectal Dis 2013;15(suppl 2): 1–38.

31. Tang LK, Berlin J, Branton P, et al. Protocol for the examination of specimens from patients with primary carcinoma of the colon and rectum. In: College of American Pathologists, Cancer Protocol Templates. 2016. Available at: http://www.cap.org/web/home/protocols-and-guidelines/cancer-reporting-tools/cancer-protocol-templates. Accessed August 15, 2017.

Persistent Problems in Colorectal Cancer Reporting

Rhonda K. Yantiss, MD

KEYWORDS

- Colorectal cancer staging • TNM • Prognostic features • Neoadjuvant

Key points

- Failure to distinguish serosal penetration (pT4a) from those confined to subserosal fat is a common problem.
- Lymph node metastases smaller than 0.2 mm in diameter are staged as pN0.
- Tumor deposits are counted and reported; an additional pN1c designation is appropriate if all other lymph nodes are negative.
- Acellular mucin is not used to assign pT or pN stage; tumor regression is assessed only in primary tumor.

ABSTRACT

Tumor stage, as determined by the Tumor, Node, Metastasis (TNM) staging system, is the single most influential factor determining treatment decisions and outcome among patients with colorectal cancer. Several stage-related elements in pathology reports consistently pose diagnostic challenges: recognition of serosal penetration by tumor (ie, pT3 vs pT4a), evaluation of regional lymph nodes, distinction between tumor deposits and effaced lymph nodes, and assessment of tumor stage in the neoadjuvant setting. This article discusses each of these issues in detail and provides practical tips regarding colorectal cancer staging.

OVERVIEW

Colorectal carcinoma is the third most frequent malignancy and second leading cause of cancer-related death in the United States; it is estimated that there were slightly more than 95,000 new colon cancer and 39,000 new rectal cancer cases diagnosed in the United States in 2016.[1] Tumor stage is the most powerful predictor of outcome and influences treatment decisions; lymph node–negative (ie, stage I and II) tumors are generally treated with surgery alone, whereas most patients with regional lymph node or distant metastases (ie, stage III or IV) are offered some form of adjuvant chemotherapy.[2] However, high-risk features (eg, colonic obstruction or perforation through the tumor, tumoral penetration of the serosa, close or positive resection margins, inadequate lymph node sampling, high-grade cytologic features associated with mismatch proficiency, lymphovascular or venous invasion, and perineural invasion) may prompt adjuvant chemotherapy among patients with stage II tumors as well.[3,4]

The Tumor, Node, Metastasis (TNM) staging system was developed by the American Joint Committee on Cancer (AJCC) and the Union for International Cancer Control to provide standardized, data-driven criteria for cancer reporting.

The author receives royalties from Elsevier, Inc for book chapter authorship.
Department of Pathology and Laboratory Medicine, Weill Cornell Medicine, 525 East 68th Street, New York, NY 10065, USA
E-mail address: rhy2001@med.cornell.edu

This classification scheme provides pathologists, clinicians, and radiologists with a common language for uniform reporting and is continually updated as new elements prove to be of prognostic and/or therapeutic importance. The most recent eighth edition of the AJCC Cancer Staging Manual defines criteria for TNM stage assessment, as well as several other clinically relevant parameters.[5] Although the manual enumerates concrete guidelines for cancer staging, it does not detail interpretive issues that arise when assessing colectomy specimens. The purpose of this article is to discuss and illustrate some of the diagnostic challenges pathologists face when applying staging criteria to colorectal cancer specimens, particularly with respect to high-risk features that influence treatment.

ASSIGNING TUMOR STAGE TO LOCALLY ADVANCED CANCERS

DEFINITIONS OF TUMOR STAGE (PT)

The T category of the TNM staging system denotes pathologic tumor stage and describes the deepest point of penetration in the colonic wall, pericolorectal fat, or adjacent structures (Table 1). Colorectal carcinomas that do not breach the muscularis mucosae are staged as in situ lesions (pTis), whereas tumors that extend into the submucosa, muscularis propria, or pericolorectal connective tissue are classified as pT1, pT2, or pT3, respectively. The pT4 category is subdivided into pT4a and pT4b to denote penetration of the visceral peritoneum and invasion into noncontiguous organs or structures, respectively. The pT4a subclassification applies only to carcinomas that occur near peritoneal surfaces; it is not relevant to tumors that invade posteriorly in the ascending and descending colon, or rectal cancers below the peritoneal reflection.[5]

DEFINITION OF SEROSAL PENETRATION (PT4A)

The most problematic aspect of pathologic tumor stage assignment is distinction between tumors confined to pericolonic adipose tissue (pT3) and those that penetrate the serosa (pT4a). Detection rates of serosal penetration depend on careful gross examination, meticulous sampling, and a clear understanding of microanatomy (Box 1).

Table 1
Summary of pathologic stage classification scheme for colorectal cancer

Definition of primary tumor stage (T)	
pT1	Tumor invades, but limited to, submucosa
pT2	Tumor invades the muscularis propria
pT3	Tumor invades through muscularis propria into pericolorectal soft tissue
pT4	Tumor penetrates visceral peritoneum or invades adjacent organs or structures
pT4a	Tumor penetrates visceral peritoneum, including gross perforation through tumor and continuous invasion of tumor through inflammation to peritoneal surface
pT4b	Tumor directly invades, or is adherent to, other organs or structures
Definition of regional lymph node stage (N)	
pN1	Metastases (tumor spanning ≥0.2 mm) in 1–3 regional lymph nodes, or tumor deposits are present when all lymph nodes are negative
pN1a	Metastases in 1 regional lymph node
pN1b	Metastases in 2–3 regional lymph nodes
pN1c	Tumor deposits in pericolic tissues without regional lymph node metastases
pN2	Metastases in 4 or more regional lymph nodes
pN2a	Metastases in 4–6 regional lymph nodes
pN2b	Metastases in 7 or more regional lymph nodes
Definition of distant metastasis (M)	
pM1	Distant metastasis to 1 or more other organs or the peritoneum
pM1a	Metastasis confined to 1 organ without peritoneal metastasis
pM1b	Metastases to more than 1 organ or site without peritoneal metastasis
pM1c	Metastasis to peritoneum alone, or in addition to other organs

Data from Jessup JM, Goldberg RM, Asare EA, et al. Colon and Rectum. In: Amin MB, editor. AJCC Cancer Staging Manual. 8th edition. Chicago (IL): Springer; 2017. 251–74.

> **Box 1**
> **Evaluating colonic adenocarcinoma for serosal penetration**
>
> - Obtain cytology preparation (smear) from serosal surface of fresh specimen
> - Examine the gross specimen
>   - Obtain at least 2 blocks from deepest extent of tumor to closest peritoneal surface
>   - Obtain at least 1 block from deepest extent of tumor to adjacent pericolonic fat
> - Look for tumor cells in clefts between fat lobules
> - Additional tissue blocks and/or levels for pT3 tumors ≤1 mm from serosal reaction
> - Elastin stains may improve detection of serosal penetration
> - No role for immunohistochemistry

Nearly 60% of cancers in colectomy specimens show serosal penetration; at least 20% of these cases are underdiagnosed.[6] Serosal penetration is readily recognized when tumor cells are present on the peritonealized surface in combination with mesothelial cell hyperplasia, fibrin deposits, erosion of the mesothelium, or an inflammatory reaction (Fig. 1). The AJCC eighth edition Cancer Staging Manual defines invasion of the visceral peritoneum as gross perforation through the tumor, tumor cells at, or on, the peritoneal surface, or continuous invasion of tumor through areas of inflammation that extend to the peritoneal surface.[5]

FEATURES OF SEROSAL PENETRATION AT THE TIME OF GROSS EXAMINATION

Accurate assessment of serosal penetration requires careful gross examination to direct appropriate sampling. The abdominal colon is normally surfaced by a minimal amount of subserosal connective tissue and epiploic fat on its antimesenteric aspect; encasement of the colon by abundant fat is an important clue to serosal penetration by tumor. Peritoneal penetration also may be evidenced by puckered or sclerotic areas on the serosa, creeping fat, plaques, and fibrinous adhesions overlying the tumor (Fig. 2). Multiple tissue sections through these areas, including the interface between the tumor and adjacent fat, can be extremely helpful in documenting extent of disease. A minimum of 2 tissue blocks obtained from the area in which tumor most closely approximates the peritoneal surface are recommended; additional sections are encouraged when histologic sections demonstrate tumor close to, but not at, the peritoneal surface.[7]

HISTOLOGIC FEATURES OF SEROSAL PENETRATION

Although the TNM criteria for pT4a designation are quite clear, their application to resection specimens can be challenging, especially when assessment is hampered by florid inflammatory changes (Box 2). The antimesenteric aspect of the abdominal colon normally contains a thin layer (1–3 mm) of connective tissue between the muscularis propria and mesothelium; lobules of pericolonic fat are surfaced by mesothelial cells.

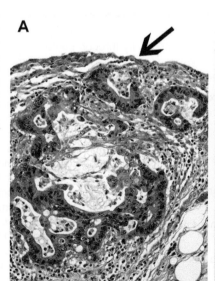
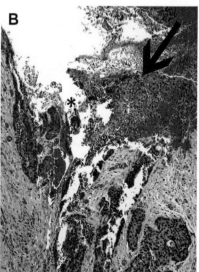

Fig. 1. Tumoral penetration of the serosa manifests as tumor cells at the peritoneal surface (*A* H&E, original magnification ×20), or free clusters of tumor cells on the peritoneal surface (*B* H&E, original magnification ×10). On the left (*A*), malignant glands extend to the mesothelium-lined serosa (*arrow*). On the right (*B*), carcinoma extends to the peritoneal surface; free-floating malignant epithelial cells (*asterisk*) are comingled with mesothelial cells (*arrow*).

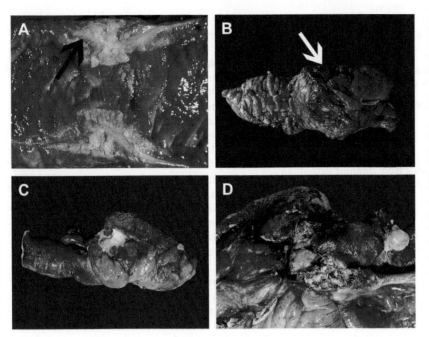

Fig. 2. Creeping fat on the antimesenteric aspect surrounds the site of serosal penetration by adenocarcinoma (*arrow*). The adjacent muscularis propria (*asterisk*) is surfaced by peritoneum (*A*). A large cancer is surrounded by fat and adhesions. Adherent omental fat is also present on the specimen (*arrow*) (*B*). White fibrin plaques on the peritoneal surface signify serosal penetration (*C*). Gross perforation through a carcinoma is associated with fibrin and fat necrosis (*D*).

Invasive carcinomas almost always elicit a tissue reaction, and extension to the visceral peritoneum is accompanied by fibrin, granulation tissue, and proliferating fibroblasts at the peritoneal surface. Thus, clues to serosal penetration by tumor include expansion of the subperitoneal connective tissue by a fibroinflammatory reaction in close proximity to the tumor and abundant fat containing cancer within expanded septa at the advancing edge of the tumor (**Fig. 3**). Close examination usually reveals comingling of tumor cells and

mesothelial cells in the granulation tissue–type reaction under the mesothelial layer, or within inflamed septa of pericolonic fat, warranting pT4a designation. Serosal penetration is frequently detected within clefts between fat lobules and, thus, at least 1 tissue section of the interface between the tumor and pericolonic fat should be obtained in all cases (**Fig. 4**).

Grossly perforated colon cancers are assigned pT4a pathologic stage, even if tumor cells are not readily demonstrable on the serosal surface in histologic sections. Although they may show free tumor cells on the peritoneal surface, tumor cells are more often embedded in granulation tissue, fibrin, or neutrophilic abscesses (**Fig. 5**). Of note, tumor cells can spread to the peritoneal cavity through peritumoral abscesses that communicate between the tumor and the serosa.[8,9] This feature is classified as pT4a in the AJCC eighth edition Cancer Staging Manual.[5]

Staging cases that show tumor cells close to, but not at, the serosal surface are problematic. Most data suggest that biologic risk of cancers ≤1 mm from a serosal reaction (ie, granulation tissue, fibrin deposits, or mesothelial hyperplasia) is intermediate between that of pT3 tumors more than 1 mm from the serosa and pT4a tumors extending to the peritoneal surface (**Fig. 6**).[9,10] Snaebjornsson and colleagues[11] evaluated 5-year survival among 889 patients with colon cancer and found 5-year survival rates to be 71% for patients with pT3 tumors distant (>1 mm) from the serosa, compared with 58%

Box 2
Clues to serosal penetration by colonic adenocarcinoma

- Fibrin plaques, fibrinous adhesions, creeping fat on serosal surface overlying tumor

- Serosal abnormalities in close proximity to tumor
  - Inflammatory reaction
  - Fibrin or hemorrhage
  - Mesothelial hyperplasia

- Mesothelial cells admixed with inflammation near serosa

- Broad, inflamed septa in pericolonic fat at advancing edge of tumor

- Peritumoral abscesses tracking to serosal surface

Fig. 3. The subserosa is expanded by a fibroin-flammatory reaction to infiltrating carcinoma near the peritoneal surface (*A*, H&E, original magnification ×2). Closer examination reveals com-ingled tumor and meso-thelial cells, signifying serosal penetration (*B*, H&E, original magnifica-tion ×40). Linear arrays of malignant glands at the advancing edge of the tu-mor (*C*, H&E, original magnification ×2) contain cancer cells (*arrow*) ad-mixed with mesothelial cells (*asterisk*) and repre-sent preexisting peritoneal surfaces (*D*, H&E, original magnification ×20).

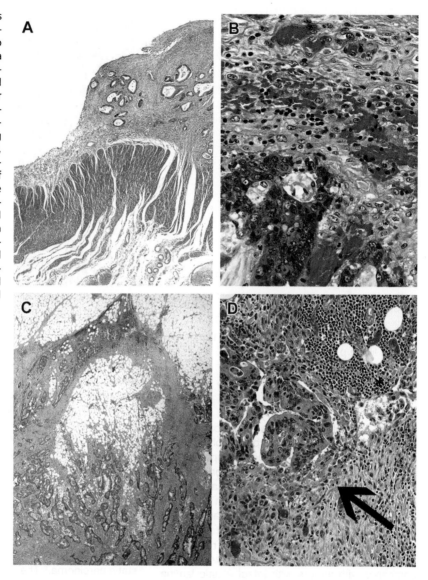

for patients with tumors ≤1 mm from a serosal re-action, 51% for patients with tumors at the serosal surface, and 20% for patients with free tumor cells on the serosal surface. In fact, cytologic tech-niques detect tumor cells on the serosal surface at similar rates among cancers that are close (<1 mm) to a serosal reaction and those that are present at the serosal surface. Panarelli and col-leagues[9] obtained cytologic smears from the serosal surfaces of 120 colon cancer resection specimens staged according to the AJCC seventh edition Cancer Staging Manual. They found that 46% of tumors close to (≤1 mm) a serosal reac-tion, but not at the serosal surface, were associ-ated with cancer cells in cytology preparations from the peritoneal surface at similar rates

compared with tumors at the peritoneal surface in histologic sections (55%). Not surprisingly, many pathologists consider tumor cells ≤1 mm from a serosal reaction to represent serosal pene-tration (Fig. 7). Kirsch and colleagues[12] surveyed 389 pathologists in North America, including 132 gastrointestinal pathologists and 257 general pa-thologists equally representing academic and community practices. They found that 34% of pa-thologists classified cancers ≤1 mm from a serosal reaction as pT4a. Subspecialists in gastro-intestinal pathology were more likely to stage such cases as pT4a than general surgical pathologists (42.4% vs 29.6%, respectively). Of note, 77% of pathologists who classified such tumors as pT3 qualified the stage by suggesting there could be

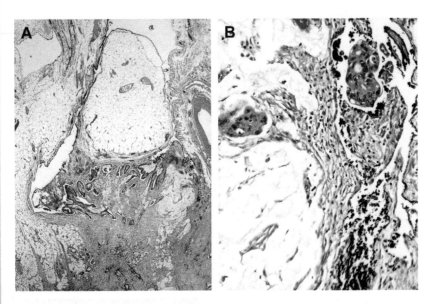

Fig. 4. Sections obtained from the interface between the advancing edge of the tumor and pericolonic help establish pathologic stage. Tumor cells aggregate in clefts between lobules of adipose tissue (*A*, H&E, original magnification ×4). Closer examination reveals growth of tumor cells on the peritoneal surface (*B*, H&E, original magnification ×20).

a breach in the peritoneum and that the tumor may behave like a pT4a lesion.

USE OF ANCILLARY TESTS TO FACILITATE DETECTION OF SEROSAL PENETRATION

Much of the colon contains a subserosal elastic lamina that can be disrupted by deeply invasive colonic carcinomas; its destruction represents a surrogate marker of serosal penetration that can be detected using elastin histochemical stains.[10] Shinto and colleagues[13] used elastin stains to classify 325 locally advanced colon cancers and found that destruction of elastic lamina was associated with increased postoperative recurrence rates (35%) and decreased 5-year survival (57%) compared with tumors with intact elastic lamina (21% and 79%, respectively). Liang and colleagues[14] evaluated 244 stage II (pT3,N0,M0) colon cancers and found that elastic lamina invasion was associated with decreased disease-specific 5-year survival (60%) compared with cases without elastic lamina invasion (88%). Although these results are promising, elastin stains do have some drawbacks: the elastic lamina may be absent, especially in the right colon, and retracted in areas of advancing tumor, thereby hampering interpretation. It may be necessary to perform elastin stains on multiple blocks to document penetration of the elastic lamina.[10]

Immunohistochemical stains have not proven useful in detection of serosal penetration.[15,16] Ambrose and colleagues[17] assessed the utility of monoclonal carcinoembryonic antigen and HFMG (milk fat globule-EGF factor 8 protein) for detecting malignant cells in peritoneal washings, and found that immunohistochemical stains failed to detect malignancy in 63% of patients with peritoneal cancer by cytology. Others have shown mesothelial markers, such as cytokeratin 7, to infrequently improve detection of serosal penetration by tumor.[14] For these reasons, ancillary stains have not gained widespread acceptance as tools to facilitate colorectal cancer staging.

STAGING REGIONAL LYMPH NODES

DEFINITIONS OF LYMPH NODE STAGE (PN)

Regional lymph nodes are staged as pN0, pN1, or pN2 depending on the number involved by metastatic carcinoma.[5] The pN1 category is subclassified as pN1a and pN1b to denote metastases in a single lymph node, or in 2 or 3 lymph nodes, respectively. The N1c category is used to describe any number of tumor deposits in the absence of regional lymph node metastases, as described later in this article. More numerous positive lymph nodes are assigned to the pN2 category and subclassified as pN2a (4 to 6 positive lymph nodes) and pN2b (7 or more positive lymph nodes). Nonregional lymph nodes containing metastases are staged as pM1 disease (see **Table 1**).

GROSS EXAMINATION OF REGIONAL LYMPH NODES

The number of lymph nodes retrieved from a resection specimen correlates with improved survival among patients with stage II and stage III

Fig. 5. A perforated colon cancer shows adenocarcinoma embedded in granulation tissue near the outer aspect of the colon (*A*, H&E, original magnification ×20). The surface (inked) of a perforated cancer reveals tumor cells embedded in organizing fibrin (*B*, H&E, original magnification ×60). Another example shows extensive tissue necrosis (*C*, H&E, original magnification ×20). Another perforated tumor is associated with peritumoral abscesses that track to the peritoneal surface (*D*, H&E, original magnification ×4).

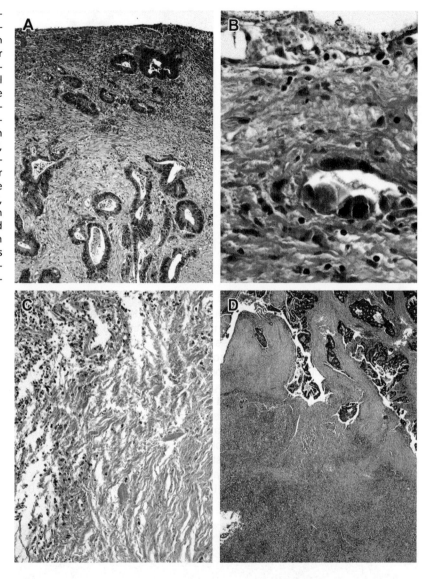

disease and, thus, surgical specimens should be carefully examined to identify as many lymph nodes as possible.[18–20] The 5-year survival rate for patients with at least 18 negative lymph nodes is approximately 76%, compared with 62% among patients with ≤7 detected lymph nodes.[21] The positive correlation between survival and number of harvested lymph nodes reflects a combination of factors. First, the likelihood of detecting metastatic deposits increases as more lymph nodes are identified, leading to classification within a higher-stage grouping that more accurately predicts outcome. Pericolonic lymph nodes are easier to detect in patients with a robust host immune response to cancer, which is independently associated with improved survival.[22]

A minimum of 12 lymph nodes is required for staging untreated carcinomas, and detection of fewer than 12 lymph nodes is not inconsequential.[23,24] Inadequate lymph node counts have therapeutic implications; lymph node counts are considered when patients are evaluated for clinical trials, and detection of fewer than 12 regional lymph nodes is a high-risk feature among patients with stage II disease. The number of retrieved lymph nodes in a curative resection specimen also represents an important quality measure for surgeons and pathologists.[25–27]

Failure to detect sufficient numbers of lymph nodes should prompt submission of additional soft tissue or use of clarifying solutions.[27,28] All grossly negative lymph nodes must be submitted

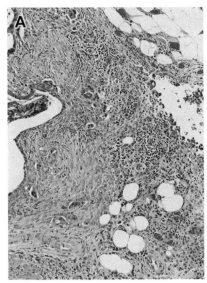
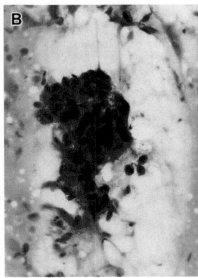

Fig. 6. Cancer (*left*) near the peritoneal surface elicits a serosal reaction (*right*), even though tumor cells are not detected on the peritoneal surface (*A* H&E, original magnification ×10). Serosal cytology preparations demonstrate malignant cells (*B* H&E, original magnification ×60).

entirely for pathologic evaluation, although representative sections of grossly positive lymph nodes adequately document extent of disease. The total number of retrieved lymph nodes is recorded in all cases, as the ratio of positive lymph nodes to the total number collected may be prognostically important.[29] Lymph nodes are difficult to detect in neoadjuvantly treated resection specimens because chemoradiation results in atrophy of lymphoid tissue and smaller lymph nodes, although at least 12 lymph nodes are still identifiable in most cases.[30] Some investigators have suggested that rigorous assessment to retrieve 12 or more lymph nodes from neoadjuvantly treated patients is not necessary, as detection of fewer lymph nodes does not affect survival.[31] In our practice, we do not report any colorectal cancer resection specimens with less than 12 lymph nodes unless all the pericolorectal soft tissue has been submitted for histologic evaluation.

MICROMETASTASES AND ISOLATED TUMOR CELLS

Micrometastases are defined as metastatic tumor deposits measuring 0.2 to 2 mm (see **Fig. 7**). Their

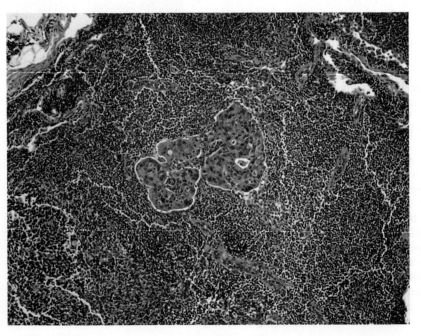

Fig. 7. A single cluster of tumor cells in the parenchyma of a lymph node represents a micrometastasis staged as a positive lymph node (H&E, original magnification ×20).

presence is associated with decreased survival and classified in the pN1 or pN2 category depending on the overall number of lymph nodes containing metastatic deposits.[32] The AJCC seventh edition of the Cancer Staging Manual classifies micrometastatic disease as pN1(mi) or pN2(mi); the "(mi)" qualifier has been eliminated in the eighth edition of the manual.[5,33]

Classification of lymph node metastases measuring smaller than 0.2 mm is problematic. Protic and colleagues[34] evaluated regional lymph nodes from 203 patients with stage II colorectal cancer, all of whom had ≥12 negative regional lymph nodes by histologic examination and multiple tissue levels. They found that patients with isolated tumor cells in lymph nodes detected by cytokeratin immunohistochemistry had a shorter disease-free survival than patients with cytokeratin-negative lymph nodes (71.8 months vs 92.9 months, respectively). Sargent and colleagues[35] evaluated histologically negative lymph nodes from 181 patients with stage II colorectal cancer using reverse-transcriptase polymerase chain reaction for guanylyl cyclase, a protein universally found in, and relatively specific for, gastrointestinal epithelium. The investigators found that patients with detectable guanylyl cyclase in lymph nodes had a higher rate of disease recurrence at 5 years compared with those who had little or no detectable guanylyl cyclase in their lymph nodes (27% vs 4%, respectively).

Although results of these studies suggest that isolated tumor cells in lymph nodes are prognostically important, clinical use of immunohistochemistry and/or molecular techniques to stage lymph nodes is not recommended at this time.[36] Single cells and metastatic deposits spanning less than 0.2 mm are currently staged in the pN0 category, and will be similarly classified when the AJCC eighth edition Cancer Staging Manual takes effect in 2018 (Fig. 8).[5,33] In our practice, however, we routinely obtain multiple tissue levels whenever tumor deposits spanning less than 0.2 mm are encountered, to ensure the small size of the focus.

ACELLULAR MUCIN IN LYMPH NODES FROM TREATMENT-NAÏVE PATIENTS

Mucin deposits without epithelium are rarely detected in regional lymph nodes of untreated colonic carcinomas. When present, they tend to be associated with mucinous adenocarcinomas of the proximal colon (Fig. 9). The AJCC Cancer Staging Manual does not directly discuss the significance of acellular mucin deposits in lymph nodes in treatment-naïve cases, although mucin in lymph nodes draining appendiceal mucinous neoplasms are considered negative for metastasis (pN0).[37] In our practice, we categorize acellular mucin deposits in lymph nodes as pN0 only after obtaining multiple tissue sections and

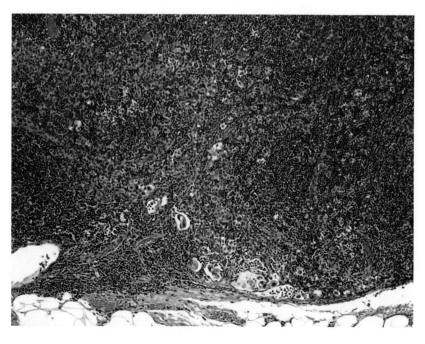

Fig. 8. A few small clusters of tumor cells span less than 0.2 mm in aggregate. Isolated tumor cells are classified in the pN0 category (H&E, original magnification ×20).

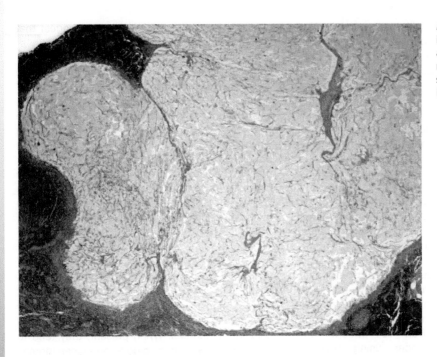

Fig. 9. Loculated mucin in a lymph node from a mucinous adenocarcinoma of the right colon is staged as pN0 (H&E, original magnification ×9).

submitting all of the pericolorectal fat for histologic evaluation.

TUMOR DEPOSITS IN PERICOLORECTAL SOFT TISSUE

Tumor deposits are discrete tumor nodules that represent lymphovascular, venous, or perineural invasion with extravascular/extraneural extension into soft tissue, or complete effacement of lymph nodes by metastatic disease.[38] They are located within the regional lymph drainage of the tumor and have a smooth or irregular contour (**Fig. 10**). Tumor deposits are associated with poor prognosis among patients with colorectal cancer, even when numerous lymph node metastases are present.[38] Ueno and colleagues[39] evaluated 695 patients with locally advanced colorectal cancer and found that 5-year disease-specific survival was 85% among patients without tumor deposits

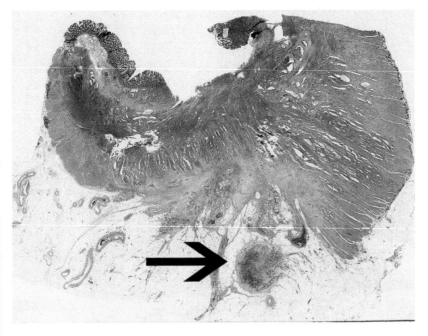

Fig. 10. A tumor deposit at the advancing edge of a carcinoma has a mostly round appearance without residual lymph node architecture (*arrow,* H&E, original magnification ×1).

Fig. 11. The AJCC sixth edition Cancer Staging Manual classified smooth, round nodules as lymph nodes in the N category (*A*, H&E, original magnification ×4), whereas irregular nodules were staged in the T category (*B*, H&E, original magnification ×2).

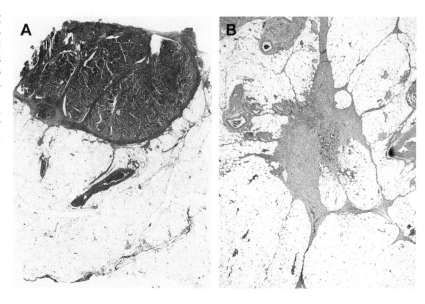

compared with 60% for patients with tumor deposits.

Tumor deposits have been variably categorized in the TNM staging system. The AJCC fifth edition Cancer Staging Manual classified tumor nodules based on size criteria: small nodules (<3 mm) were considered to represent vascular invasion, perineural invasion, or extension of the primary tumor and staged in the T category; larger nodules were classified as effaced lymph nodes and staged in the N category.[40] Although highly reproducible, the "3-mm rule" was clinically irrelevant. The AJCC sixth edition Cancer Staging Manual classified round tumor nodules as effaced lymph nodes and staged them as pN1 or pN2, whereas ill-defined tumor nodules were staged in the T category (**Fig. 11**).[33] Unfortunately, classifying nodules based on contour is subjective, and "upstaging" a tumor otherwise confined to the colonic wall as pT3 based solely on tumor nodules is problematic.

The AJCC seventh edition Cancer Staging Manual introduced a novel classification scheme for tumor deposits. Tumor nodules interpreted to represent effaced lymph nodes are classified as pN1 or pN2 regardless of size or shape; nodules that are not considered to represent lymph nodes are classified as tumor deposits and counted.[33] Given that cancers with tumor deposits are prognostically comparable to stage III disease, tumor deposits are reported in the N category, thereby upstaging patients for potential adjuvant chemotherapy. The "N1c" category is used for tumor deposits to facilitate long-term follow-up of affected patients in large, multi-institutional studies. Tumor deposits are similarly handled in the AJCC eighth edition Cancer Staging Manual.[5]

Distinction between completely replaced lymph nodes and satellite tumor deposits is subjective and reproducibility is poor.[41] Rock and colleagues[42] circulated 25 virtual slides of tumor nodules and asked 7 gastrointestinal pathologists to classify each as a tumor deposit or effaced lymph node. All 7 pathologists agreed on the diagnosis in 11 (44%) cases, including similar numbers of nodules classified as effaced lymph nodes and tumor deposits. Features the investigators felt to be suggestive of effaced lymph nodes included round shape, peripheral rim of lymphoid tissue, capsule, and subcapsular sinus (**Box 3**).

Box 3
Features that aid distinction between lymph nodes and tumor deposits

- Effaced lymph node
  - Round shape
  - Peripheral rim of lymphocytes
  - Peripheral lymphoid follicles
  - Capsule
  - Subcapsular sinus
- Tumor deposits
  - Irregular contour
  - No organized lymphoid tissue
  - Not surrounded by capsule
  - Sometimes near arteries
  - Peripheral rim of lymphocytes

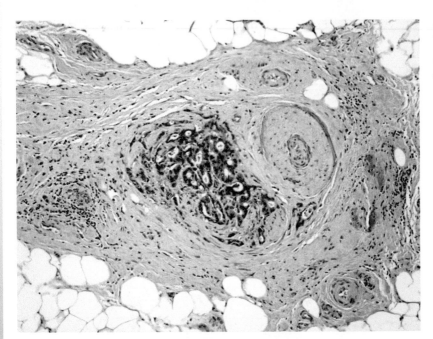

Fig. 12. An ill-defined aggregate of tumor cells located next to an artery represents venous invasion (H&E, original magnification ×10).

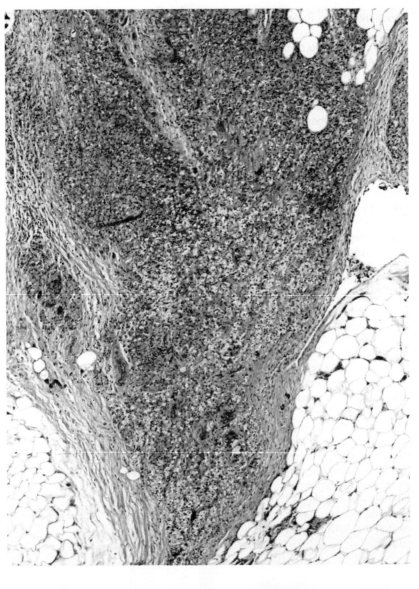

Fig. 13. Discontinuous tumor nodules on the peritoneal surface are classified as distant metastases in the M category (H&E, original magnification ×10).

Tumor nodules that can be recognized as other types of lesions should not be classified as tumor deposits. Nodules close to (<1 mm) the advancing edge of the tumor may represent irregular extensions of the primary mass; if tissue levels demonstrate continuity between the tumor and a nodule, then it should be staged in the T category rather than as a tumor deposit. Round or serpiginous aggregates of tumor cells in close proximity to arteries likely represent venous invasion rather than tumor deposits (**Fig. 12**). Tumor nodules that can be classified as lymphatic vessel or perineural invasion are reported as such, but not denoted as tumor deposits.[33] Discontinuous tumor nodules at the peritoneal surface probably represent peritoneal carcinomatosis (pM1c), rather than tumor deposits (**Fig. 13**).

Several criteria govern pathologic reporting of tumor deposits. When present in association with positive lymph nodes, the number of tumor deposits is recorded in the body of the report, but do not contribute to the T or N staging categories. The number of tumor deposits should not be added to the total number of positive lymph nodes. The N1c category is used only when tumor deposits are detected in patients without metastases in regional lymph nodes. Of note, N1c does not imply a more advanced stage than N1a or N1b.[5,33]

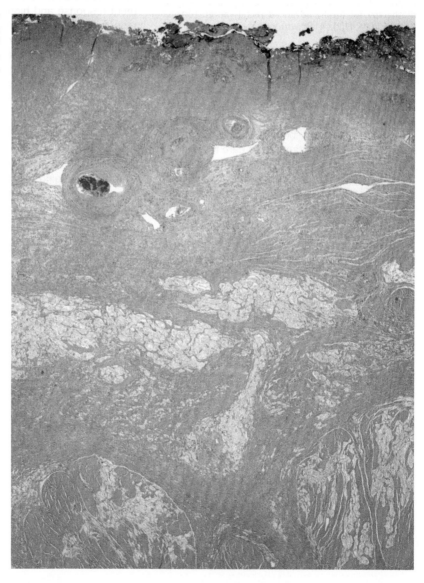

Fig. 14. A neoadjuvantly treated rectal carcinoma shows residual pools of acellular mucin extending into the prostate (*top*, H&E, original magnification ×2).

Table 2
Classification of tumor regression among treated rectal cancers

Tumor Regression Grade	Grade Definition
Grade 0	Complete regression: No viable cancer cells
Grade 1	Near complete regression: Single cells or small groups of tumor cells
Grade 2	Moderate regression: Residual cancer outgrown by fibrosis
Grade 3	No regression: Minimal or no tumor cells killed

From Ryan R, Gibbons D, Hyland JM, et al. Pathological response following long-course neoadjuvant chemoradiotherapy for locally advanced rectal cancer. Histopathology 2005;47(2):141–6; with permission.

PROGNOSTIC IMPORTANCE OF RESPONSE TO NEOADJUVANT THERAPY

Neoadjuvant therapy before definitive surgical resection is now the standard of care for patients with locally advanced rectal carcinoma. Preoperative treatment offers an opportunity to downstage the tumor, improve surgical outcome, and enhance quality of life.[43] Treated rectal carcinomas show therapy-related cellular changes as well as tumor regression with dense fibrosis, dystrophic calcifications, and pools of mucin without viable tumor cells.[44] The extent of therapy-related tumor regression is predictive of prognosis.[45] An extensive therapeutic response with little residual viable tumor is associated with improved outcome, whereas survival is poorer among patients with abundant viable tumor remaining after neoadjuvant treatment.[46,47]

Neoadjuvantly treated rectal cancers are designated with a "y" prefix to denote prior therapy. Assignment of T and N stages is based on extent of viable tumor; acellular mucin and dystrophic calcifications are not used to determine pathologic stage (Fig. 14). Extent of tumor regression can be assessed using a variety of methods, although the system endorsed by the AJCC Cancer Staging Manual applies the lowest grade to the best treatment response and highest grade to the poorest response (Table 2).[48] Tumor regression is evaluated only in the primary tumor. Lymph node deposits that show a therapeutic response are not considered when grading tumor regression, nor are they counted toward the assignment of N stage unless viable tumor is identified within the lymph node (Fig. 15).[36]

SUMMARY

Pathologic staging information is one of the most important factors in determining postsurgical management of patients with colorectal carcinoma.

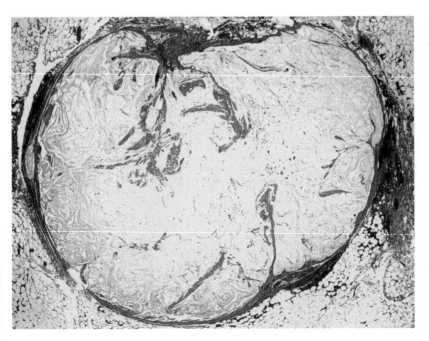

Fig. 15. Mucin pools in regional lymph nodes of treated carcinomas are not classified as positive lymph nodes (H&E, original magnification ×4).

Although the AJCC Cancer Staging Manual provides helpful guidelines, pathologists still have difficulty applying staging criteria. Serosal penetration (pT4a) by cancer is frequently underdiagnosed, although assessment of regional lymph nodes and classification of tumor deposits also can be problematic. Acellular mucin is a common finding in the tumor bed and regional lymph nodes of neoadjuvantly treated patients, and does not contribute to overall stage assignment.

REFERENCES

1. Siegel RL, Miller KD, Jemal A. Cancer statistics, 2016. CA Cancer J Clin 2016;66(1):7–30.
2. Benson AB 3rd, Schrag D, Somerfield MR, et al. American Society of Clinical Oncology recommendations on adjuvant chemotherapy for stage II colon cancer. J Clin Oncol 2004;22(16):3408–19.
3. Benson AB 3rd, Choti MA, Cohen AM, et al. NCCN practice guidelines for colorectal cancer. Oncology (Williston Park) 2000;14(11A):203–12.
4. Williams CD, Grady WM, Zullig LL. Use of NCCN guidelines, other guidelines, and biomarkers for colorectal cancer screening. J Natl Compr Canc Netw 2016;14(11):1479–85.
5. Jessup JM, Goldberg RM, Asare EA, et al. Colon and rectum. In: Amin MB, editor. AJCC cancer staging manual. 8th edition. Chicago: Springer; 2017. p. 251–74.
6. Shepherd NA, Baxter KJ, Love SB. The prognostic importance of peritoneal involvement in colonic cancer: a prospective evaluation. Gastroenterology 1997;112(4):1096–102.
7. Ludeman L, Shepherd NA. Serosal involvement in gastrointestinal cancer: its assessment and significance. Histopathology 2005;47(2):123–31.
8. Petersen VC, Baxter KJ, Love SB, et al. Identification of objective pathological prognostic determinants and models of prognosis in Dukes' B colon cancer. Gut 2002;51(1):65–9.
9. Panarelli NC, Schreiner AM, Brandt SM, et al. Histologic features and cytologic techniques that aid pathologic stage assessment of colonic adenocarcinoma. Am J Surg Pathol 2013;37(8):1252–8.
10. Kojima M, Nakajima K, Ishii G, et al. Peritoneal elastic laminal invasion of colorectal cancer: the diagnostic utility and clinicopathologic relationship. Am J Surg Pathol 2010;34(9):1351–60.
11. Snaebjornsson P, Coupe VM, Jonasson L, et al. pT4 stage II and III colon cancers carry the worst prognosis in a nationwide survival analysis. Shepherd's local peritoneal involvement revisited. Int J Cancer 2014;135(2):467–78.
12. Kirsch R, Messenger D, Shepherd N, et al. Widespread variability in assessment and reporting of colorectal cancer specimens among North American pathologists: results of a Canada-US survey. Mod Pathol 2015;28(S2):170A.
13. Shinto E, Ueno H, Hashiguchi Y, et al. The subserosal elastic lamina: an anatomic landmark for stratifying pT3 colorectal cancer. Dis Colon Rectum 2004; 47(4):467–73.
14. Liang WY, Chang WC, Hsu CY, et al. Retrospective evaluation of elastic stain in the assessment of serosal invasion of pT3N0 colorectal cancers. Am J Surg Pathol 2013;37(10):1565–70.
15. Leather AJ, Kocjan G, Savage F, et al. Detection of free malignant cells in the peritoneal cavity before and after resection of colorectal cancer. Dis Colon Rectum 1994;37(8):814–9.
16. Zuna RE, Mitchell ML. Cytologic findings in peritoneal washings associated with benign gynecologic disease. Acta Cytol 1988;32(2):139–47.
17. Ambrose NS, MacDonald F, Young J, et al. Monoclonal antibody and cytological detection of free malignant cells in the peritoneal cavity during resection of colorectal cancer–can monoclonal antibodies do better? Eur J Surg Oncol 1989;15(2):99–102.
18. Le Voyer TE, Sigurdson ER, Hanlon AL, et al. Colon cancer survival is associated with increasing number of lymph nodes analyzed: a secondary survey of intergroup trial INT-0089. J Clin Oncol 2003; 21(15):2912–9.
19. Cserni G, Vinh-Hung V, Burzykowski T. Is there a minimum number of lymph nodes that should be histologically assessed for a reliable nodal staging of T3N0M0 colorectal carcinomas? J Surg Oncol 2002;81(2):63–9.
20. Kim J, Huynh R, Abraham I, et al. Number of lymph nodes examined and its impact on colorectal cancer staging. Am Surg 2006;72(10):902–5.
21. Goldstein NS. Lymph node recoveries from 2427 pT3 colorectal resection specimens spanning 45 years: recommendations for a minimum number of recovered lymph nodes based on predictive probabilities. Am J Surg Pathol 2002;26(2): 179–89.
22. George S, Primrose J, Talbot R, et al. Will Rogers revisited: prospective observational study of survival of 3592 patients with colorectal cancer according to number of nodes examined by pathologists. Br J Cancer 2006;95(7):841–7.
23. Swanson RS, Compton CC, Stewart AK, et al. The prognosis of T3N0 colon cancer is dependent on the number of lymph nodes examined. Ann Surg Oncol 2003;10(1):65–71.
24. Prandi M, Lionetto R, Bini A, et al. Prognostic evaluation of stage B colon cancer patients is improved by an adequate lymphadenectomy: results of a secondary analysis of a large scale adjuvant trial. Ann Surg 2002;235(4):458–63.
25. Fujita S, Shimoda T, Yoshimura K, et al. Prospective evaluation of prognostic factors in patients with

colorectal cancer undergoing curative resection. J Surg Oncol 2003;84:127–31.

26. Chapuis PH, Dent OF, Bokey EL, et al. Adverse histopathological findings as a guide to patient management after curative resection of node-positive colonic cancer. Br J Surg 2004;91(3):349–54.

27. Dillman RO, Aaron K, Heinemann FS, et al. Identification of 12 or more lymph nodes in resected colon cancer specimens as an indicator of quality performance. Cancer 2009;115(9):1840–8.

28. Scott KW, Grace RH. Detection of lymph node metastases in colorectal carcinoma before and after fat clearance. Br J Surg 1989;76(11):1165–7.

29. Sugimoto K, Sakamoto K, Tomiki Y, et al. Proposal of new classification for stage III colon cancer based on the lymph node ratio: analysis of 4,172 patients from multi-institutional database in Japan. Ann Surg Oncol 2015;22(2):528–34.

30. Miller ED, Robb BW, Cummings OW, et al. The effects of preoperative chemoradiotherapy on lymph node sampling in rectal cancer. Dis Colon Rectum 2012;55(9):1002–7.

31. Govindarajan A, Gonen M, Weiser MR, et al. Challenging the feasibility and clinical significance of current guidelines on lymph node examination in rectal cancer in the era of neoadjuvant therapy. J Clin Oncol 2011;29(34):4568–73.

32. Sloothaak DA, Sahami S, van der Zaag-Loonen HJ, et al. The prognostic value of micrometastases and isolated tumour cells in histologically negative lymph nodes of patients with colorectal cancer: a systematic review and meta-analysis. Eur J Surg Oncol 2014;40(3):263–9.

33. Edge SB, American Joint Committee on Cancer. AJCC cancer staging manual. 7th edition. New York: Springer; 2010.

34. Protic M, Stojadinovic A, Nissan A, et al. Prognostic effect of ultra-staging node-negative colon cancer without adjuvant chemotherapy: a prospective National Cancer Institute-sponsored clinical trial. J Am Coll Surg 2015;221(3):643–51, [quiz: 783–5].

35. Sargent DJ, Resnick MB, Meyers MO, et al. Evaluation of guanylyl cyclase C lymph node status for colon cancer staging and prognosis. Ann Surg Oncol 2011;18(12):3261–70.

36. Washington MK. Colorectal carcinoma: selected issues in pathologic examination and staging and determination of prognostic factors. Arch Pathol Lab Med 2008;132(10):1600–7.

37. Overman MJ, Asare EA, Compton CC, et al. Appendix-carcinoma. In: Amin MB, editor. AJCC cancer staging manual. Chicago: Springer; 2017. p. 237–50.

38. Puppa G, Maisonneuve P, Sonzogni A, et al. Pathological assessment of pericolonic tumor deposits in advanced colonic carcinoma: relevance to prognosis and tumor staging. Mod Pathol 2007;20(8): 843–55.

39. Ueno H, Hashiguchi Y, Shimazaki H, et al. Peritumoral deposits as an adverse prognostic indicator of colorectal cancer. Am J Surg 2014;207(1):70–7.

40. Colon and rectum. In: Fleming ID, Cooper JS, Henson DE, et al, editors. AJCC cancer staging manual. 5th edition. Philadelphia: Lippincott-Raven; 1997. p. 83–90.

41. Nagtegaal ID, Tot T, Jayne DG, et al. Lymph nodes, tumor deposits, and TNM: are we getting better? J Clin Oncol 2011;29(18):2487–92.

42. Rock JB, Washington MK, Adsay NV, et al. Debating deposits: an interobserver variability study of lymph nodes and pericolonic tumor deposits in colonic adenocarcinoma. Arch Pathol Lab Med 2014; 138(5):636–42.

43. Kapiteijn E, Marijnen CA, Nagtegaal ID, et al. Preoperative radiotherapy combined with total mesorectal excision for resectable rectal cancer. N Engl J Med 2001;345(9):638–46.

44. Shia J, Tickoo SK, Guillem JG, et al. Increased endocrine cells in treated rectal adenocarcinomas: a possible reflection of endocrine differentiation in tumor cells induced by chemotherapy and radiotherapy. Am J Surg Pathol 2002;26(7):863–72.

45. Kuo LJ, Liu MC, Jian JJ, et al. Is final TNM staging a predictor for survival in locally advanced rectal cancer after preoperative chemoradiation therapy? Ann Surg Oncol 2007;14(10):2766–72.

46. Abdul-Jalil KI, Sheehan KM, Kehoe J, et al. The prognostic value of tumour regression grade following neoadjuvant chemoradiation therapy for rectal cancer. Colorectal Dis 2014;16(1):O16–25.

47. Ruo L, Tickoo S, Klimstra DS, et al. Long-term prognostic significance of extent of rectal cancer response to preoperative radiation and chemotherapy. Ann Surg 2002;236(1):75–81.

48. Ryan R, Gibbons D, Hyland JM, et al. Pathological response following long-course neoadjuvant chemoradiotherapy for locally advanced rectal cancer. Histopathology 2005;47(2):141–6.

Immunohistochemical Pitfalls

Common Mistakes in the Evaluation of Lynch Syndrome

Michael Markow, MD, Wei Chen, MD, PhD,
Wendy L. Frankel, MD*

KEYWORDS

• Lynch syndrome • Immunohistochemistry • Pitfalls • Staining pattern

Key points

• A diagnostic algorithm for screening newly diagnosed colorectal cancer for Lynch syndrome is discussed.

• Usual staining patterns of mismatch repair protein immunohistochemistry are discussed.

• Unusual staining patterns of mismatch repair protein immunohistochemistry are discussed.

• Pitfalls in interpreting mismatch repair protein immunohistochemistry are discussed.

ABSTRACT

At least 15% of colorectal cancers diagnosed in the United States are deficient in mismatch repair mechanisms. Most of these are sporadic, but approximately 3% of colorectal cancers result from germline alterations in mismatch repair genes and represent Lynch syndrome. It is critical to identify patients with Lynch syndrome to institute appropriate screening and surveillance for patients and their families. Exclusion of Lynch syndrome in sporadic cases is equally important because it reduces anxiety for patients and prevents excessive spending on unnecessary surveillance. Immunohistochemistry is one of the most widely used screening tools for identifying patients with Lynch syndrome.

OVERVIEW

Lynch syndrome is the most common hereditary colorectal cancer syndrome; it accounts for approximately 3% of colorectal cancers and affects approximately 1 in 35 unselected patients with colorectal cancer.[1–3] Patients with Lynch syndrome carry a germline mutation in one of the mismatch repair genes (MLH1, PMS2, MSH2, MSH6) or an EPCAM mutation.[4] In the latter situation, germline deletion of the 3′ end of EPCAM silences MSH2 from transcription; EPCAM is located just upstream to MSH2, and its inactivation leads to methylation and inactivation of MSH2. Patients with this genetic alteration have Lynch syndrome and loss of immunostaining for MSH2 and MSH6, as discussed later.

Patients with Lynch syndrome are at an increased risk for several other types of malignancy, including endometrial, gastric, ovarian, pancreas, ureter, renal pelvis, biliary tract, and brain tumors.[5] Universal screening of patients with colorectal carcinoma for Lynch syndrome is recommended by multiple sources, including Evaluation of Genomic Applications in Practice and Prevention,[6] National Comprehensive Cancer Network,[7] US Multi-Society Task Force,[8] the

Disclosure for All Authors: None.
Department of Pathology, The Ohio State University Wexner Medical Center, 129 Hamilton Hall, 1645 Neil Avenue, Columbus, OH 43210, USA
* Corresponding author.
E-mail address: Wendy.Frankel@osumc.edu

Surgical Pathology 10 (2017) 977–1007
http://dx.doi.org/10.1016/j.path.2017.07.012
1875-9181/17/© 2017 Elsevier Inc. All rights reserved.

American College of Gastroenterology,[9] and the American Society of Clinical Oncology.[10] Screening for Lynch syndrome is cost-effective for the US health care system[11–13] and helps determine appropriate lifetime screening regimens for patients and their family members. Identification of microsatellite instability (MSI) is also important because cancers with MSI do not respond well to 5-fluorouracil[14] and may be more amenable to anti–programmed cell death 1 immunotherapy.[15]

Families are smaller than in the past; many patients undergo preventive colonoscopy with polypectomy, so family and personal history of cancer do not reliably detect all affected patients. In fact, approximately 50% of patients with Lynch syndrome are not detected by Amsterdam and Bethesda criteria.[2] Histologic features, including tumor-infiltrating lymphocytes, mucinous or high-grade features, and a Crohnlike peritumoral lymphocytic response, are suggestive of MSI but are not entirely sensitive or specific.

MISMATCH REPAIR PROTEIN IMMUNOHISTOCHEMISTRY AND MICROSATELLITE INSTABILITY

Analysis for MSI by polymerase chain reaction (PCR) and mismatch repair protein immunohistochemistry facilitates screening for mismatch repair deficiency, but each method has advantages and disadvantages.[16,17] If only one test is used, immunohistochemistry is preferred by most because it is more cost-effective and readily available than

PCR and the results can be used to guide further testing of the germline. However, it is likely and may be true in some cases that decreasing costs of next-generation sequencing will reach the point at which the cost of analyzing multiple genes is comparable with that of single-gene testing. If this time comes, then solid tumor immunohistochemistry and MSI analysis may become largely obsolete for Lynch syndrome screening.

There is a high degree of concordance (>90%) between mismatch repair deficiency by immunohistochemistry and MSI,[2,18–20] although tumors with MSH6 mutations may not show MSI, particularly if the Bethesda panel is used. Immunohistochemical stain results implicating deficient MSH2, MSH6, and PMS2 proteins generally suggest Lynch syndrome. However, results showing MLH1 deficiency are not specific for Lynch syndrome; most cases are sporadic and result from MLH1 hypermethylation.[16,21] Tests for BRAF V600E mutations and MLH1 methylation are used to identify these sporadic tumors, as shown in the algorithm later.

DIAGNOSTIC ALGORITHM FOR SCREENING NEWLY DIAGNOSED COLORECTAL CANCER FOR LYNCH SYNDROME

Multiple algorithms are available to screen for Lynch syndrome, but most are fairly similar. Loss of staining for one or more mismatch repair proteins indicates the need for additional testing. Fig. 1 demonstrates the authors' algorithm:

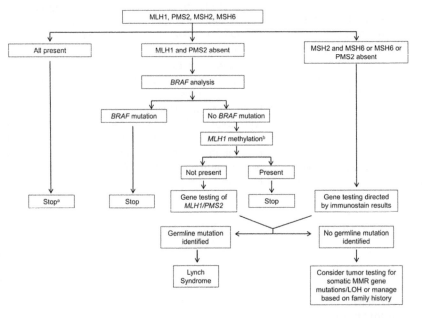

Fig. 1. Diagnostic algorithm for screening newly diagnosed colorectal cancer for Lynch syndrome. [a]Consider referral to genetics and MSI testing if concerning family history and age. [b]Consider gene testing rather than methylation if suspicious for Lynch syndrome by age or patient history LOH, Loss of heterozygosity.

- All newly diagnosed colorectal cancer cases are subjected to mismatch repair protein (MLH1, PMS2, MSH2, MSH6) immunohistochemistry.
- No further workup is necessary if staining for all proteins is preserved (Fig. 2), unless there is a strong clinical suspicion for Lynch syndrome.
- Combined loss of MLH1 and PMS2 staining is followed by mutational analysis of BRAF[22,23] to determine whether a tumor is sporadic (positive for BRAF mutation) or should be further evaluated for Lynch syndrome (negative for BRAF mutation). If a BRAF V600E mutation is found, the tumor is likely sporadic and no further testing is required. The V600E BRAF mutation occurs in about 10% to 15% of all colorectal carcinomas and is associated with epigenetic methylation of several promoter regions throughout the genome, including the

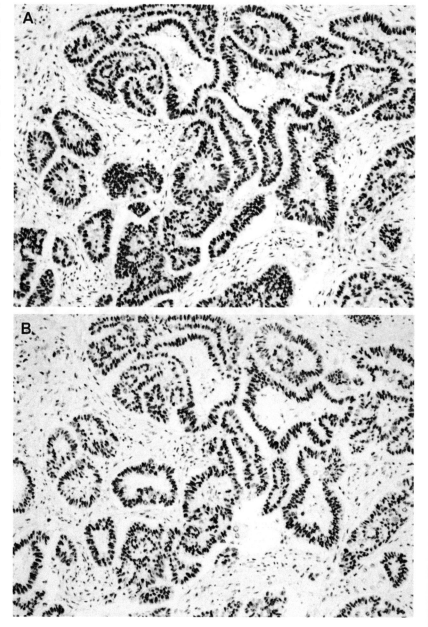

Fig. 2. Mismatch repair protein immunohistochemistry: intact staining of all 4 proteins. This mismatch repair proficient tumor shows intact nuclear staining and is microsatellite stable by PCR. (*A*) MLH1, (*B*) PMS2, (*C*) MSH2, (*D*) MSH6. Note the positive internal controls for all images [original magnification, ×200].

Fig. 2. (continued).

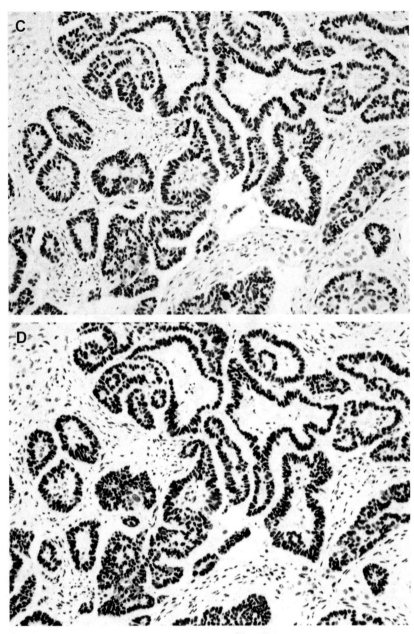

promoter region of the *MLH1* gene. Promoter hypermethylation impairs transcription to mRNA, effectively silencing *MLH1* expression and MLH1 protein formation. Of note, *BRAF* mutational testing has no role in the evaluation of extracolonic cancers with MSI because of deficient MLH1; sporadic endometrial and ovarian cancers do not harbor *BRAF* mutations.[24]

- If a *BRAF* mutation is not detected, evaluation of the tumor for *MLH1* promoter hypermethylation is performed when suspicion for Lynch syndrome is low or genetic sequencing of *MLH1* or *PMS2* is undertaken when there is a clinical suspicion for Lynch syndrome. Some laboratories use *MLH1* methylation testing rather than *BRAF* mutational analysis to evaluate tumors with combined loss of MLH1 and PMS2 staining. Similar to *BRAF* mutated cases, those with *MLH1* methylation are presumed to represent sporadic tumors and require no further testing.

- Cases with loss of MSH2 and MSH6, isolated MSH6 loss, and isolated PMS2 loss require genetic testing for Lynch syndrome after appropriate informed consent.

Once mismatch-deficient tumors are identified by immunohistochemistry, the underlying mechanism of mismatch repair deficiency must be determined. Hereditary cancers result from germline mutations in one of the mismatch repair genes (Table 1). Sporadic mismatch repair deficiency can be due to *MLH1* hypermethylation or double somatic mutations of any mismatch repair gene. Patients and family members with sporadic tumors do not need lifelong screening, alleviating much anxiety and cost.

USUAL AND UNUSUAL STAINING PATTERNS OF MISMATCH REPAIR PROTEINS

The common patterns of mismatch repair protein expression can be explained by the biology of their function. The mismatch repair proteins form 2 heterodimer complexes, MLH1 and PMS2 and MSH2 and MSH6, that facilitate repair in DNA sequences. Both PMS2 and MSH6 require their binding partners to be expressed so they can form a stable

heterodimer. As a result, defective MLH1 is manifest by combined loss of MLH1 and PMS2 (Fig. 3A–D), whereas MSH2 and MSH6 are lost when MSH2 is defective (see Fig. 3E–H). However, both MLH1 and MSH2 can form heterodimers with other proteins; thus, MLH1 and MSH2 are expressed despite loss of PMS2 or MSH6 function (Table 2).[25,26] Occasionally, unusual staining scenarios occur (Fig. 4 and Table 3).

REPORTING AND INTERPRETATION PITFALLS FOR MISMATCH REPAIR PROTEIN IMMUNOHISTOCHEMISTRY

The College of American Pathologists' biomarker protocol[27] recommends that the pattern of immunohistochemical staining should be described as lost and intact. This terminology is preferred over the terms *negative* and *positive*, because the latter may be ambiguously interpreted to mean negative or positive for Lynch syndrome rather than negative or positive for mismatch repair protein expression. Colectomy specimens are commonly used for Lynch syndrome screening; however, screening can be performed on biopsies and other samples (Table 4). Corresponding warnings/suggestions when using other specimens are provided.

Mismatch proficient tumors typically show diffuse strong nuclear staining in the tumor cells as well as staining of proliferative epithelial cells

---

Table 1
Comparison of mismatch repair protein-deficient colorectal cancers

| | Hereditary Mismatch Repair Deficiency | | Sporadic Mismatch Repair Deficiency | |
	Lynch Syndrome	Constitutional Mismatch Repair Deficiency	*MLH1* Promoter Hypermethylation	Somatic Mismatch Repair Mutations
Germline mutation	One allele of a mismatch repair gene (*MLH1, PMS2, MSH2, MSH6*)	Both alleles of a mismatch repair gene (*MLH1, PMS2, MSH2, MSH6*)	None	None
Somatic mutation	Second allele of the mutated mismatch repair gene	None	*BRAF* V600E	Both alleles of a mismatch repair gene (*MLH1, PMS2, MSH2, MSH6*)
Epigenetic alteration	Germline deletion in 3′ end of *EPCAM* leads to *MSH2* methylation	None	Somatic biallelic promoter methylation of *MLH1*	None
Lifelong Screening	Yes	Yes	No	No

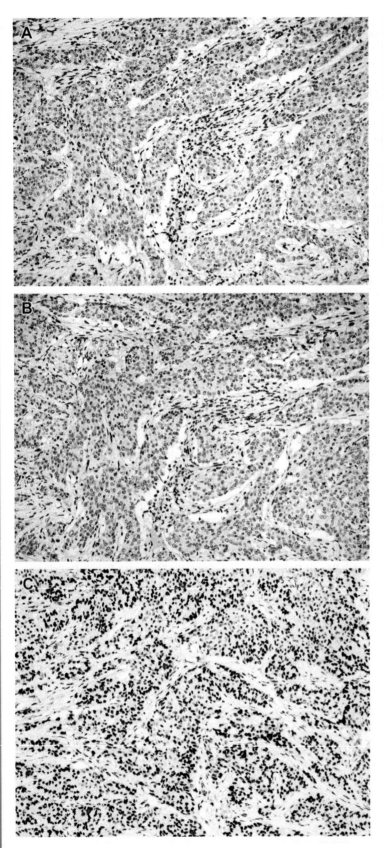

Fig. 3. Mismatch repair protein immunohistochemistry: usual patterns (typical losses). The most common abnormal staining pattern is the loss of MLH1 (*A*) and PMS2 (*B*) staining, as illustrated in this patient who had a *MLH1* mutation. Notice the intact expression of MSH2 (*C*) and MSH6 (*D*). In this patient with *MSH2* mutation, expression of MLH1 (*E*) and PMS2 (*F*) is intact, whereas MSH2 (*G*) and MSH6 (*H*) are lost together. Other common lost patterns include isolated loss of MSH6 and isolated loss of PMS2 (not shown) [original magnification, ×200].

Fig. 3. (continued).

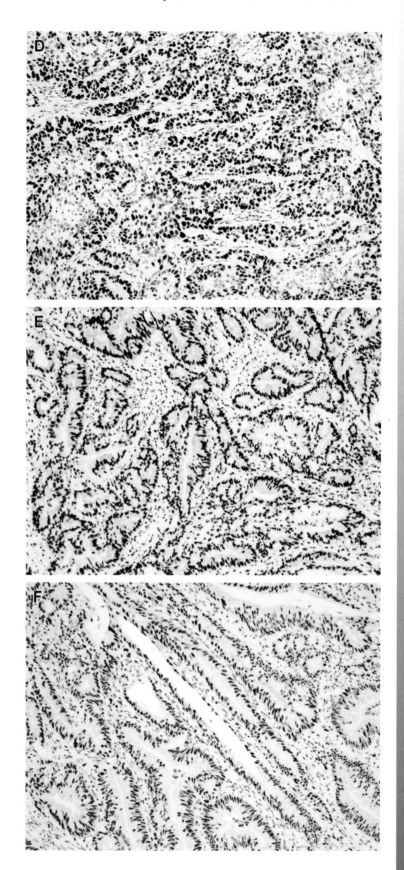

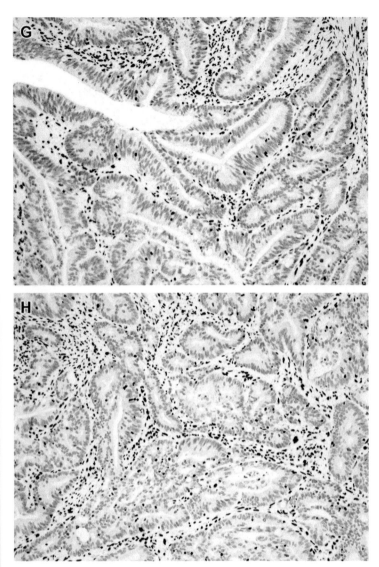

Fig. 3. (*continued*).

Table 2
Mismatch repair protein immunohistochemistry: usual patterns and causes

Mismatch Repair Protein Staining Pattern	Frequency	Most Common Causes
MLH1, PMS2, MSH2, and MSH6 intact	85%	Microsatellite stable
MLH1/PMS2 loss MSH2/MSH6 intact	~13%	Somatic *MLH1* promotor hypermethylation (12%)[58] Germline *MLH1* mutation and epimutation (<1%)[a]
MLH1/PMS2 intact MSH2/MSH6 loss	1%	Germline *MSH2* mutation or *EPCAM* mutation[a]
Isolated PMS2 loss	<1%	Germline *PMS2* mutation[a]
Isolated MSH6 loss	<1%	Germline *MSH6* mutation[a]

[a] Somatic double mutations of MLH1, PMS2, MSH2, and MSH6 have been reported in microsatellite unstable colorectal and endometrial cancers.[31,32]

Fig. 4. Mismatch repair protein immunohistochemistry: unusual scenarios. Intact expression of all 4 proteins are present (*A*, MLH1 shown here), in this case of a missense mutation in *MLH1* that leads to nonfunctional protein with retained antigenicity. Rarely, null pattern/loss of all 4 proteins are seen (*B*, MSH2 shown here) because of concurrent somatic *MLH1* hypermethylation and germline *MSH2* mutation leading to the loss of their partners. In this *MLH1/PMS2*-deficient medullary tumor (*C*, MLH1), there is heterogeneous loss of MSH6 (*D*, *E*) due to secondary mutation in *MSH6*. Similarly, (*F*) demonstrates another case of heterogeneous MSH6 loss in an *MLH1/PMS2*-deficient tumor with glandular morphology. Both patients were found to have *MLH1* hypermethylation together with a secondary mutation in *MSH6*. In D, E, and F, the internal control is intact in areas of the tumor with (*arrows in D, E, and F*) and without (*arrowheads in D, E, and F*) expression [original magnification, (*A, E, F*) ×400, (*B, C, D*) x200].

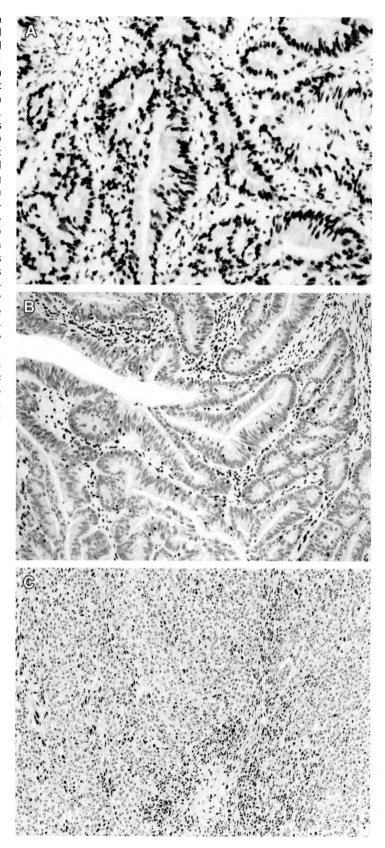

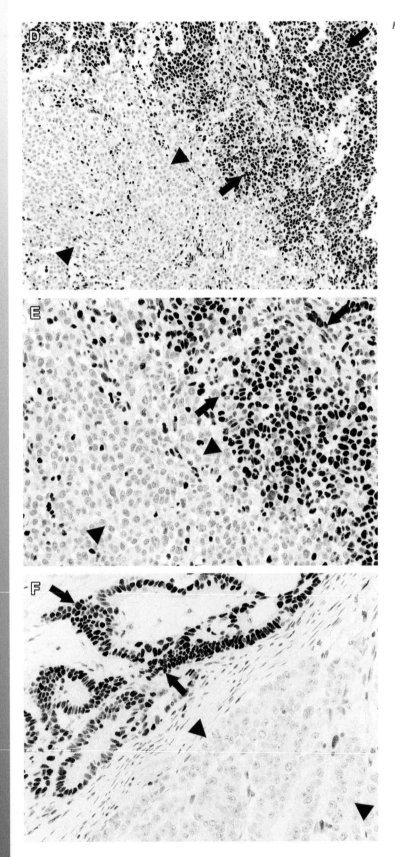

Fig. 4. (*continued*).

Table 3
Mismatch repair protein immunohistochemistry: unusual scenarios and explanation

Mismatch Repair Protein Staining Pattern	Molecular Abnormality	Frequency	Explanation
Normal expression of all 4 proteins	Missense mutation present (especially in *MLH1*)	5% of Lynch syndrome families	Mutation leads to a nonfunctional protein with retained antigenicity.
Isolated loss of PMS2	No *PMS2* mutation detected Germline *MLH1* mutation or *MLH1* promotor hypermethylation	24% of cases with isolated loss of PMS2 expression	Germline *MLH1* mutation results in functionally inactive and unstable MLH1 protein that is antigenically intact, compromised stability of MLH1-PMS2 complex, and loss of PMS2 staining.[59–61]
Null pattern (all 4 stains are lost)	Somatic *MLH1* hypermethylation and germline *MSH2* mutation	Rare	A somatic MLH1 hypermethylation (causing absent MLH1/PMS2) is present, in addition to germline *MSH2* mutation (causing absent MSH2/MSH6).[51]
Abnormal MSH6 (complete loss or heterogeneous staining) in addition to loss of MLH1, PMS2	Somatic *MLH1* hypermethylation or germline *MLH1/PMS2* mutation Secondary mutation in *MSH6*	Rare	Secondary mutation in a coding mononucleotide tract in *MSH6* causes loss of expression of MSH6 in tumors with *MLH1/PMS2* deficiency.[43,44]

and lymphocytes that serve as a positive internal control (**Fig. 5**A, B). The following staining patterns are considered abnormal and may warrant additional investigation: punctate/speckled nuclear staining, nuclear membranous staining, and nucleolar staining (**Table 5**).[25] Patchy immunostaining for mismatch repair proteins is not uncommon and may be related to tissue hypoxia and variable fixation conditions (see **Fig. 5**C, D).[28,29]

In the authors' practice, if more than 5% tumor nuclei show unequivocal nuclear staining, they sign out the case as present/intact mismatch repair protein expression. Some investigators use different cutoff values, such as greater than 10%,[25] greater than 1%,[27] or any degree of convincing staining.[27] In the authors' experience, variability in expression may occur; but most cases are diffusely positive and show staining of more than 50% of the tumor cells. If equivocal staining is detected, additional workup could include repeating the stain, choosing another

block, choosing another sample (ie, pretreatment biopsy for postneoadjuvant rectal cancer), or additional testing (MSI or other molecular testing). Stain interpretation can be complicated by abundant tumor-infiltrating lymphocytes that express mismatch repair proteins; their staining can be misinterpreted as staining of tumor cells in some instances (**Fig. 6**A, B). Nuclear staining can also be difficult to evaluate in signet ring cells (see **Fig. 6**C, D).

MISMATCH REPAIR-DEFICIENT COLORECTAL CANCERS

The most common cause of mismatch repair deficiency is sporadic hypermethylation of the *MLH1* promoter. Once hypermethylation is excluded, the possibility of germline alterations in mismatch repair genes requires investigation; these tests can be performed on patients' blood. Although germline mutations are detected in most cases,

Table 4
Mismatch repair protein immunohistochemistry: pitfalls in samples

Sample Type	Pitfalls and Warning	Suggestions
Inadequate biopsy (crush artifact, insufficient tumor cells) of colorectal cancer	A false positive is possible (loss of staining in a small biopsy could represent a no-staining area in a heterogeneous staining case).	Biopsy specimens work well for mismatch repair immunohistochemistry.[45–47] If there is clinical concern, repeat on the resection specimen or larger biopsy.
Adenoma	A false negative is possible (adenoma of a Lynch syndrome patient may show intact staining, especially in small adenoma without villous component or high-grade dysplasia).	Test cancer from patients or families if available. If the test is on adenoma, add a disclaimer: whereas absent staining may be seen in Lynch syndrome and the pattern of loss useful in directing gene testing, intact expression does not exclude the diagnosis.
Serrated polyp	Serrated polyps without dysplasia do not have mismatch repair deficiency; Lynch syndrome–associated colorectal cancer does not typically arise from serrated polyps.	Do not perform mismatch repair protein immunohistochemistry on serrated polyps for Lynch syndrome screening or to classify most serrated polyp.
Metastatic colorectal cancer	None	Metastatic cancer can be used for screening[62]
Synchronous/metachronous carcinoma	Synchronous and/or metachronous neoplasms in patients with Lynch syndrome can show discordant mismatch repair protein immunoreactivity.	Perform mismatch repair protein immunohistochemistry in all primary, synchronous, and metachronous Lynch syndrome–associated neoplasms if a previous tumor screened is intact.[63]
Tumor from autopsy	A false positive is possible (weak and/or patchy nuclear staining in the tumor due to autolysis or inferior preservation of tissue).	Review internal controls in autolyzed or poorly fixed tissue, and compare the tumor with internal control.

analysis may fail to identify Lynch syndrome in a minority of tumors. These cases should be tested for double somatic mutations or other alterations to help explain the mismatch repair deficiency. If molecular changes are limited to neoplastic cells, they can be considered to represent sporadic cancers and further evaluation for Lynch syndrome is unnecessary. Universal screening of colorectal cancers for mismatch repair deficiency has revealed several other causes of mismatch repair deficiency. The Spanish EPICOLON study identified 2.5% of cases that were termed Lynchlike syndrome because they showed MSI and immunostaining profiles typical of Lynch syndrome (ie, combined loss of MSH6/MSH2, isolated loss of MSH6, isolated loss of PMS2) but were not associated with detectable germline mutations.[30] They and other investigators have reported Lynch-like cases resulting from several causes, including

- Double somatic mutations[31,32]
- Incorrect interpretation of immunohistochemical results (false positive cases)
- Failure to detect germline alterations in mismatch repair genes using currently available tests (for example: inversion of *MSH2* exons 1–7 is not tested by many commercial laboratories)

Fig. 5. Mismatch repair protein immunohisto-chemistry: intact staining. In most cases the staining is diffusely present in almost all tumor nuclei (*A*) albeit with slight variation in staining intensity (*B*) [original magnification, (*A*) x100, (*B-D*) x400].

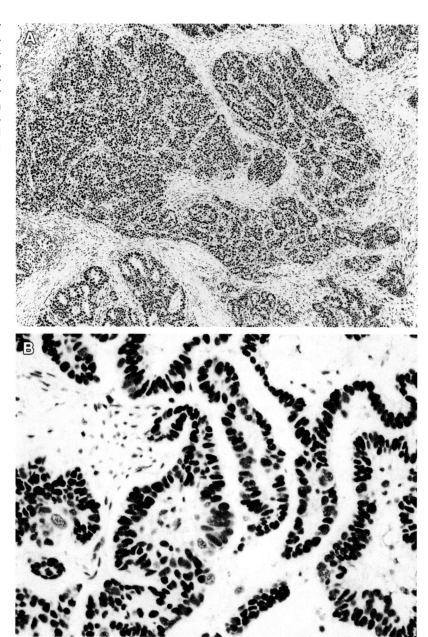

- Other germline genetic defects that also cause MSI, such as biallelic *MUTYH* mutation[33–35]
- Somatic mosaicism[36–38]
- Constitutional epi-mutation of *MLH1* (germline mono-allelic hypermethylation of the *MLH1* promoter region; no alteration to the genetic sequence of *MLH1*)[39–41]

Thus, Lynchlike cases result from several causes, most of which are not related to germline mutations and familial cancer risk. They are best referred by the cause; the ambiguous term *Lynch-like* should be avoided.

COMMONLY ENCOUNTERED MISTAKES IN INTERPRETING MISMATCH REPAIR PROTEIN EXPRESSION USING IMMUNOHISTOCHEMISTRY

- Misinterpreting cytoplasmic staining as intact expression of mismatch repair proteins

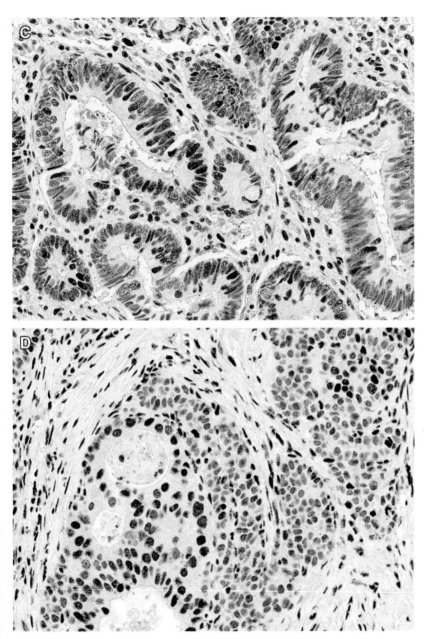

Fig. 5. *(continued).* Of note, areas of patchy staining (C, D) are not uncommon. Patchy staining is considered present/intact staining, and these patients were found to be microsatellite stable by PCR confirming that the stains should be interpreted as intact.

The mismatch repair proteins are expressed in nuclei of proliferating cells, including cancer cells, crypt epithelial cells, and lymphocytes. Therefore, only nuclear staining should be evaluated. Cytoplasmic staining may reflect high background staining and can be so strong that it obscures the nuclei, but it should not be considered for interpretation (**Fig. 7**). Repeat staining should be considered when strong cytoplasmic staining is encountered and, if persistent, should prompt further investigation. Exclusive cytoplasmic staining for MSH2 has been described in a patient with Lynch syndrome resulting from an *EPCAM-MSH2* fusion.[42]

- Interpreting a tumor as mismatch repair proficient when weaker than control staining is present

Table 5
Mismatch repair protein immunohistochemistry: interpretation pitfalls and how to avoid them

Error	Pitfalls	Possible Causes	Suggestions
Interpret as absent when present	Negative or weak internal positive control	Tumor not fixed well Technical immunohistochemistry	Repeat Stain other block Consider MSI by PCR
Interpret as absent in setting of neoadjuvant therapy	Nucleolar or decreased/ equivocal staining interpreted as absent	Post neoadjuvant therapy	Repeat Stain pretreatment biopsy
Interpret as present when absent	Cytoplasmic staining only	Technical immunohistochemistry (high background)	Repeat and call absent
Interpret as present when abnormal	Staining intensity in the tumor that is significantly weaker than internal positive control	Mismatch repair abnormality Technical problem in immunohistochemistry	Repeat and call absent If still equivocal, consider MSI by PCR

Occasional tumors show mismatch repair protein staining in tumor nuclei that differs in intensity from that of control nuclei of lymphocytes, stroma, or epithelium. Cases that show similar or stronger staining of tumor cell nuclei than internal controls are readily interpreted as mismatch repair proficient. Weak or absent staining of tumor cell nuclei associated with weak or negative staining of controls cannot be interpreted; the stain should be repeated in such cases. If the control remains negative after repeating the immunohistochemistry, analysis for MSI by PCR should be considered. Of note, some mismatch repair protein-deficient cancers do not show complete absence of nuclear staining. Weak or equivocal staining of tumor cell nuclei accompanied by stronger staining of the internal controls may reflect an underlying mutation (**Fig. 8**). In the authors' practice, they repeat the stain in such cases and, if the results are similar, suggest additional testing.

- Interpreting heterogeneous tumor staining as decreased or absent expression
  Heterogeneous staining of the tumor can be due to focal immunohistochemistry failure owing to technical issues accompanied by lack of staining in control (**Fig. 9**). However, occasional cases show loss of staining in some areas of the tumor alternating with regions of tumor staining combined with intact staining of the internal control (see example in **Fig. 4D–F** and **Table 3**). In some cases, the areas of tumor with different staining patterns shows distinctive morphologic variation, whereas in others, different staining patterns occur in areas that are morphologically similar. This heterogeneity can reflect molecular variation among subclones within the tumor. These cancers are generally mismatch repair proficient and occur in patients without germline mutations.[43,44] Tumor heterogeneity could be a potential problem with small biopsies, although staining patterns in biopsy material generally show excellent correlation with those of resection specimens.[45–47]

- Misinterpreting weak or nucleolar staining as absent in posttreatment rectal cancers
  Neoadjuvantly treated rectal cancers may show nearly complete loss of MSH6 staining or only nucleolar staining (**Figs. 10** and **11**).[48,49] Decreased PMS2 staining has also been reported in 30% of posttreatment rectal carcinomas.[50] Most of these cases do not have a germline mutation. If the stain is equivocal, performing immunohistochemical stains on the pretreatment biopsy usually resolves the problem (see **Fig. 10E, F**).

- Overstating the likelihood of Lynch syndrome
  It used to be assumed that all mismatch repair deficiencies unassociated with

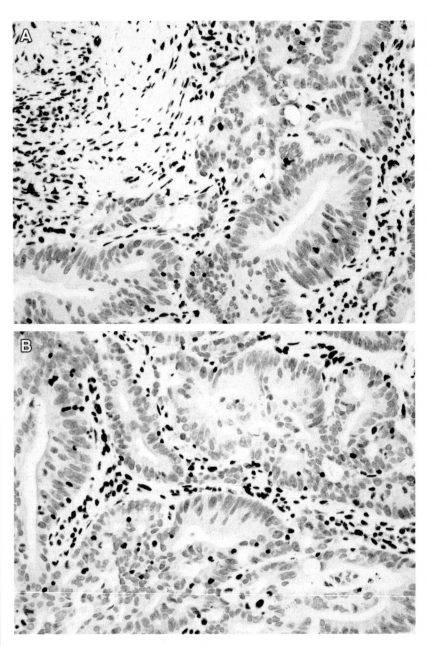

Fig. **6.** Interpretation challenges: tumor infiltrating lymphocytes and signet ring cell carcinoma. In this MSH2- (*A*) and MSH6-deficient (*B*) tumor, abundant brown-staining lymphocytes may be mistaken for immunoreactive tumor cells. Interpretation of a signet ring cell tumor can be challenging because of the discohesive cells with signet-shaped nuclei. The MLH1 stain (*C*) is lost in the scattered signet ring cells (*arrows*), which are surrounded by immunoreactive lymphocytes and benign epithelial cells (*arrowheads*). In the same case, MSH6 (*D*) is intact. Notice the tumor nuclei are larger and more atypical (*arrows*) than the background lymphocytes (*arrowheads*) [original magnification, (*A-D*) ×400].

MLH1 hypermethylation were due to Lynch syndrome, even if a germline mutation could not be confirmed with molecular testing. Family members were counseled to have lifelong surveillance. It is now clear that mismatch repair deficiency in cancers lacking both *MLH1* methylation and detectable germline mutations can often be explained by acquired, double somatic mutations in the tumor.[31,32] Recognizing somatic mutations and excluding possible Lynch syndrome alleviate patient anxiety and avoid unnecessary lifetime surveillance of patients and family members.

• Overlooking Lynch syndrome because of an erroneous assumption that intact mismatch

Fig. 6. (*continued*).

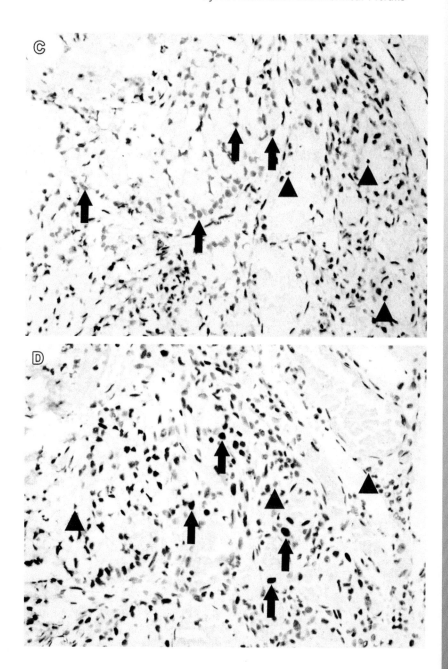

repair staining can never be seen in Lynch syndrome

Some germline alterations in mismatch repair genes produce nonfunctional proteins that retain their antigenicity. Lynch syndrome is rarely caused by a missense mutation that impairs protein function but does not induce intracellular protein degradation. The result is a dysfunctional protein with intact epitopes for antibody binding. Affected patients have a Lynch syndrome phenotype with defective mismatch repair mechanisms and elevated carcinoma risk, but their tumors

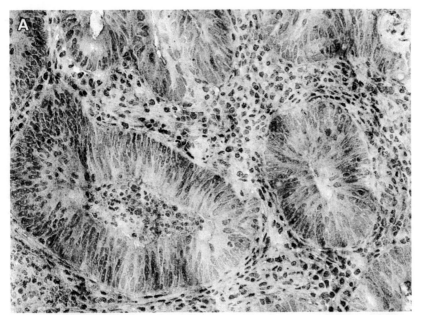

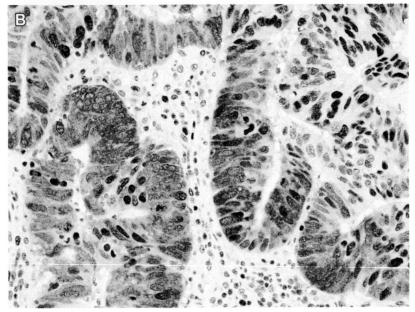

Fig. 7. Mismatch repair protein immunohisto-chemistry: cytoplasmic staining. Cytoplasmic staining sometimes oc-curs because of the high background (*A*); this should not be inter-preted as intact staining, unless accompanied by nuclear staining. When this case was repeated, nuclear staining was confirmed. This MSH6 stain (*B*) shows both cyto-plasmic and nuclear staining in the tumor cells, which represents intact MSH6 expression. This patient was found to be microsatellite sta-ble by PCR [original magnification, ×400].

show intact immunohistochemical stain-ing for all mismatch repair proteins (see example in **Fig. 4**A and **Table 3**). Molecu-lar testing of clinically suspected patients should be considered even if staining of all markers is intact.

- Attributing unusual patterns to failure of immunohistochemical stains

If all 4 mismatch repair proteins show lack of staining, the possibility of stain failure due to fixation or technical issues should be addressed by evaluating the control (see example in **Fig. 9**A, B). A null pattern of expression with loss of all 4 mismatch repair proteins in the presence of adequate controls has been described

Fig. *8.* Interpretation challenges: tumor staining weaker than internal control. This tumor shows weaker than control MLH1 staining in the tumor nuclei (*A, B*), whereas another tumor shows weaker than control MSH6 staining in the tumor nuclei (*C, D*). Both patients were found to have a germline mutation (MLH1 and MSH6, respectively) with additional workup [original magnification, (*A, C*) ×200, (*B, D*) ×400].

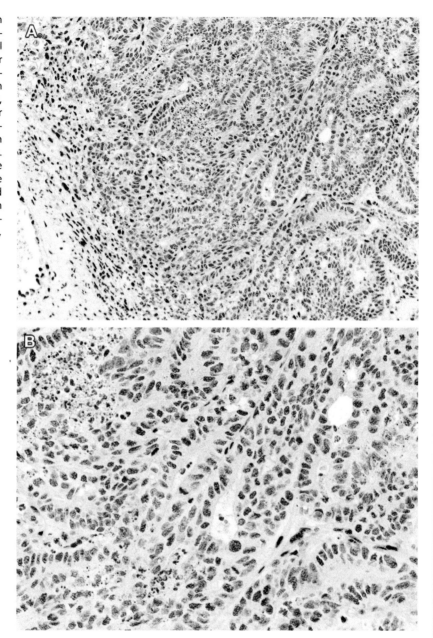

(see example in **Fig. 4**B). This pattern is due to a combination of a germline *MSH2* mutation (causing MSH2 and MSH6 loss) and sporadic *MLH1* methylation (leading to loss of MLH1 and PMS2 expression).[51] Another unusual pattern is loss of MLH1 and PMS2 staining together with either total or heterogeneous loss of MSH6 staining (see example in **Fig. 4**C–F). Clonal loss of MSH6 staining can be explained by a secondary mutation of mononucleotide repeats located in the coding region of *MSH6*. MSI resulting from defective *MLH1* causes a secondary mutation in *MSH6*, silencing it from expression.[43,44] If the controls are intact, these patterns should not be dismissed as a failure of

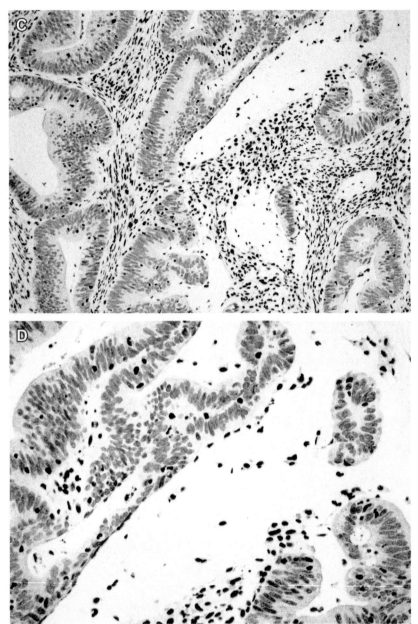

Fig. 8. (continued).

immunohistochemistry but described in the report. Examples of unusual staining patterns are listed in Table 3.

- Assuming adenomas are as useful as adenocarcinoma specimens to screen for Lynch syndrome

    Ideally, screening for Lynch syndrome using mismatch repair protein immunohistochemistry should be performed on adenocarcinomas, although the authors are sometimes asked to evaluate adenomas. With the exception of the extremely rare biallelic germline loss of mismatch repair genes (constitutional mismatch repair deficiency), Lynch syndrome is due to heterozygous germline mutations. Therefore, adenomas in Lynch syndrome may not yet have acquired a second event leading to loss of mismatch repair protein expression (Fig. 12). Halvarsson and

Fig. 9. Mismatch repair protein immunohisto-chemistry: technical problems. In this MLH1 stain, apparent hetero-geneous staining is present with areas showing complete loss with no staining in both tumor and background stroma (*A*) adjacent to areas with intact staining (*B*). MLH1 loss should not be diagnosed when the in-ternal positive control is negative as illustrated in (*A*). In some cases, the staining is variable because of uneven anti-body diffusion into the tissue. Notice the periph-ery of the tissue (*C, D, right*) stains darker than the tumor nuclei in the inner portion of the tis-sue (*C, D, left*). Both cases were found to be micro-satellite stable by PCR [original magnification, (*A-D*) ×400].

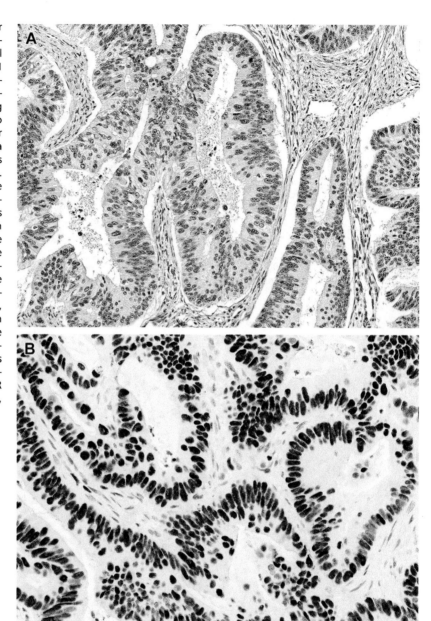

colleagues[52] found that 66% of ade-nomas from patients with Lynch syn-drome show loss of mismatch repair protein expression, with an even higher percentage (88%) in large adenomas (>5 mm). Adenomas with high-grade dysplasia, a villous component, or size greater than 10 mm are more likely to have the second mutation leading to loss of protein expression.[53–55] There-fore, patients with Lynch syndrome can have adenomas with intact mismatch repair protein expression. When reporting results for intact mismatch repair immu-nohistochemistry on adenomas, a comment should always be included that Lynch syndrome cannot be excluded.

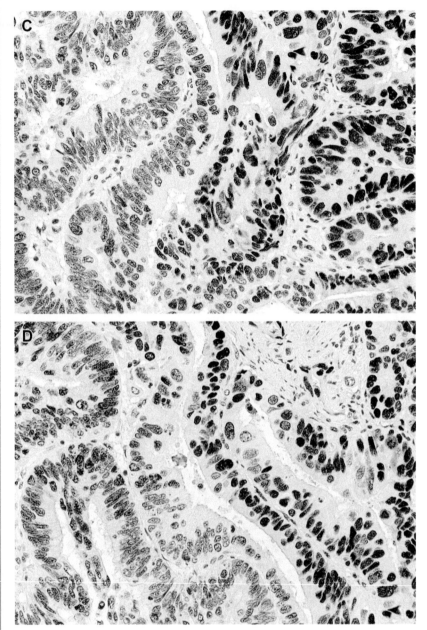

Fig. 9. (continued).

- Using sessile serrated adenomas to screen for Lynch syndrome or to help categorize the type of serrated polyp

    Sessile serrated adenomas should not be used to screen for Lynch syndrome. The adenoma is the cancer precursor lesion of Lynch syndrome, not a serrated polyp.[54,56,57] Some serrated polyps follow the serrated pathway to microsatellite unstable carcinoma through sporadic *BRAF* mutation and *MLH1* methylation. However, these changes are not typically found until the serrated polyps become dysplastic and dysplasia is usually recognizable using routine histochemical stains. Mismatch repair protein expression is not routinely suggested when subclassifying serrated polyps.[55]

- Not considering constitutional mismatch repair deficiency (CMMRD) when tumor and

Fig. 10. Mismatch repair protein immunohistochemistry: rectal cancer after neoadjuvant treatment. Intact staining is present with MLH1 (*A*), PMS2 (*B*), and MSH2 (*C*) in this rectal tumor treated with neoadjuvant chemoradiation therapy. However, MSH6 (*D*) shows a peculiar nucleolar staining pattern. MSH6 stain repeated on the pre-treatment rectal biopsy reveals intact nuclear staining (*E*, hematoxylin and eosin; *F*, MSH6). In addition, the tumor was found to be microsatellite stable by PCR [original magnification, ×200].

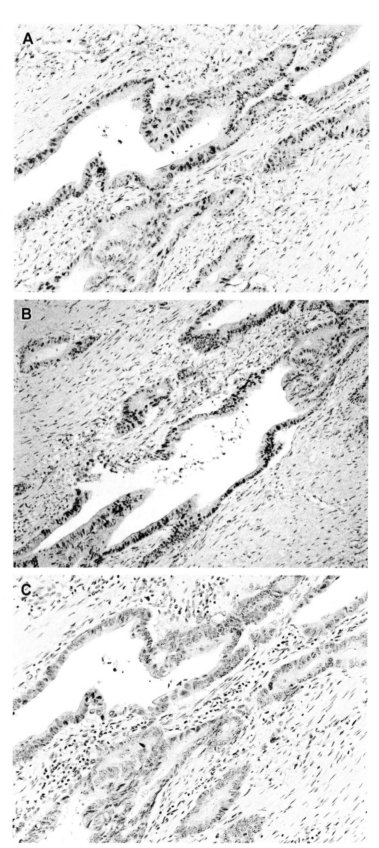

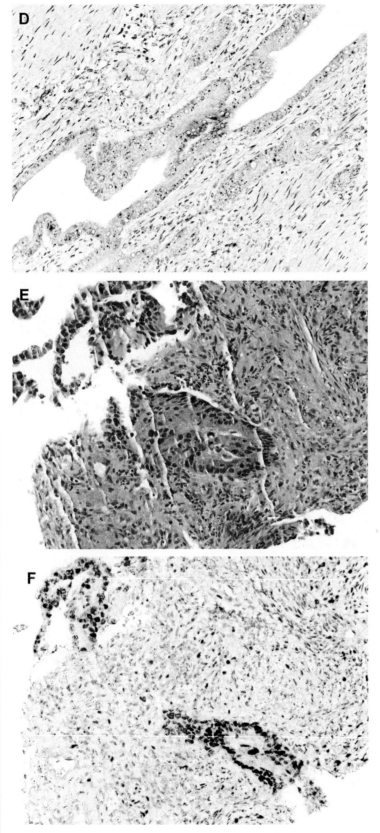

Fig. 10. (*continued*).

Fig. 11. Mismatch repair protein immunohistochemistry: rectal cancer after neoadjuvant treatment, challenging examples. Another example of treated rectal cancer with intact MLH1, MSH2, and PMS2 staining (*A,* MLH1) but apparently decreased MSH6 staining (*B, arrows* pointing to the occasional, variable, immunoreactive tumor nuclei). (*C, D*) Other examples of abnormal MSH6 staining in treated tumor. Image (*C*) shows predominantly nucleolar staining. Image (*D*) demonstrates decreased staining (*arrow* pointing to one immuno-reactive tumor nucleus, *arrowheads* pointing to decreased/ lost staining in tumor nuclei; notice the appropriate positive internal control). All cases should be interpreted as intact MSH6 staining. These cases were found to be microsatellite stable by PCR [original magnification, (*A-D*) ×400].

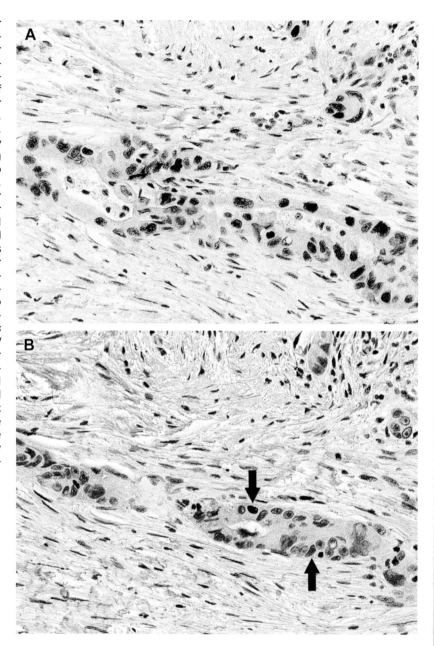

internal control fail to stain even after mismatch repair immunohistochemistry is repeated

Mismatch repair immunohistochemistry failure due to technical issues with the stain or tissue is the most likely reason for absent mismatch repair staining in both tumor and background non-neoplastic tissue. However, this can also be seen in CMMRD, due to biallelic germline mutation of a mismatch repair gene. In these cases, the external positive control will still stain and can suggest either a problem with the tissue or

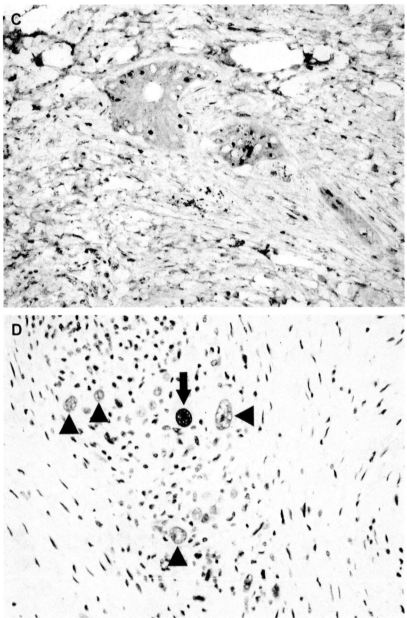

Fig. 11. (continued).

CMMRD. Therefore, if internal (but not external) controls fail to stain after repeat immunohistochemistry, additional testing either on other tissue and/or molecular testing should be recommended. The rare possibility of CMMRD should be included in the differential for these cases.

SUMMARY

Approximately 15% of all colorectal cancers are mismatch repair deficient. Most of these are sporadic, but a minority result from germline alterations in mismatch repair genes. The latter represent Lynch syndrome, which is important to recognize

Fig. 12. Mismatch repair protein immunohistochemistry: adenoma and adenocarcinoma. A case with *MSH2* germline mutation shows (*A–D*) an adenocarcinoma (*arrowheads*) arising in a tubular adenoma (*arrows*). MLH1 expression (*B*) is intact in both adenoma and adenocarcinoma, whereas MSH2 (*C, D*) is lost in adenocarcinoma while retained in the adenoma. PMS2 stains similarly to MLH1 and MSH6 similarly to MSH2 (not shown) [original magnification, (*A-C*) ×100, *D* ×400].

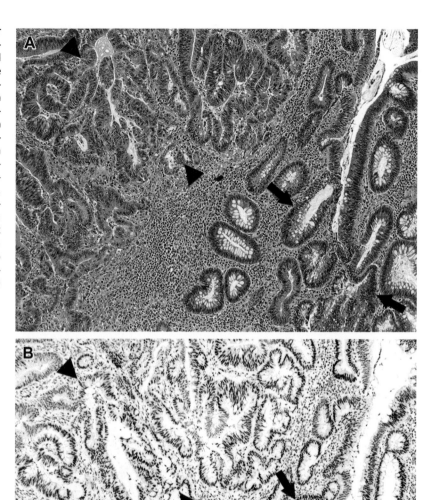

in order to institute appropriate screening and surveillance for affected patients and their families. Recognition of sporadic cases is also important because it averts costs associated with unnecessary surveillance. Mismatch repair protein immunohistochemistry is widely used to detect mismatch repair deficiency and is a valuable screening tool for identifying patients with Lynch syndrome. Interpretation of immunohistochemical stains can be challenging because of technical issues as well as unusual staining patterns. Avoiding interpretive pitfalls is crucial for practicing surgical pathologists to

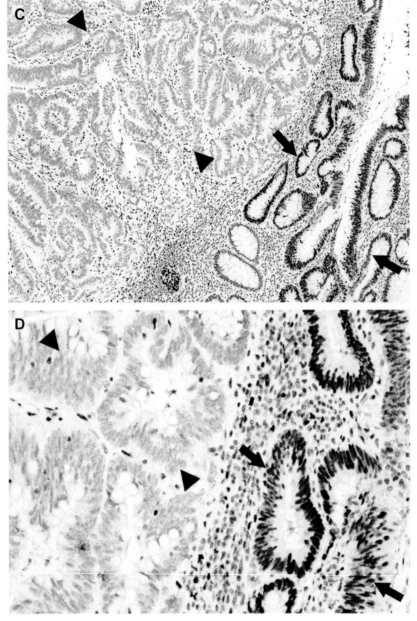

Fig. 12. (*continued*).

accurately identify possible patients with Lynch syndrome and helps to save cost and anxiety for patients and family members.

REFERENCES

1. Hampel H, Frankel WL, Martin E, et al. Feasibility of screening for Lynch syndrome among patients with colorectal cancer. J Clin Oncol 2008;26(35):5783–8.

2. Hampel H, Frankel WL, Martin E, et al. Screening for the Lynch syndrome (hereditary nonpolyposis colorectal cancer). N Engl J Med 2005;352(18):1851–60.

3. Lynch HT, Lynch PM, Lanspa SJ, et al. Review of the Lynch syndrome: history, molecular genetics, screening, differential diagnosis, and medicolegal ramifications. Clin Genet 2009;76(1):1–18.

4. Ligtenberg MJ, Kuiper RP, Chan TL, et al. Heritable somatic methylation and inactivation of MSH2 in

families with Lynch syndrome due to deletion of the 3' exons of TACSTD1. Nat Genet 2009;41(1):112–7.

5. Lynch HT, Snyder CL, Shaw TG, et al. Milestones of Lynch syndrome: 1895-2015. Nat Rev Cancer 2015; 15(3):181–94.

6. Evaluation of Genomic Applications in Practice and Prevention (EGAPP) Working Group. Recommendations from the EGAPP Working Group: genetic testing strategies in newly diagnosed individuals with colorectal cancer aimed at reducing morbidity and mortality from Lynch syndrome in relatives. Genet Med 2009;11(1):35–41.

7. Hampel H. NCCN increases the emphasis on genetic/familial high-risk assessment in colorectal cancer. J Natl Compr Canc Netw 2014;12(5 Suppl): 829–31.

8. Giardiello FM, Allen JI, Axilbund JE, et al. Guidelines on genetic evaluation and management of Lynch syndrome: a consensus statement by the US Multi-Society Task Force on colorectal cancer. Gastroenterology 2014;147(2):502–26.

9. Syngal S, Brand RE, Church JM, et al. ACG clinical guideline: genetic testing and management of hereditary gastrointestinal cancer syndromes. Am J Gastroenterol 2015;110(2):223–62, [quiz: 263].

10. Stoffel EM, Mangu PB, Gruber SB, et al, American Society of Clinical Oncology, European Society for Medical Oncology. Hereditary colorectal cancer syndromes: American Society of Clinical Oncology clinical practice guideline endorsement of the familial risk-colorectal cancer: European society for medical oncology clinical practice guidelines. J Clin Oncol 2015;33(2):209–17.

11. Lynch HT, Lynch J. Lynch syndrome: genetics, natural history, genetic counseling, and prevention. J Clin Oncol 2000;18(21 Suppl):19S–31S.

12. Mvundura M, Grosse SD, Hampel H, et al. The cost-effectiveness of genetic testing strategies for Lynch syndrome among newly diagnosed patients with colorectal cancer. Genet Med 2010;12(2):93–104.

13. Palomaki GE, McClain MR, Melillo S, et al. EGAPP supplementary evidence review: DNA testing strategies aimed at reducing morbidity and mortality from Lynch syndrome. Genet Med 2009;11(1):42–65.

14. Kawakami H, Zaanan A, Sinicrope FA. Microsatellite instability testing and its role in the management of colorectal cancer. Curr Treat Options Oncol 2015; 16(7):30.

15. Le DT, Uram JN, Wang H, et al. PD-1 blockade in tumors with mismatch-repair deficiency. N Engl J Med 2015;372(26):2509–20.

16. Shia J. Immunohistochemistry versus microsatellite instability testing for screening colorectal cancer patients at risk for hereditary nonpolyposis colorectal cancer syndrome. Part I. The utility of immunohistochemistry. J Mol Diagn 2008;10(4):293–300.

17. Zhang L. Immunohistochemistry versus microsatellite instability testing for screening colorectal cancer patients at risk for hereditary nonpolyposis colorectal cancer syndrome. Part II. The utility of microsatellite instability testing. J Mol Diagn 2008;10(4): 301–7.

18. de Jong AE, van Puijenbroek M, Hendriks Y, et al. Microsatellite instability, immunohistochemistry, and additional PMS2 staining in suspected hereditary nonpolyposis colorectal cancer. Clin Cancer Res 2004;10(3):972–80.

19. Lindor NM, Burgart LJ, Leontovich O, et al. Immunohistochemistry versus microsatellite instability testing in phenotyping colorectal tumors. J Clin Oncol 2002;20(4):1043–8.

20. Southey MC, Jenkins MA, Mead L, et al. Use of molecular tumor characteristics to prioritize mismatch repair gene testing in early-onset colorectal cancer. J Clin Oncol 2005;23(27):6524–32.

21. Salahshor S, Koelble K, Rubio C, et al. Microsatellite Instability and hMLH1 and hMSH2 expression analysis in familial and sporadic colorectal cancer. Lab Invest 2001;81(4):535–41.

22. Domingo E, Laiho P, Ollikainen M, et al. BRAF screening as a low-cost effective strategy for simplifying HNPCC genetic testing. J Med Genet 2004; 41(9):664–8.

23. Jin M, Hampel H, Zhou X, et al. BRAF V600E mutation analysis simplifies the testing algorithm for Lynch syndrome. Am J Clin Pathol 2013;140(2): 177–83.

24. Mills AM, Longacre TA. Lynch syndrome: female genital tract cancer diagnosis and screening. Surg Pathol Clin 2016;9(2):201–14.

25. Pai RK, Pai RK. A practical approach to the evaluation of gastrointestinal tract carcinomas for Lynch syndrome. Am J Surg Pathol 2016;40(4):e17–34.

26. Peltomaki P. Update on Lynch syndrome genomics. Fam Cancer 2016;15(3):385–93.

27. Bartley AN, Hamilton SR, Alsabeh R, et al. Template for reporting results of biomarker testing of specimens from patients with carcinoma of the colon and rectum. Arch Pathol Lab Med 2014;138(2): 166–70.

28. Chang CL, Marra G, Chauhan DP, et al. Oxidative stress inactivates the human DNA mismatch repair system. Am J Physiol Cell Physiol 2002;283(1): C148–54.

29. Mihaylova VT, Bindra RS, Yuan J, et al. Decreased expression of the DNA mismatch repair gene Mlh1 under hypoxic stress in mammalian cells. Mol Cell Biol 2003;23(9):3265–73.

30. Rodriguez-Soler M, Perez-Carbonell L, Guarinos C, et al. Risk of cancer in cases of suspected lynch syndrome without germline mutation. Gastroenterology 2013;144(5):926–32.e1, [quiz: e13–4].

31. Geurts-Giele WR, Leenen CH, Dubbink HJ, et al. Somatic aberrations of mismatch repair genes as a cause of microsatellite-unstable cancers. J Pathol 2014;234(4):548–59.

32. Haraldsdottir S, Hampel H, Tomsic J, et al. Colon and endometrial cancers with mismatch repair deficiency can arise from somatic, rather than germline, mutations. Gastroenterology 2014;147(6): 1308–16.e1.

33. Al-Tassan N, Chmiel NH, Maynard J, et al. Inherited variants of MYH associated with somatic G: C–>T: a mutations in colorectal tumors. Nat Genet 2002; 30(2):227–32.

34. Morak M, Heidenreich B, Keller G, et al. Biallelic MUTYH mutations can mimic Lynch syndrome. Eur J Hum Genet 2014;22(11):1334–7.

35. Nielsen M, de Miranda NF, van Puijenbroek M, et al. Colorectal carcinomas in MUTYH-associated polyposis display histopathological similarities to microsatellite unstable carcinomas. BMC Cancer 2009;9:184.

36. Buchanan DD, Rosty C, Clendenning M, et al. Clinical problems of colorectal cancer and endometrial cancer cases with unknown cause of tumor mismatch repair deficiency (suspected Lynch syndrome). Appl Clin Genet 2014;7:183–93.

37. Pastrello C, Fornasarig M, Pin E, et al. Somatic mosaicism in a patient with Lynch syndrome. Am J Med Genet A 2009;149A(2):212–5.

38. Sourrouille I, Coulet F, Lefevre JH, et al. Somatic mosaicism and double somatic hits can lead to MSI colorectal tumors. Fam Cancer 2013;12(1): 27–33.

39. Hitchins M, Williams R, Cheong K, et al. MLH1 germline epimutations as a factor in hereditary nonpolyposis colorectal cancer. Gastroenterology 2005; 129(5):1392–9.

40. Hitchins MP, Rapkins RW, Kwok CT, et al. Dominantly inherited constitutional epigenetic silencing of MLH1 in a cancer-affected family is linked to a single nucleotide variant within the 5'UTR. Cancer Cell 2011;20(2):200–13.

41. Ward RL, Dobbins T, Lindor NM, et al. Identification of constitutional MLH1 epimutations and promoter variants in colorectal cancer patients from the Colon Cancer Family Registry. Genet Med 2013;15(1):25–35.

42. Sekine S, Ogawa R, Saito S, et al. Cytoplasmic MSH2 immunoreactivity in a patient with Lynch syndrome with an EPCAM-MSH2 fusion. Histopathology 2017;70(4):664–9.

43. Graham RP, Kerr SE, Butz ML, et al. Heterogenous MSH6 loss is a result of microsatellite instability within MSH6 and occurs in sporadic and hereditary colorectal and endometrial carcinomas. Am J Surg Pathol 2015;39(10):1370–6.

44. Shia J, Zhang L, Shike M, et al. Secondary mutation in a coding mononucleotide tract in MSH6 causes loss of immunoexpression of MSH6 in colorectal carcinomas with MLH1/PMS2 deficiency. Mod Pathol 2013;26(1):131–8.

45. Kumarasinghe AP, de Boer B, Bateman AC, et al. DNA mismatch repair enzyme immunohistochemistry in colorectal cancer: a comparison of biopsy and resection material. Pathology 2010;42(5):414–20.

46. Shia J, Stadler Z, Weiser MR, et al. Immunohistochemical staining for DNA mismatch repair proteins in intestinal tract carcinoma: how reliable are biopsy samples? Am J Surg Pathol 2011;35(3):447–54.

47. Vilkin A, Leibovici-Weissman Y, Halpern M, et al. Immunohistochemistry staining for mismatch repair proteins: the endoscopic biopsy material provides useful and coherent results. Hum Pathol 2015; 46(11):1705–11.

48. Bao F, Panarelli NC, Rennert H, et al. Neoadjuvant therapy induces loss of MSH6 expression in colorectal carcinoma. Am J Surg Pathol 2010;34(12): 1798–804.

49. Radu OM, Nikiforova MN, Farkas LM, et al. Challenging cases encountered in colorectal cancer screening for Lynch syndrome reveal novel findings: nucleolar MSH6 staining and impact of prior chemoradiation therapy. Hum Pathol 2011;42(9):1247–58.

50. Vilkin A, Halpern M, Morgenstern S, et al. How reliable is immunohistochemical staining for DNA mismatch repair proteins performed after neoadjuvant chemoradiation? Hum Pathol 2014;45(10): 2029–36.

51. Hagen CE, Lefferts J, Hornick JL, et al. "Null pattern" of immunoreactivity in a Lynch syndrome-associated colon cancer due to germline MSH2 mutation and somatic MLH1 hypermethylation. Am J Surg Pathol 2011;35(12):1902–5.

52. Halvarsson B, Lindblom A, Johansson L, et al. Loss of mismatch repair protein immunostaining in colorectal adenomas from patients with hereditary nonpolyposis colorectal cancer. Mod Pathol 2005; 18(8):1095–101.

53. Kalady MF, Kravochuck SE, Heald B, et al. Defining the adenoma burden in lynch syndrome. Dis Colon Rectum 2015;58(4):388–92.

54. Walsh MD, Buchanan DD, Pearson SA, et al. Immunohistochemical testing of conventional adenomas for loss of expression of mismatch repair proteins in Lynch syndrome mutation carriers: a case series from the Australasian site of the colon cancer family registry. Mod Pathol 2012;25(5):722–30.

55. Yurgelun MB, Goel A, Hornick JL, et al. Microsatellite instability and DNA mismatch repair protein deficiency in Lynch syndrome colorectal polyps. Cancer Prev Res (Phila) 2012;5(4):574–82.

56. Bae JM, Kim JH, Kang GH. Molecular subtypes of colorectal cancer and their clinicopathologic features, with an emphasis on the serrated neoplasia pathway. Arch Pathol Lab Med 2016;140(5): 406–12.

57. Jass JR. Classification of colorectal cancer based on correlation of clinical, morphological and molecular features. Histopathology 2007;50(1): 113–30.

58. Boland CR, Goel A. Microsatellite instability in colorectal cancer. Gastroenterology 2010;138(6): 2073–87.e3.

59. Dudley B, Brand RE, Thull D, et al. Germline MLH1 mutations are frequently identified in Lynch syndrome patients with colorectal and endometrial carcinoma demonstrating isolated loss of PMS2 immunohistochemical expression. Am J Surg Pathol 2015;39(8):1114–20.

60. Kato A, Sato N, Sugawara T, et al. Isolated loss of PMS2 immunohistochemical expression is frequently caused by heterogenous MLH1 promoter hypermethylation in Lynch syndrome screening for endometrial cancer patients. Am J Surg Pathol 2016;40(6):770–6.

61. Rosty C, Clendenning M, Walsh MD, et al. Germline mutations in PMS2 and MLH1 in individuals with solitary loss of PMS2 expression in colorectal carcinomas from the colon cancer family registry cohort. BMJ Open 2016;6(2):e010293.

62. Haraldsdottir S, Roth R, Pearlman R, et al. Mismatch repair deficiency concordance between primary colorectal cancer and corresponding metastasis. Fam Cancer 2016;15(2):253–60.

63. Roth RM, Haraldsdottir S, Hampel H, et al. Discordant mismatch repair protein immunoreactivity in Lynch syndrome-associated neoplasms: a recommendation for screening synchronous/metachronous neoplasms. Am J Clin Pathol 2016;146(1):50–6.

Molecular Testing of Colorectal Cancer in the Modern Era
What Are We Doing and Why?

Efsevia Vakiani, MD, PhD

KEYWORDS

• Molecular testing • Colorectal cancer • Next-generation sequencing

---

Key points

- Microsatellite instability testing is recommended for all patients with colorectal cancer. It is important in identifying patients with Lynch syndrome in addition to guiding therapeutic decisions.

- Extended RAS gene mutation testing is recommended for patients who are being considered for therapy with inhibitors of the epidermal growth factor receptor.

- Next-generation sequencing assays are increasingly used in clinical molecular pathology laboratories; in addition to detecting specific genetic events they can provide information about microsatellite instability status.

ABSTRACT

A plethora of tests are routinely ordered and interpreted by pathologists to assist the management of colorectal cancer patients. Many of these tests are immunohistochemistry assays using antibodies against prognostically relevant proteins, some of which predict therapeutic response. This review focuses on tissue DNA-based tests. It presents novel methodologies for assessing well-established biomarkers, updates the expanding spectrum of genetic alterations that are associated with resistance to inhibition of epidermal growth factor receptor signaling, and briefly discusses emerging actionable alterations that may translate into new therapeutic options for colorectal cancer patients. The utility of next-generation sequencing is emphasized.

OVERVIEW

Colorectal cancer is the fourth most frequently diagnosed cancer in the United States, affecting approximately 8% of women and men.[1] A majority of adenocarcinomas arise from conventional adenomas; histologic progression is accompanied by accumulation of molecular changes.[2] Most commonly, the initiating event is a mutation in *APC*, which results in activation of the WNT/β-catenin pathway. Mutations in *RAS/RAF* constitutively activate the mitogen-activated protein kinase (MAPK) pathway to promote tumor growth. Subsequent clonal expansion results from alterations in several genes, including *TP53* and *SMAD4*, and is usually associated with chromosomal instability.[3] A minority of cancers develop through a different pathway characterized by microsatellite instability (MSI); these tumors may be sporadic or associated with Lynch syndrome.[4]

Despite improvements in detection, prevention, and management, colorectal carcinoma remains the second leading cause of cancer-related death with more than 50,000 deaths reported in 2014.[5] Targeted therapies for patients with unresectable metastatic colorectal cancer consist of bevacizumab, a monoclonal antibody against vascular

---

The author has no conflicts of interest to disclose.
Department of Pathology, Memorial Sloan Kettering Cancer Center, 1275 York Avenue, New York, NY 10065, USA
E-mail address: vakianie@mskcc.org

Surgical Pathology 10 (2017) 1009–1020
http://dx.doi.org/10.1016/j.path.2017.07.013
1875-9181/17/© 2017 Elsevier Inc. All rights reserved.

endothelial growth factor A, as well as cetuximab and panitumumab, 2 monoclonal antibodies against the epidermal growth factor receptor (EGFR).[6] Clinical trials assessing novel molecules and drugs that are effective in other tumor types are currently under way.

ESTABLISHED BIOMARKERS

MICROSATELLITE INSTABILITY

Microsatellites are short sequences of genomic DNA containing repeats that are prone to mistakes during replication. Defective DNA mismatch repair mechanisms result in alterations of microsatellite length, which can be used to assess for mismatch repair proficiency. Approximately 15% of colorectal cancers show MSI, and most of these arise sporadically through hypermethylation of the *MLH1* promoter. Approximately 3% of microsatellite unstable colon cancers occur in patients with deleterious germline alterations in *MLH1*, *MSH2*, *MSH6* and *PMS2*, or *EPCAM*. *EPCAM* is located immediately upstream of *MSH2*; deletions in its terminal region result in *MSH2* promoter hypermethylation and inactivation.[7]

MSI can be assessed in several ways. The approach most familiar to surgical pathologists is immunohistochemical staining with antibodies directed against MLH1, MSH2, MSH6, and PMS2, as detailed in Michael Markow and colleagues' article, "Immunohistochemical Pitfalls: Common Mistakes in the Evaluation of Lynch Syndrome," in this issue. Polymerase chain reaction (PCR) using fluorescently labeled primers against select microsatellites is the principal DNA-based method used when testing for MSI. The currently recommended panel of microsatellites consists of 5 mononucleotide repeats. Both tumor and normal DNA are required for analysis (**Fig. 1**). Microsatellite stable tumors show similar peak profiles when tumor DNA is compared with that of non-neoplastic tissue from the same patient, whereas unstable tumors show expansion or contraction of greater than or equal to 30% of examined loci (≥2 when a panel of 5 microsatellites is used). Instability at only 1 locus is classified as indeterminate, because this finding may be seen in some patients with Lynch syndrome; low-frequency MSI has been used to describe instability at 1 locus but is appropriate terminology only when the Bethesda panel (ie, 2 dinucleotide and 3 mononucleotide repeats) is used.

Next-generation sequencing (NGS) is increasingly used to assess for MSI. Stadler and colleagues[8] evaluated 224 tumors sequenced with a 341-gene NGS panel and found that all tumors with less than 20 mutations were mismatch repair proficient, whereas those with 20 mutations to 150 mutations were mismatch repair deficient. Three cases with greater than 150 mutations were microsatellite stable but had hotspot mutations in the central catalytic subunit of the DNA polymerase epsilon (*POLE*) gene, consistent with the ultramutator phenotype described in both colorectal and endometrial carcinomas.[8–10] Bioinformatics tools can also be used to analyze NGS data and predict microsatellite status. Niu and colleagues[11] developed MSIsensor, a software program that uses paired tumor-normal NGS data to predict MSI and found an excellent correlation between results obtained from PCR using 5 microsatellite sequences. Salipante and colleagues[12] developed a method (mSINGS) to infer microsatellite status

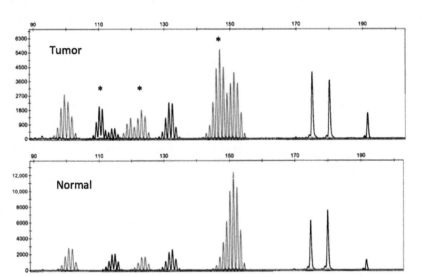

Fig. 1. Example of a tumor showing microsatellite instability using the PCR method. Capillary electrophoresis tracings afer PCR of 5 microsatellites markers show that 3 of the 5 markers (*asterisks*) show variability in their length in the tumor DNA compared with what is seen in normal DNA.

based on a comparison between the number of differently sized repeats in microsatellites of a tumor and a population of normal controls. They found that the sensitivity and specificity of their approach were highest when using whole-exome sequencing data, although data from targeted NGS panels showed greater than 95% sensitivity and specificity for detection of MSI. More recently, Kautto and colleagues[13] introduced a new tool, MANTIS, which, similar to MSIsensor, uses data from normal-tumor NGS, but, unlike MSIsensor, assesses aggregate instability instead of individual loci differences.

The 2016 NCCN guidelines recommend universal testing for all patients with colorectal cancer.[14] The most well-established indication for determining microsatellite status is identification of families with Lynch syndrome. Results of microsatellite stability testing, however, are also incorporated into management decisions regarding patients with

colorectal cancer (Table 1). Tumors with MSI have an improved stage-specific prognosis compared with microsatellite stable tumors,[15] and affected patients do not derive benefit from 5-fluorouracil–based chemotherapy.[16–18] MSI is also a positive predictor of response to immunotherapy. Pembrolizumab is an anti–PD-1 (programmed cell death protein 1) immune checkpoint inhibitor that induces an objective response in 40% of patients with treatment-refractory metastatic, microsatellite unstable colorectal cancers.[19] Immunoexpression of PD-1 ligands on tumor cells does not seem to be a predictive marker of response to PD-1 blockade.[19]

MLH1 PROMOTER HYPERMETHYLATION

Given that most microsatellite unstable tumors occur sporadically, detecting MSI in a given tumor is only a first step toward establishing the presence of Lynch syndrome. The diagnosis is

Table 1
Selected biomarkers in colorectal cancer

Biomarker	Indication for Testing	Colorectal Cancer Patients who Should Be Tested
MSI	• Identification of Lynch syndrome patients • Predictor of resistance to 5-fluorouracil-based therapy in stage II patients • Predictor of response to immunotherapy	Universal testing recommended
MLH1 promoter hypermethylation	• Identification of sporadic microsatellite unstable tumors	Patients with microsatellite unstable tumors
Mutations in KRAS codons 12 and 13	• Predictor of resistance to EGFR inhibition	Patients with stage IV disease who are candidates for treatment with EGFR inhibitors
Mutations in other KRAS and NRAS codons	• Predictor of resistance to EGFR inhibition	Patients with stage IV disease who are candidates for treatment with EGFR inhibitors
BRAF V600E mutation	• Identification of sporadic microsatellite unstable tumors • Predictor of resistance to EGFR inhibition • Predictor of response to BRAF V600E inhibitors (investigational)	Patients with microsatellite unstable tumors Recommended for patients with stage IV disease who are candidates for treatment with EGFR inhibitors
PIK3CA mutations	• Predictor of resistance to EGFR inhibition • Predictor of response to prophylactic aspirin use	Currently investigational
HER2 amplification; HER2 mutations	• Predictor of resistance to EGFR inhibition • Response to HER2 inhibitors	Currently investigational

ultimately based on identifying germline pathogenic events, which is costly and time consuming. Testing for *MLH1* promoter hypermethylation can reduce the number of patients referred for germline testing. Methylation of *MLH1* is responsible for most sporadic cancers with MSI and often reflects more widespread methylation affecting multiple genes, a process termed, *CpG island methylator phenotype*. These CpG islands are stretches of DNA rich in CG dinucleotide sequences found in many gene promoters and aberrant methylation results in silencing of several important genes. The mechanisms underlying aberrant methylation are not entirely clear but may result from increased DNA methyltransferase activity via genetic or epigenetic mechanisms.[20] Although *MLH1* promoter hypermethylation usually implies a sporadic tumor, Lynch syndrome can result from germline *MLH1* promoter hypermethylation.[21,22] *MLH1* hypermethylation is reportedly only 66% specific for a sporadic tumor according to some investigators.[23] Thus, patients with tumors that show *MLH1* promoter hypermethylation may be considered for germline testing when there is a strong clinical suspicion for Lynch syndrome.[24]

RAS MUTATIONS

Members of the RAS family are small guanine nucleotide-binding proteins that alternate between an inactive GDP-bound and an active GTP-bound state. They regulate many cellular processes, including proliferation and apoptosis, and are encoded by 3 genes *KRAS*, *NRAS*, and *HRAS*. RAS proteins are tightly regulated, but mutations in key regions result in constitutive activation and uncontrolled cell growth. Such mutations are observed frequently in a variety of human tumor types, including colorectal carcinoma: 30% to 40% of cases harbor *KRAS* exon 2 mutations in codons 12 and 13.[25,26] Another 15% to 20% of tumors have mutations in *KRAS* exons 3 (codon 61) and 4 (codons 117 and 146) as well as mutations in *NRAS* exons 2 to 4 (**Fig. 2**).[25,26]

The RAS proteins act as a key signal transducer for several cellular receptors, including EGFR (**Fig. 3**). As such, the presence of *RAS* mutations downstream of EGFR render tumors insensitive to inhibitors of EGFR-mediated cell signaling. Mutations in KRAS codons 12 and 13 predict a lack of response when cetuximab or panitumumab was given as a single agent or in combination with chemotherapy.[27–29] Not all exon 2 mutations are equivalent, however. Data from retrospective studies indicate that KRAS G13D mutant tumors show a modest response to anti-EGFR therapy, although the degree of tumor response is unlikely sufficient to warrant use of EGFR inhibitors in this setting.[30] The Food and Drug Administration has restricted use of cetuximab and panitumumab to patients whose tumors did not harbor mutations in *KRAS* exon 2; testing for these mutations is mandatory among patients considered candidates for anti-EGFR therapy. Nonetheless, approximately 40% of patients with KRAS codons 12 and 13 wild-type tumors fail to respond to cetuximab and panitumumab.[31,32] In some of these patients resistance was attributed to the presence of RAS mutations affecting other codons.[33–35] The most recent 2016 National Comprehensive Cancer Network (NCCN) guidelines state that patients with any known *KRAS* or *NRAS* mutation should not receive an EGFR inhibitor, and this opinion is shared by the American Society of Clinical Oncology.[14,36]

BRAF V600E MUTATION

BRAF is a serine/threonine protein similar to RAS proteins and an integral mediator of EGFR

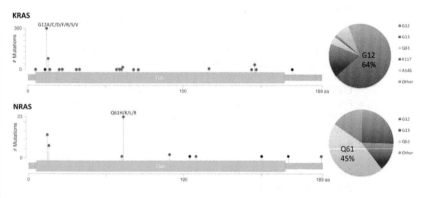

Fig. 2. Distribution of mutations in the *KRAS* (*top*) and *NRAS* (*bottom*) genes in a cohort of 1274 colorectal adenocarcinomas that underwent NGS at Memorial Sloan Kettering Cancer Center. KRAS mutations were seen in 45% of cases, whereas NRAS mutations were seen in 4% of cases. Pie charts show the percentage of RAS mutations in each codon. Mutations at the G12 codon are the most common ones in KRAS, in NRAS Q61 is the most commonly mutated codon.

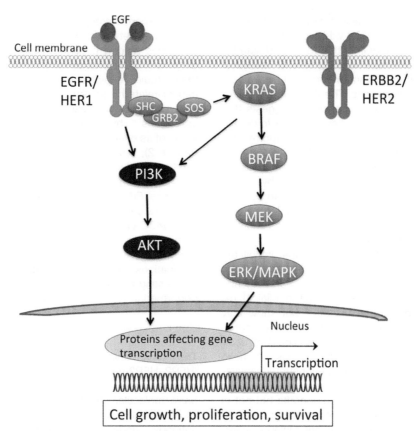

Fig. 3. Schematic representation of the EGFR signaling pathway. Binding of growth factors to the extracellular part of EGFR activates the receptor, which in turn turns on cytoplasmic proteins that are part of important signaling pathways, including the KRAS/BRAF/MAPK and PI3K/AKT pathways. Ultimately, several factors are activated within the nucleus, which regulate the transcription of key genes regulating cell growth, proliferation, and survival. Cetuximab and panitumumb are antibodies that bind the extracellular portion of EGFR preventing ligand binding. HER2 has a similar structure to EGFR although it does not have a known endogenous ligand. It also signals through the KRAS/BRAF/MAPK and PI3K/AKT pathways. Trastuzumab is a is an antibody that binds the extracellular part of HER2 preventing activation, whereas molecules like lapatinib and neratinib bind the intracellular portion of HER2 also blocking activation.

signaling (see **Fig. 3**). Mutations in *BRAF* are detected in 10% to 15% of colorectal carcinomas. The most prevalent mutation is a T to A transversion at nucleotide 1799 that results in a valine to glutamate change at residue 600 (V600E) that leads to a constitutively active protein. The presence of a BRAF V600E mutation can be useful in categorizing a microsatellite unstable tumor as sporadic or familial.[37] The mutation is present in approximately 50% of sporadic colorectal carcinomas with MSI but is generally lacking in colorectal cancers from patients with Lynch syndrome. Occasional patients with tumors that show MSI and *BRAF* mutations still prove, however, to have Lynch syndrome, emphasizing the importance of interpreting test results in the context of all available clinical data, including family history.[38]

Detection of BRAF V600E mutation influences prognosis and may affect treatment decisions. Many studies have shown BRAF V600E mutations to confer a poor prognosis among all stage IV patients as well as patients with stage II–III microsatellite stable tumors.[39–41] Given that BRAF mediates EGFR signaling, the V600E mutation might be expected to predict lack of response to EGFR inhibitors. Several studies have shown a lack of response to cetuximab or panitumumab among patients with BRAF mutant tumors.[34,41] Investigators of a recent meta-analysis of data from 9 phase III trials and 1 phase II trial concluded that the addition of an EGFR inhibitor does not improve progression-free survival or objective response rates among patients with *BRAF* mutant tumors.[42] On the other hand, data from another meta-analysis based on 7 randomized controlled trials suggest there are insufficient data to justify exclusion of patients with *RAS* wild-type/*BRAF* mutant tumors from anti-EGFR therapy.[43] Admittedly, the latter analysis used different statistical methods and inclusion criteria that may have affected the conclusions. The 2016 NCCN guidelines state, "evidence increasingly suggests that BRAF V600E mutation makes response to cetuximab or panitumumab highly unlikely" and recommend *BRAF* genotyping of tumor tissue in patients with stage IV disease.[14] This recommendation was not put forth, however, by recent guidelines from the American Society for Clinical Pathology, College of American Pathologists, Association for Molecular Pathology, and American Society for Clinical Oncology.[44]

The advent of small molecules that inhibit the BRAF V600E protein raised hope for patients with aggressive *BRAF*-mutated tumors. Agents, such as vemurafenib, induce good clinical responses in melanoma patients[45] but show only limited activity in patients with colorectal carcinoma.[46] Laboratory experiments aimed at deciphering the biological underpinnings of these clinical observations have demonstrated activation of an EGFR feedback loop in *BRAF*-mutated colon cancer cell lines and xenografts but not in melanoma cell lines.[47,48] These findings resulted in the initiation of clinical trials combining vemurafenib and cetuximab with or without irinotecan.[49,50] Early data suggest better results with combination therapy compared with vemurafenib alone, although the response rates have not exceeded 35%.[50]

EMERGING BIOMARKERS

PIK3CA MUTATIONS

The *PIK3CA* gene encodes the catalytic subunit of phosphatidylinositol 3-kinase (PI3K), a downstream effector of EGFR signaling (see **Fig. 3**). Mutations in *PIK3CA* occur in 15% to 20% of colorectal carcinomas and usually affect helical (exon 9) or catalytic (exon 20) domains, resulting in the functional activation of PI3K. Initial studies provided conflicting results regarding the response of *PIK3CA* mutant tumors to EGFR inhibitor therapy. Some investigators have shown resistance to panitumumab or cetuximab,[51] whereas others have failed to find a correlation between *PIK3CA* mutational status and therapeutic response.[52] De Roock and colleagues[34] separately examined the effects of exon 9 and exon 20 mutations and found that only the latter were associated with resistance to EGFR inhibitors.

Two recent retrospective studies reported an association between *PIK3CA* mutations and better outcomes among patients taking aspirin after a diagnosis of colorectal carcinoma.[53,54] Prior to these studies, aspirin had been reported to reduce cancer-related mortality among colorectal cancer patients through unclear mechanisms.[55] Liao and colleagues[54] hypothesized that aspirin exerts some of its effects by inhibiting PTSG2 (cyclooxygenase 2), resulting in decreased prostaglandin synthesis and suppression of PI3K signaling activity. They correlated regular aspirin use with the presence *PIK3CA* mutations in a cohort of 964 colorectal cancer patients and found that patients with *PIK3CA* mutant tumors had improved survival compared with patients with wild-type tumors. Prospective studies addressing the therapeutic implications of *PIK3CA* mutations are needed and testing for *PIK3CA* mutations is not currently performed in standard clinical practice.

HER2 GENETIC ALTERATIONS

The human epidermal growth factor receptor 2 (HER2, HER2/neu, or ERBB2) is a transmembrane tyrosine kinase receptor protein with the same basic molecular structure as EGFR. Inhibition of HER2 signaling with trastuzumab, an anti-HER2 antibody, and/or a tyrosine kinase inhibitor (eg, lapatinib, afatinib, or neratinib) is an established therapeutic approach for patients with breast cancer, gastroesophageal adenocarcinoma, and gastric carcinoma whose tumors show overexpression of HER2. Overexpression of HER2 usually results from *HER2* gene amplification. In clinical practice, cancers are routinely assessed for HER2 status using immunohistochemistry and, in select cases, fluorescence in situ hybridization. Some investigators have also used data from NGS to determine HER2 status. Ross and colleagues[56] found good concordance with respect to *HER2* amplification calls when comparing immunohistochemistry, in situ hybridization, and NGS data.

Amplification of *HER2* is observed in 3% of colorectal cancers. Another 4% to 5% of cases harbor somatic mutations, including the hotspot kinase domain mutations V777L and V824I, which activate HER2 signaling.[10,57] Preclinical models of *HER2* amplified colorectal tumors have shown that monotherapy with either HER2 tyrosine kinase inhibitors or anti-HER2 antibodies are not effective, but the combination of an antibody and a tyrosine kinase inhibitor leads to sustained tumor shrinkage.[58] The ongoing HERACLES clinical trial is aimed at assessing the activity of trastuzumab and lapatinib in patients with HER2-positive, *KRAS* exon 2 wild-type metastatic colorectal cancer. Phase II of the

HERACLES trial enrolled 27 patients who were refractory to standard-of-care treatment, including EGFR inhibitors. Investigators observed an objective response in 8 (30%) patients, whereas 12 patients had stable disease.[59,60]

Both *HER2*-amplified and *HER2*-mutated cancers can show de novo and acquired resistance to EGFR inhibitors,[61,62] resulting in persistent signaling in the presence of an EGFR inhibitor (see **Fig. 3**). Most studies, however, assessing the role of *HER2* alterations in colorectal cancer have been small and/or retrospective. The 2016 NCCN guidelines do not recommend HER2 testing for treatment planning, citing the need for larger confirmatory studies.[14]

PRACTICAL CONSIDERATIONS

APPROACHES TO GENOTYPING

Clinical molecular testing has been largely based on conventional dideoxy sequencing/Sanger sequencing, a reliable, fast, cost-effective tool that assesses individual gene regions for single nucleotide polymorphisms and small insertions/deletions.[63] This approach cannot be scaled up to asses a large number of genes and has limited sensitivity for detecting genetic alterations. It is not quantitative, so it cannot yield information regarding the percentage of altered tumor cells. Copy number abnormalities and genomic rearrangements cannot be detected. Alternative techniques that overcome these limitations include mass-spectrometry genotyping, allele-specific PCR, real-time PCR with melt-curve analysis, and pyrosequencing.[33,64,65] These methods require less DNA and have higher sensitivity than Sanger sequencing, but many of them only detect prespecified hotspot mutations. For example, allele-specific PCR kits include primers that correspond to potential mutant DNA sequences and only detection of these sequences yields a positive result. False-negative results can result if a tumor harbors a different mutation than that for which the kit was designed.

NGS uses parallel sequencing of millions of fragments of DNA and can be performed on formalin-fixed, paraffin-embedded tissue.[66] Multiple genes can be interrogated simultaneously and a given DNA region can be independently sequenced many times (often >300×) resulting in high sensitivity. This method also allows detection of copy number alterations and structural rearrangements in some cases. The technique can be used to sequence selected genes, whole exomes, or the entire genome of a tumor. In general, the larger the amount of genetic material covered, the lower the sequencing depth. Most clinical assays consist of targeted sequencing panels that examine a limited number of genes covered at high depth,[67–70] although some institutions perform whole-exome sequencing that queries approximately 20,000 genes at a lower depth.[71,72]

NGS poses several challenges. Performance of the assay and interpretation of data require several weeks and, despite declining sequencing costs, NGS-based assays entail other expenses related to equipment and bioinformatics support. The vast amount of data generated complicates data processing and interpretation. Distinguishing passenger genetic events (ie, changes that do not have a deleterious effect) from driver alterations that influence tumor biology or determine therapeutic response is difficult. High sensitivity also leads to detection of genetic events that are present in only a small fraction of tumor cells; the significance of such alterations even when present in established cancer genes may be unclear.

TYPE OF SPECIMEN

Pathologists are often responsible for choosing the best material for molecular profiling and need to consider several factors when making their selection (**Box 1**). Tumor content and quantity are among the most critical factors that affect DNA

Box 1
Considerations in specimen selection for molecular profiling

- Choosing a tumor sample with the highest tumor content (% of tumor cells) can facilitate downstream analysis and avoid false-negative results.

- Acceptable tumor content depends on the characteristics of the assay used for genotyping; in general a minimum of 10% tumor content is recommended with sensitive assays.

- Specimens with tumor cells within dense lymphoid tissue (eg, lymph node) should be avoided as they are associated with lower tumor content.

- Pretreatment biopsies are often the preferred sample in cases of rectal tumors undergoing neoadjuvant therapy with good treatment response.

- Efforts should be made to minimize the adenoma component if present.

- Cytology specimens may be good source of tumor DNA and should be considered, especially if other material is suboptimal.

yield, positive predictive value, and negative predictive value. Tumor containing tissue is often dissected to enrich for tumor content. Neoadjuvantly treated rectal tumors often contain tumor cells widely separated by fibrosis; pretreatment biopsy samples are preferable in these cases. Many patients with metastatic carcinoma are not surgically treated and thus, small biopsies and/or cytology specimens represent the only tumor material available for ancillary testing. Core needle or surgical biopsies have been preferred to cytologic material for DNA for molecular testing in the past, but cytology samples are often adequate and, sometimes even superior to paraffin-embedded tissue.[73,74] Formalin fixation leads to nucleic acid degradation that can result in sequencing artifacts, whereas cytology samples are collected in non–formalin-based fixatives that yield higher-quality DNA.[75]

There has been some controversy as to whether testing of the primary lesion is sufficient to correctly characterize the genetics of extracolonic tumors when patients have distant metastatic disease. Some clinical trials using targeted therapeutics have required biopsy of metastatic tumor to increase the likelihood that an agent will be effective, although there is no evidence that this approach is necessary.[76] Molecular heterogeneity within a tumor, or between the primary tumor and metastatic deposit, is common among tumors; however, the extent and the relevance of this heterogeneity seems to vary among different cancer types.[77] Early studies reported a significant rate of discordance between primary colorectal carcinomas and metastases with respect to KRAS mutational status, leading some investigators to recommend testing the metastasis rather than the primary tumor.[78,79] Nonetheless, recent data using NGS show a high rate of concordance in KRAS mutational status between primary and metastatic tumors using NGS.[80–83]

The current NCCN guidelines state that either primary tumor or metastasis may be used for RAS/BRAF testing prior to initiation of treatment with cetuximab or panitumumab.[14] In patients undergoing EGFR inhibitor therapy, RAS-mutant metastases associated with RAS wild-type tumors are well documented, presumably as a mechanism of resistance.[84,85] In some cases, primary tumors initially believed to be KRAS wild type were shown to harbor minor populations of KRAS mutant cells detected by ultrasensitive sequencing techniques. These findings suggest that EGFR inhibitor therapy applies selective pressure to expand small subclones in the primary tumor, giving rise to metastases that show KRAS mutations. Mutations can also arise de novo as a result of ongoing mutagenesis.

In contrast to genetic events that are acquired early, higher rates of discordance between primary tumors and metastases have been reported for genes altered late in the pathogenesis of colorectal carcinoma, such as TP53, SMAD4, and PIK3CA.[82,83,86] Whether or not mutational heterogeneity is clinically important remains to be seen; additional studies are needed if the protein products of these genes prove to be druggable targets or biomarkers predictive of therapeutic response.

SUMMARY

Currently, standard molecular testing in colorectal carcinoma is aimed at identifying patients with Lynch syndrome and detecting mutations that predict for resistance to EGFR inhibitor therapy. Testing all tumors for MSI is the first step toward the first goal, whereas testing for MLH1 promoter hypermethylation and/or BRAF V600E mutation provides important information in patients whose tumors show MSI. Patients who are candidates to receive an EGFR inhibitor should have their tumors tested for mutations in KRAS and NRAS codons 12, 13, 59, 61, 117, and 164. The BRAF V600E is not yet universally accepted as a negative predictor of response to EGFR inhibitor therapy.

Many clinical trials are currently under way using both compounds that target specific molecular alterations and immunomodulators. These trials often require a specific genotype for inclusion and may only be available to patients that had molecular testing that is more comprehensive than what is currently required as part of standard of care. An increasing number of laboratories are turning into NGS assays that have the capability to detect many different types of genetic alterations using small amounts of DNA in a single assay. Surgical pathologists play a pivotal role in selecting the most appropriate tissue source for molecular profiling and should be familiar with the downstream assays used by their institutions.

REFERENCES

1. Siegel RL, Miller KD, Jemal A. Cancer statistics, 2016. CA Cancer J Clin 2016;66:7–30.
2. Fearon ER, Vogelstein B. A genetic model for colorectal tumorigenesis. Cell 1990;61:759–67.
3. Diep CB, Kleivi K, Ribeiro FR, et al. The order of genetic events associated with colorectal cancer progression inferred from meta-analysis of copy number changes. Genes Chromosomes Cancer 2006;45:31–41.

4. Kalady MF. Sessile serrated polyps: an important route to colorectal cancer. J Natl Compr Canc Netw 2013;11:1585–94.

5. Siegel R, Desantis C, Jemal A. Colorectal cancer statistics, 2014. CA Cancer J Clin 2014;64:104–17.

6. Siegfried JM, Gillespie AT, Mera R, et al. Prognostic value of specific KRAS mutations in lung adenocarcinomas. Cancer Epidemiol Biomarkers Prev 1997; 6:841–7.

7. Ligtenberg MJ, Kuiper RP, Geurts van Kessel A, et al. EPCAM deletion carriers constitute a unique subgroup of Lynch syndrome patients. Fam Cancer 2013;12:169–74.

8. Stadler ZK, Battaglin F, Middha S, et al. Reliable detection of mismatch repair deficiency in colorectal cancers using mutational load in next-generation sequencing panels. J Clin Oncol 2016;34:2141–7.

9. Cancer Genome Atlas Research Network, Kandoth C, Schultz N, Cherniack AD, et al. Integrated genomic characterization of endometrial carcinoma. Nature 2013;497:67–73.

10. Cancer Genome Atlas Network. Comprehensive molecular characterization of human colon and rectal cancer. Nature 2012;487:330–7.

11. Niu B, Ye K, Zhang Q, et al. MSIsensor: microsatellite instability detection using paired tumor-normal sequence data. Bioinformatics 2014;30:1015–6.

12. Salipante SJ, Scroggins SM, Hampel HL, et al. Microsatellite instability detection by next generation sequencing. Clin Chem 2014;60:1192–9.

13. Kautto EA, Bonneville R, Miya J, et al. Performance evaluation for rapid detection of pan-cancer microsatellite instability with MANTIS. Oncotarget 2016; 8(5):7452–63.

14. Network NCC. Clinical practice guidelines in oncology: colon cancer (Version 1.2017). 2016. Available at: https://www.nccn.org/professionals/ physician_gls/pdf/colon.pdf. Accessed January 18, 2017.

15. Samowitz WS, Curtin K, Ma KN, et al. Microsatellite instability in sporadic colon cancer is associated with an improved prognosis at the population level. Cancer Epidemiol Biomarkers Prev 2001;10:917–23.

16. Sargent DJ, Marsoni S, Monges G, et al. Defective mismatch repair as a predictive marker for lack of efficacy of fluorouracil-based adjuvant therapy in colon cancer. J Clin Oncol 2010;28:3219–26.

17. Ribic CM, Sargent DJ, Moore MJ, et al. Tumor microsatellite-instability status as a predictor of benefit from fluorouracil-based adjuvant chemotherapy for colon cancer. N Engl J Med 2003;349: 247–57.

18. Sinicrope FA, Foster NR, Thibodeau SN, et al. DNA mismatch repair status and colon cancer recurrence and survival in clinical trials of 5-fluorouracil-based adjuvant therapy. J Natl Cancer Inst 2011;103: 863–75.

19. Le DT, Uram JN, Wang H, et al. PD-1 blockade in tumors with mismatch-repair deficiency. N Engl J Med 2015;372:2509–20.

20. Nosho K, Shima K, Irahara N, et al. DNMT3B expression might contribute to CpG island methylator phenotype in colorectal cancer. Clin Cancer Res 2009;15:3663–71.

21. Rahner N, Friedrichs N, Steinke V, et al. Coexisting somatic promoter hypermethylation and pathogenic MLH1 germline mutation in Lynch syndrome. J Pathol 2008;214:10–6.

22. Niessen RC, Hofstra RM, Westers H, et al. Germline hypermethylation of MLH1 and EPCAM deletions are a frequent cause of Lynch syndrome. Genes Chromosomes Cancer 2009;48:737–44.

23. Gausachs M, Mur P, Corral J, et al. MLH1 promoter hypermethylation in the analytical algorithm of Lynch syndrome: a cost-effectiveness study. Eur J Hum Genet 2012;20:762–8.

24. Hitchins MP, Lynch HT. Dawning of the epigenetic era in hereditary cancer. Clin Genet 2014;85:413–6.

25. Douillard JY, Oliner KS, Siena S, et al. Panitumumab-FOLFOX4 treatment and RAS mutations in colorectal cancer. N Engl J Med 2013;369:1023–34.

26. Van Cutsem E, Lenz HJ, Kohne CH, et al. Fluorouracil, leucovorin, and irinotecan plus cetuximab treatment and RAS mutations in colorectal cancer. J Clin Oncol 2015;33:692–700.

27. Bokemeyer C, Bondarenko I, Makhson A, et al. Fluorouracil, leucovorin, and oxaliplatin with and without cetuximab in the first-line treatment of metastatic colorectal cancer. J Clin Oncol 2009;27:663–71.

28. Karapetis CS, Khambata-Ford S, Jonker DJ, et al. K-ras mutations and benefit from cetuximab in advanced colorectal cancer. N Engl J Med 2008; 359:1757–65.

29. Amado RG, Wolf M, Peeters M, et al. Wild-type KRAS is required for panitumumab efficacy in patients with metastatic colorectal cancer. J Clin Oncol 2008;26:1626–34.

30. Tejpar S, Celik I, Schlichting M, et al. Association of KRAS G13D tumor mutations with outcome in patients with metastatic colorectal cancer treated with first-line chemotherapy with or without cetuximab. J Clin Oncol 2012;30:3570–7.

31. Van Cutsem E, Kohne CH, Hitre E, et al. Cetuximab and chemotherapy as initial treatment for metastatic colorectal cancer. N Engl J Med 2009;360:1408–17.

32. Douillard JY, Siena S, Cassidy J, et al. Randomized, phase III trial of panitumumab with infusional fluorouracil, leucovorin, and oxaliplatin (FOLFOX4) versus FOLFOX4 alone as first-line treatment in patients with previously untreated metastatic colorectal cancer: the PRIME study. J Clin Oncol 2010;28: 4697–705.

33. Janakiraman M, Vakiani E, Zeng Z, et al. Genomic and biological characterization of exon 4 KRAS

mutations in human cancer. Cancer Res 2010;70: 5901–11.

34. De Roock W, Claes B, Bernasconi D, et al. Effects of KRAS, BRAF, NRAS, and PIK3CA mutations on the efficacy of cetuximab plus chemotherapy in chemotherapy-refractory metastatic colorectal cancer: a retrospective consortium analysis. Lancet Oncol 2010;11(8):753–62.

35. Sorich MJ, Wiese MD, Rowland A, et al. Extended RAS mutations and anti-EGFR monoclonal antibody survival benefit in metastatic colorectal cancer: a meta-analysis of randomized, controlled trials. Ann Oncol 2015;26:13–21.

36. Allegra CJ, Rumble RB, Hamilton SR, et al. Extended RAS gene mutation testing in metastatic colorectal carcinoma to predict response to anti-epidermal growth factor receptor monoclonal antibody therapy: American society of clinical oncology provisional clinical opinion update 2015. J Clin Oncol 2016;34:179–85.

37. Domingo E, Laiho P, Ollikainen M, et al. BRAF screening as a low-cost effective strategy for simplifying HNPCC genetic testing. J Med Genet 2004;41: 664–8.

38. Walsh MD, Buchanan DD, Walters R, et al. Analysis of families with Lynch syndrome complicated by advanced serrated neoplasia: the importance of pathology review and pedigree analysis. Fam Cancer 2009;8:313–23.

39. Phipps AI, Limburg PJ, Baron JA, et al. Association between molecular subtypes of colorectal cancer and patient survival. Gastroenterology 2015;148: 77–87.e2.

40. Roth AD, Tejpar S, Delorenzi M, et al. Prognostic role of KRAS and BRAF in stage II and III resected colon cancer: results of the translational study on the PETACC-3, EORTC 40993, SAKK 60-00 trial. J Clin Oncol 2010;28:466–74.

41. Van Cutsem E, Kohne CH, Lang I, et al. Cetuximab plus irinotecan, fluorouracil, and leucovorin as first-line treatment for metastatic colorectal cancer: updated analysis of overall survival according to tumor KRAS and BRAF mutation status. J Clin Oncol 2011; 29:2011–9.

42. Pietrantonio F, Petrelli F, Coinu A, et al. Predictive role of BRAF mutations in patients with advanced colorectal cancer receiving cetuximab and panitumumab: a meta-analysis. Eur J Cancer 2015;51: 587–94.

43. Rowland A, Dias MM, Wiese MD, et al. Meta-analysis of BRAF mutation as a predictive biomarker of benefit from anti-EGFR monoclonal antibody therapy for RAS wild-type metastatic colorectal cancer. Br J Cancer 2015;112:1888–94.

44. Sepulveda AR, Hamilton SR, Allegra CJ, et al. Molecular biomarkers for the evaluation of colorectal cancer: guideline from the American Society for Clinical Pathology, College of American Pathologists, Association for Molecular Pathology, and the American Society of Clinical Oncology. J Clin Oncol 2017;35(13):1453–86.

45. Chapman PB, Hauschild A, Robert C, et al. Improved survival with vemurafenib in melanoma with BRAF V600E mutation. N Engl J Med 2011; 364:2507–16.

46. Kopetz S, Desai J, Chan E, et al. Phase II pilot study of vemurafenib in patients with metastatic BRAF-mutated colorectal cancer. J Clin Oncol 2015;33: 4032–8.

47. Prahallad A, Sun C, Huang S, et al. Unresponsiveness of colon cancer to BRAF(V600E) inhibition through feedback activation of EGFR. Nature 2012; 483:100–3.

48. Corcoran RB, Ebi H, Turke AB, et al. EGFR-mediated re-activation of MAPK signaling contributes to insensitivity of BRAF mutant colorectal cancers to RAF inhibition with vemurafenib. Cancer Discov 2012;2: 227–35.

49. Yaeger R, Cercek A, O'Reilly EM, et al. Pilot trial of combined BRAF and EGFR inhibition in BRAF-mutant metastatic colorectal cancer patients. Clin Cancer Res 2015;21:1313–20.

50. Hong DS, Morris VK, El Osta B, et al. Phase 1B study of vemurafenib in combination with irinotecan and cetuximab in patients with metastatic colorectal cancer with BRAF V600E mutation. Cancer Discov 2016; 6(12):1352–65.

51. Sartore-Bianchi A, Martini M, Molinari F, et al. PIK3CA mutations in colorectal cancer are associated with clinical resistance to EGFR-targeted monoclonal antibodies. Cancer Res 2009;69: 1851–7.

52. Prenen H, De Schutter J, Jacobs B, et al. PIK3CA mutations are not a major determinant of resistance to the epidermal growth factor receptor inhibitor cetuximab in metastatic colorectal cancer. Clin Cancer Res 2009;15:3184–8.

53. Domingo E, Church DN, Sieber O, et al. Evaluation of PIK3CA mutation as a predictor of benefit from nonsteroidal anti-inflammatory drug therapy in colorectal cancer. J Clin Oncol 2013;31:4297–305.

54. Liao X, Lochhead P, Nishihara R, et al. Aspirin use, tumor PIK3CA mutation, and colorectal-cancer survival. N Engl J Med 2012;367:1596–606.

55. Rothwell PM, Wilson M, Elwin CE, et al. Long-term effect of aspirin on colorectal cancer incidence and mortality: 20-year follow-up of five randomised trials. Lancet 2010;376:1741–50.

56. Ross DS, Zehir A, Cheng DT, et al. Next-generation assessment of ERBB2 (Human epidermal growth factor receptor 2) amplification status: clinical validation in the context of a hybrid capture-based, comprehensive solid tumor genomic profiling assay. J Mol Diagn 2017;19(2):244–54.

57. Kavuri SM, Jain N, Galimi F, et al. HER2 activating mutations are targets for colorectal cancer treatment. Cancer Discov 2015;5:832–41.

58. Bertotti A, Migliardi G, Galimi F, et al. A molecularly annotated platform of patient-derived xenografts ("xenopatients") identifies HER2 as an effective therapeutic target in cetuximab-resistant colorectal cancer. Cancer Discov 2011;1:508–23.

59. Sartore-Bianchi A, Trusolino L, Martino C, et al. Dual-targeted therapy with trastuzumab and lapatinib in treatment-refractory, KRAS codon 12/13 wild-type, HER2-positive metastatic colorectal cancer (HERACLES): a proof-of-concept, multicentre, open-label, phase 2 trial. Lancet Oncol 2016;17:738–46.

60. Valtorta E, Martino C, Sartore-Bianchi A, et al. Assessment of a HER2 scoring system for colorectal cancer: results from a validation study. Mod Pathol 2015;28:1481–91.

61. Bertotti A, Papp E, Jones S, et al. The genomic landscape of response to EGFR blockade in colorectal cancer. Nature 2015;526:263–7.

62. Yonesaka K, Zejnullahu K, Okamoto I, et al. Activation of ERBB2 signaling causes resistance to the EGFR-directed therapeutic antibody cetuximab. Sci Transl Med 2011;3:99ra86.

63. Sanger F, Nicklen S, Coulson AR. DNA sequencing with chain-terminating inhibitors. Proc Natl Acad Sci U S A 1977;74:5463–7.

64. Herreros-Villanueva M, Chen CC, Yuan SS, et al. KRAS mutations: analytical considerations. Clin Chim Acta 2014;431:211–20.

65. Harrington CT, Lin EI, Olson MT, et al. Fundamentals of pyrosequencing. Arch Pathol Lab Med 2013;137:1296–303.

66. Wagle N, Berger MF, Davis MJ, et al. High-throughput detection of actionable genomic alterations in clinical tumor samples by targeted, massively parallel sequencing. Cancer Discov 2012;2:82–93.

67. Cheng DT, Mitchell TN, Zehir A, et al. Memorial sloan kettering-integrated mutation profiling of actionable cancer targets (MSK-IMPACT): a hybridization capture-based next-generation sequencing clinical assay for solid tumor molecular oncology. J Mol Diagn 2015;17:251–64.

68. Cottrell CE, Al-Kateb H, Bredemeyer AJ, et al. Validation of a next-generation sequencing assay for clinical molecular oncology. J Mol Diagn 2014;16:89–105.

69. Pritchard CC, Salipante SJ, Koehler K, et al. Validation and implementation of targeted capture and sequencing for the detection of actionable mutation, copy number variation, and gene rearrangement in clinical cancer specimens. J Mol Diagn 2014;16:56–67.

70. Frampton GM, Fichtenholtz A, Otto GA, et al. Development and validation of a clinical cancer genomic profiling test based on massively parallel DNA sequencing. Nat Biotechnol 2013;31:1023–31.

71. Roychowdhury S, Iyer MK, Robinson DR, et al. Personalized oncology through integrative high-throughput sequencing: a pilot study. Sci Transl Med 2011;3:111ra21.

72. Van Allen EM, Wagle N, Stojanov P, et al. Whole-exome sequencing and clinical interpretation of formalin-fixed, paraffin-embedded tumor samples to guide precision cancer medicine. Nat Med 2014;20:682–8.

73. Roy-Chowdhuri S, Stewart J. Preanalytic variables in cytology: lessons learned from next-generation sequencing-the MD Anderson experience. Arch Pathol Lab Med 2016, [Epub ahead of print].

74. Tian SK, Killian JK, Rekhtman N, et al. Optimizing workflows and processing of cytologic samples for comprehensive analysis by next-generation sequencing: memorial sloan kettering cancer center experience. Arch Pathol Lab Med 2016, [Epub ahead of print].

75. Williams C, Ponten F, Moberg C, et al. A high frequency of sequence alterations is due to formalin fixation of archival specimens. Am J Pathol 1999;155:1467–71.

76. Le Tourneau C, Delord JP, Goncalves A, et al. Molecularly targeted therapy based on tumour molecular profiling versus conventional therapy for advanced cancer (SHIVA): a multicentre, open-label, proof-of-concept, randomised, controlled phase 2 trial. Lancet Oncol 2015;16:1324–34.

77. McGranahan N, Swanton C. Biological and therapeutic impact of intratumor heterogeneity in cancer evolution. Cancer Cell 2015;27:15–26.

78. Albanese I, Scibetta AG, Migliavacca M, et al. Heterogeneity within and between primary colorectal carcinomas and matched metastases as revealed by analysis of Ki-ras and p53 mutations. Biochem Biophys Res Commun 2004;325:784–91.

79. Molinari F, Martin V, Saletti P, et al. Differing deregulation of EGFR and downstream proteins in primary colorectal cancer and related metastatic sites may be clinically relevant. Br J Cancer 2009;100:1087–94.

80. Santini D, Loupakis F, Vincenzi B, et al. High concordance of KRAS status between primary colorectal tumors and related metastatic sites: implications for clinical practice. Oncologist 2008;13:1270–5.

81. Vignot S, Lefebvre C, Frampton GM, et al. Comparative analysis of primary tumour and matched metastases in colorectal cancer patients: evaluation of concordance between genomic and transcriptional profiles. Eur J Cancer 2015;51:791–9.

82. Brannon AR, Vakiani E, Sylvester BE, et al. Comparative sequencing analysis reveals high genomic concordance between matched primary and metastatic colorectal cancer lesions. Genome Biol 2014;15:454.

83. Vakiani E, Janakiraman M, Shen R, et al. Comparative genomic analysis of primary versus metastasis in colorectal carcinomas. J Clin Oncol 2011;29: 10500.

84. Diaz LA Jr, Williams RT, Wu J, et al. The molecular evolution of acquired resistance to targeted EGFR blockade in colorectal cancers. Nature 2012;486: 537–40.

85. Misale S, Yaeger R, Hobor S, et al. Emergence of KRAS mutations and acquired resistance to anti-EGFR therapy in colorectal cancer. Nature 2012; 486:532–6.

86. Goswami RS, Patel KP, Singh RR, et al. Hotspot mutation panel testing reveals clonal evolution in a study of 265 paired primary and metastatic tumors. Clin Cancer Res 2015;21:2644–51.

Lymphoproliferative Diseases of the Gut
A Survival Guide for the General Pathologist

Scott R. Owens, MD

KEYWORDS

• Gastrointestinal • Lymphoma • Lymphoproliferative • B cell • T cell

Key points

- Although uncommon in comparison with epithelial neoplasms, lymphomas in the gastrointestinal tract are seen on a regular basis by pathologists examining gastrointestinal tissues.

- B-cell lymphomas are far more common than T-cell lymphomas in the gastrointestinal tract, but there are a few T-cell neoplasms that have characteristic presentations and/or associations.

- The most common lymphoma throughout the gastrointestinal tract is diffuse large B-cell lymphoma.

- A pragmatic approach to lymphoma diagnosis as outlined in this article will allow the pathologist to approach most cases encountered on a regular basis.

ABSTRACT

The gastrointestinal tract is the most common extranodal site of involvement by lymphoma, with B-cell tumors outnumbering T-cell tumors by a wide margin. Diffuse large B-cell lymphoma is the most common lymphoid neoplasm involving the gastrointestinal tract; but a variety of other B- and T-cell neoplasms occur in the gastrointestinal organs, often with characteristic associations and/or manifestations. Although the diagnosis of gastrointestinal lymphomas can sometimes seem daunting to general pathologists, a knowledge of the most commonly encountered entities, in combination with a reasoned and pragmatic approach to the diagnostic workup, makes it possible to approach most cases with confidence.

OVERVIEW

Although the gastrointestinal (GI) tract gives rise to many different types of neoplasia, perhaps nothing strikes fear into the heart of the pathologist the way that an atypical lymphoid infiltrate can. The specter of multiple immunohistochemical stains, correlation with gene rearrangement studies, and decisions regarding the need for additional tissue to send for flow cytometry makes it tempting to package up the entire case and send it to a hematolymphoid specialist. Although lymphomas are uncommon compared with epithelial neoplasms of the GI tract, this organ system is the most common extranodal site of involvement by lymphoma; up to 20% of all lymphomas occur in the GI tract, and they often present with characteristic findings.[1] Despite inherent complexities in lymphoma classification, any pathologist who reviews GI specimens can make a confident diagnosis or at least begin the process, using a rational and pragmatic approach. This article begins with a review of normal and reactive GI tract lymphoid populations followed by specific examples of GI lymphomas. The emphasis is on lymphomas of mature B- and T-cell phenotypes, as these entities are most commonly encountered.

Disclosure Statement: No disclosures.
Department of Pathology, University of Michigan Medical School, M5224 Medical Science I, 1301 Catherine Street, Ann Arbor, MI 48109, USA
E-mail address: srowens@med.umich.edu

Surgical Pathology 10 (2017) 1021–1037
http://dx.doi.org/10.1016/j.path.2017.07.014
1875-9181/17/

GASTROINTESTINAL LYMPHOID TISSUE

The normal and acquired lymphoid populations of the GI tract vary in a site-specific fashion depending on the nature of stimuli. The terminal ileum, for example, normally contains a large population of organized lymphoid tissue that is most prominent in children and young adults. These Peyer patches consist of lymphoid follicles/germinal centers surrounded by B-cell containing mantle zones and marginal zones with T lymphocytes in the interfollicular areas. The architecture recapitulates that of a lymph node and represents one type of native mucosa-associated lymphoid tissue (MALT).[2] Peyer patches may appear as an endoscopically visible mucosal nodularity or even appear as small polyps that prompt endoscopic biopsy. The lymphoid population in Peyer patches may push aside the normal crypts, flatten the overlying villi (Fig. 1), and interdigitate with fibers of the muscularis mucosae (Fig. 2); these features should not be overinterpreted as atypical. Similar aggregates are scattered throughout the GI tract.

Acquired MALT refers to lymphoid infiltrates that develop in response to a stimulus, such as chronic gastritis associated with Helicobacter pylori.[2] Infection with H pylori elicits a dense, bandlike infiltrate of plasma cells and lymphocytes in the superficial (foveolar or pit) compartment of the gastric mucosa (Fig. 3A). Organized lymphoid

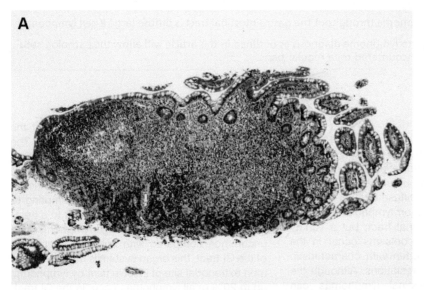

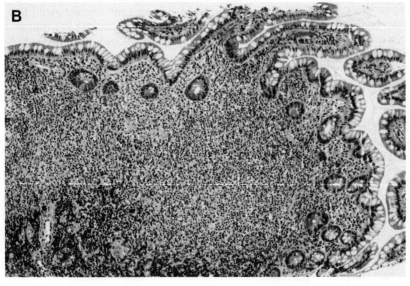

Fig. 1. A typical Peyer patch is seen in a biopsy from the terminal ileum. (A) Note the flattened area of mucosa toward the left of the lymphoid aggregate (H&E, original magnification ×40). (B) At higher magnification, the benign lymphoid infiltrate can be see among the intestinal crypts, which are otherwise intact (H&E, original magnification ×100).

Fig. 2. The lymphocytes in normal, non-neoplastic lymphoid aggregates may also interdigitate with fibers of the muscularis mucosae. Note the presence of a mantle zone surrounding the well-developed follicular structure (H&E, original magnification ×200).

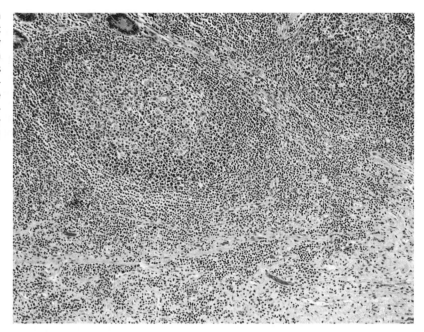

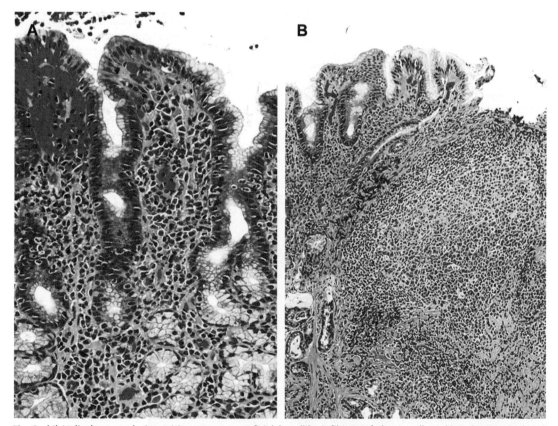

Fig. 3. (*A*) *Helicobacter pylori* gastritis creates a superficial, bandlike infiltrate of plasma cells and lymphocytes in the pit compartment of the gastric mucosa. Note the presence of neutrophils in the epithelium of the deep pit/mucus neck region of the mucosa (H&E, original magnification ×200). (*B*) Commonly, the superficial gastritis will be accompanied by deeper lymphoid aggregates containing germinal centers. Note the tendency of this aggregate to push apart the mucosal structures; although this distorts the mucosal architecture, there is no true destructive character to the infiltrate (H&E, original magnification ×100).

follicles and germinal centers are commonly encountered in the deeper mucosa, distorting the mucosa and separating the normally dense population of gastric pits and glands (see **Fig.** 3B). Chronic *H pylori*–associated gastritis is a risk factor for lymphoid neoplasia, particularly extranodal marginal zone lymphoma of MALT type; distinction between acquired MALT and lymphoma can be challenging.[1,3]

Lymphoid hyperplasia in the rectum is another, relatively common acquired MALT that mimics lymphoma, which has been referred to as the rectal tonsil or rectal lymphoid polyp.[4–6] Polypoid collections of organized lymphoid tissue may span up to 1 cm; they harbor germinal centers that contain B cells as well as surrounding T cells in the interfollicular areas (**Fig. 4**). Some reports suggest that lymphoid hyperplasia in the rectum may reflect underlying infection with *Chlamydia* or Epstein-Barr virus (EBV). This type of lymphoid process is nondestructive and has an immunophenotype that usually allows distinction from MALT lymphoma and follicular lymphoma.

SPECIFIC GASTROINTESTINAL LYMPHOMAS

Most lymphomas occurring in the GI tract are B-cell lymphomas, although a few lymphomas of T-cell lineage have characteristic presentations and/or associations that merit discussion.[2,7,8] Most GI lymphomas occur in the stomach, followed by the small intestine and colon. Primary lymphomas of the esophagus, anus, liver, and pancreas are uncommon. This section discusses key features of the most commonly encountered B- and T-cell neoplasms, emphasizing a practical approach to their workup and diagnosis. The intent is not to provide a comprehensive discussion of each entity but rather to provide a survival guide for the general pathologist to approach them in daily practice.

B-CELL LYMPHOMAS

Diffuse Large B-Cell Lymphoma

This lymphoma is the most common type of lymphoma affecting the GI tract. It is composed of sheets of large (or occasionally medium-sized) cells with vesicular nuclei, scant cytoplasm, and a high proliferative rate (often >50%).[1,7,9] Discohesive tumor cells have a destructive pattern of infiltration, obliterating the normal structures and architecture, resulting in ulcers, masses, or even perforation of a viscus (**Fig. 5**). Diffuse large B cell lymphoma (DLBCL) may arise de novo or evolve from an underlying, low-grade neoplasm, such as MALT lymphoma or follicular lymphoma.[10] It is clinically important to search for such a low-grade component and to report it if found; DLBCL can often be cured with therapy, whereas low-grade lymphoma may be refractory and persist after treatment. Subtypes of DLBCL related to EBV

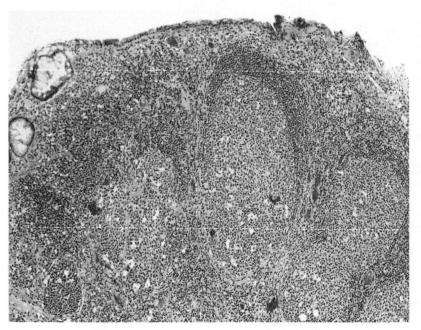

Fig. 4. The rectal tonsil is a benign collection of lymphoid tissue that can be found in the distal rectum, sometimes leading to confusion with lymphoma. Several well-formed germinal centers with surrounding mantle zones occupy the mucosa and submucosa, in a pattern similar to that seen in the Waldeyer ring tissue of the head and neck region (H&E, original magnification ×100).

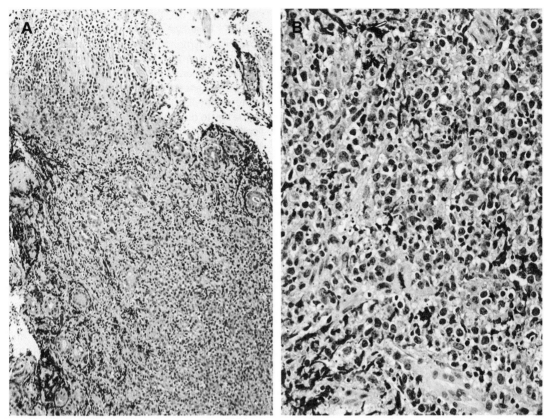

Fig. 5. (*A*) This gastric DLBCL has destroyed much of the mucosal structure in the stomach, leading to an ulcer (H&E, original magnification ×200). (*B*) At high magnification, the lymphoma cells can be discerned as being of large size (in comparison with the nuclei of the endothelial cells in the traversing capillaries), with vesicular nuclei that have one or more nucleoli. A mitotic figure is visible near the center of the image (H&E, original magnification ×400).

infection show a predilection for the elderly and immunosuppressed patients.[11] Iatrogenic immunocompromise following solid-organ transplantation predisposes to a lymphoma that is very often morphologically and immunophenotypically consistent with DLBCL but is more properly classified as monomorphic posttransplant lymphoproliferative disorder (PTLD).[12,13]

The large cells of DLBCL contain nuclei that are comparable in size with normal endothelial cells. These tumors express pan-B cell markers, including CD20, CD79a, and PAX-5. Most tumors also aberrantly express BCL-2, and a subset of cases display a germinal center cell phenotype with CD10 and frequent BCL-6 expression. T-cell markers are negative, although approximately 10% of DLBCLs express CD5. Cyclin-D1 is also usually negative. Nongerminal center DLBCLs lack CD10 and BCL-6 staining and may be classified as activated B-cell type, a distinction that may

be used to guide therapy and prognosis. Distinction between these two types of DLBCL is definitively made at the molecular level, and data regarding the utility of immunohistochemistry as a surrogate are conflicting.[14,15] If immunohistochemistry is used, staining of at least 30% of cells is considered a positive result. Staining for CD10 indicates germinal center cell phenotype, whereas lack of CD10 and BCL-6 staining indicates a nongerminal center phenotype. Tumors that are CD10 negative and positive for BCL-6 can be further evaluated for MUM-1 staining; positivity in more than 30% of cells indicates a nongerminal center phenotype.

Although DLBCL is clinically aggressive, it is potentially curable with chemotherapy. Regimens typically include a combination of cyclophosphamide, vincristine, doxorubicin, and dexamethasone (CHOP therapy), frequently with the addition of anti-CD20 immunotherapy (rituximab).[16]

Key Features

- Most common GI lymphoma

- Diffuse, destructive infiltrate of large cells (compare with macrophage and/or endothelial cell nuclei)

- May arise de novo or from another low-grade lymphoma

- Aggressive clinical course but potentially curable

- Cases in immunocompromised and/or elderly may be EBV related

- May be important to distinguish between germinal center and nongerminal center types

Pitfalls

! Cases occurring in patients after transplantation should be considered PTLD by definition.

! Do not misdiagnose aggressive subtypes of mantle cell lymphoma (pleomorphic and/or blastoid) as DLBCL.

! Do not fail to identify/report any low-grade lymphoma component from which DLBCL may have arisen.

Mucosa-Associated Lymphoid Tissue Lymphoma

Like DLBCL, MALT lymphoma can occur anywhere in the GI tract, although it is most common in the stomach. In fact, 85% of cases occur in the stomach, often in association with *H pylori*–associated gastritis.[1,3] Bacterial strains that harbor the *CagA* gene are particularly associated with the development of lymphoma.

Several cell types comprise MALT lymphomas, and their numbers are variable. The predominant cell type in most cases is a small, mature-appearing lymphocyte that is essentially indistinguishable from the small cells of a normal germinal center (centrocytes).[12,17] Variable numbers of somewhat larger cells with more ample cytoplasm and slightly indented nuclei are also present; these monocytoid B cells recapitulate normal lymphocytes in the marginal zone of a germinal center (Fig. 6A). Finally, a small proportion of large cells recapitulate centroblasts of a germinal center. These large cells should not predominate or form large

sheets; if they do, the lesion is best classified as DLBCL. Reactive germinal centers commonly accompany lymphoma; they may be invaded or disrupted by the lymphoma cells, creating a moth-eaten or naked appearance (see Fig. 6B). This appearance can be enhanced when immunostains for follicle center cells (CD10 and/or BCL-6) are used.

The key to diagnosis of MALT lymphoma is identification of a destructive growth pattern. Macroscopically, this can come in the form of an ulcer or thickened and full-appearing mucosal folds. The histologic hallmark of MALT lymphoma is the presence of destructive epithelial infiltration by lymphoma cells, creating lymphoepithelial lesions (see Fig. 6A). This feature is not absolutely specific for MALT lymphoma, but it is very characteristic. Unlike most other B cell lymphomas MALT lymphoma has no distinctive immunophenotype.[3] In combination with its lack of unequivocally malignant cells, this can make distinction between benign acquired MALT and low-grade lymphoma frustratingly difficult.

Up to 50% of MALT lymphomas coexpress CD43, which is normally found on T cells and plasma cells; convincing coexpression of this antigen on B cells can be a helpful feature. Some MALT lymphomas show plasmacytic differentiation, and occasional tumors are composed entirely of plasma cells or nearly so.[1,12,17] Establishing kappa or lambda light chain restriction using immunohistochemistry can prove clonality such cases. Like their normal counterparts, neoplastic plasma cells express CD138.

Importantly, up to 80% of MALT lymphomas are responsive to conservative therapy aimed at eradication of the inciting entity. For example, *H pylori*–related MALT lymphomas can completely resolve following treatment with a combination of antibiotic and acid-suppressive therapy, even if the organism is not identified. A minority of gastric MALT lymphomas harbor the *API2-MALT1* fusion resulting from a t(11;18) (q21;q21) translocation. They occur independent of *H pylori* infection and are resistant to conservative therapy.[3] For this reason, some investigators recommend testing for this translocation a priori for all MALT lymphomas, although it is probably reasonable to attempt *H pylori* eradication therapy for most cases. Full resolution of the atypical lymphoid infiltrate can take months or even more than a year in some cases. Routine reexamination and biopsy six-to-eight weeks after successful treatment is expected to reveal an atypical lymphoid infiltrate that may be largely unchanged but should not necessarily be interpreted as a treatment failure. Comparisons between serial biopsies may be reported as residual MALT lymphoma with a statement noting improvement or similarity to prior samples.

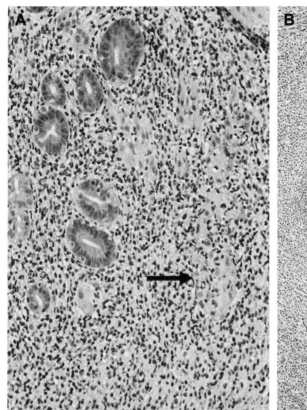

Fig. 6. (A) In contrast to *H pylori* gastritis, gastric MALT lymphoma has a truly destructive pattern of infiltration, with disruption of mucosal structures by small lymphocytes that often have ample, pale cytoplasm. Just to the right of center, a lymphoepithelial lesion is visible (*arrow*), created when the neoplastic lymphocytes infiltrate and destroy the glands of the gastric mucosa. This type of lesion is characteristic of MALT lymphoma and confirms the destructive nature of the infiltrate; but this appearance is not specific for MALT lymphoma, occurring in other types of lymphoma as well (H&E, original magnification ×200). (B) Residual, reactive germinal centers may be included in the infiltrate, often with a moth-eaten appearance indicating that they have been colonized by the lymphoma cells (H&E, original magnification ×100).

Key Features

- They most commonly occur in the stomach.

- Gastric cases are usually related to underlying infection with *H pylori*.

- They are composed of predominantly small lymphocytes, some with monocytoid appearance.

- Many cases can be cured with therapy aimed at *H pylori* eradication.

- They may have plasmacytic differentiation.

Pitfalls

! Lymphoepithelial lesions are characteristic but not specific for MALT lymphoma.

! No specific immunohistochemical marker identifies MALT lymphoma.

! Cases with extensive plasmacytic differentiation may be misdiagnosed as plasmacytoma or plasma cell myeloma.

! Lymphoid infiltrate may take months to disappear after *H pylori* eradication therapy.

Follicular lymphoma

Follicular lymphoma may involve the GI tract either secondarily (such as when GI organs are involved by a systemic lymphoma arising in the retroperitoneal lymph nodes) or, occasionally, primarily.[18,19] It usually appears as a nodular infiltrate of small, mature-appearing lymphocytes that recapitulate the follicle center B cells, specifically, centrocytes and centroblasts (**Fig. 7**A and B). The proportions of each cell population determine the grade of the lymphoma with a larger number of centroblast-like cells imparting a higher grade (**Table 1**). Grades 1 and 2 are considered low grade. The individual cells of grade 3 are morphologically indistinguishable from those of DLBCL. Grade 3 tumors that contain a significant component of diffuse involvement with such cells (around 25% or more) should be regarded as DLBCL, and any background component of follicular lymphoma should be reported secondarily.[18]

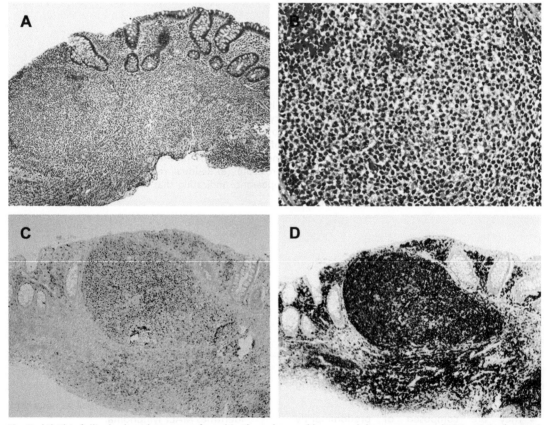

Fig. 7. (*A*) This follicular lymphoma was found in the colon and has a nodular appearance (H&E, original magnification ×100), (*B*) with predominantly small, centroblastlike lymphoid cells predominating in the nodules (H&E, original magnification ×400). The monotonous appearance of these cells helps to distinguish these structures from reactive follicles, which typically have a polarized appearance divided into light (centrocyte-containing) and dark (centroblast-containing) zones. (*C*) The diagnosis can be confirmed using immunohistochemical markers to prove that the follicular structures contain follicle center-type cells (BCL-6 stain, original magnification ×100) that aberrantly express BCL-2 (*D*; original magnification ×100).

Table 1
Follicular lymphoma grades

Grade	Histologic Features	
1	0–5 centroblasts/HPF	Low grade
2	6–15 centroblasts/HPF	
3A	>15 centroblasts/HPF with centrocytes in follicular structures	High grade
3B	>15 centroblasts/HPF without centrocytes (ie, only centroblasts in follicular structures)	

When available, 10 high-power field should be counted and the result divided by 10 to obtain the average centroblast count.

Abbreviation: HPF, high-power field (40× microscope objective).

Key Features

- Most cases involve the GI tract secondarily as part of systemic disease.
- A primary GI (specifically duodenal) form is restricted to the GI tract and seems to have very indolent clinical course.
- Grading (1–3) is based on the number of centroblast cells in follicular structures.
- BCL-2 staining is helpful in distinguishing neoplastic (positive) from reactive (negative) follicles.

Follicular lymphomas express pan-B cell markers, including CD20, and also the markers of follicle center cell differentiation, CD10 and BCL-6 (see **Fig. 7**C). Follicular lymphoma typically has a nodular pattern, recapitulating the nodularity seen in follicular hyperplasia. Neoplastic follicular structures have a dendritic cell meshwork, which can be highlighted by CD21 and CD23. The cells of follicular lymphoma express BCL-2, whereas non-neoplastic, reactive germinal centers are negative (see **Fig. 7**D). However, BCL-2 is not specific for follicular lymphoma and is expressed by many B cell lymphomas as well as normal lymphoid cells, including T cells, plasma cells, and primary follicles.

Follicular lymphoma is typically indolent, especially when low grade, although it frequently involves bone marrow and can be difficult to cure.[19–23] Recently, a subset of follicular lymphomas has been described arising primarily in the GI tract. These primary intestinal follicular lymphomas (or, in the most recent World Health Organization's [WHO] classification, *duodenal-type follicular lymphoma*) appear as nodules or polyps and most commonly occur in the duodenum. They have a very indolent clinical course and may require no additional therapy beyond local excision. All forms of follicular lymphoma are associated with a t(14;18) (q32;q21) translocation involving *IGH* and *BCL2*.

Mantle Cell Lymphoma

Mantle cell lymphoma (MCL) classically produces lymphomatous polyposis characterized by multiple (sometimes hundreds) of polyps that can widely involve the GI tract, mimicking an

Pitfalls

! BCL-2 expression is not specific for follicular lymphoma; many different lymphomas as well as normal lymphoid cells, including T cells, primary follicles, and plasma cells, express this antigen.

! Diagnosis of primary GI/duodenal-type follicular lymphoma cannot be made based on histology alone; formal clinical staging workup is necessary.

Key Features
FOLLICULAR LYMPHOMA VERSUS FOLLICULAR HYPERPLASIA

Follicular Lymphoma	Follicular Hyperplasia
Nodular architecture	Nodular architecture
Diffuse lymphoma cells among follicles	T cells between follicles
Monotonous cells in follicles	Polarized follicles (light and dark zones)
Few or no tingible-body macrophages	Tingible-body macrophages present
BCL-2 positive	BCL-2 negative

inherited polyposis syndrome.[1,24] It is a systemic lymphoma that, despite its population of small and mature-appearing lymphocytes, has a relatively aggressive clinical course with overall survival of 3 to 5 years. It occurs in middle-aged or older patients and involves the GI tract in one-third of cases. Hepatosplenomegaly and lymphadenopathy are common, as is peripheral blood involvement. Tumor cells have dark, angulated nuclei and may infiltrate diffusely or in a nodular pattern (Fig. 8A). Thick-walled capillaries and epithelioid, eosinophilic histiocytes are often interspersed in the infiltrate (see Fig. 8B). Occasional cases show a mantle zone pattern with lymphoma cells arranged around non-neoplastic germinal centers. Unlike many of the other lymphomas, mantle cell lymphoma does not generally transform to DLBCL, although aggressive subtypes can contain larger cells that mimic B lymphoblasts (blastoid variant) or show nuclear pleomorphism (pleomorphic variant). Distinction between these variants and the neoplasms that they mimic (ie, acute lymphoblastic leukemia/lymphoma and DLBCL) is important; the latter are potentially curable, whereas mantle cell lymphoma typically is not.[25]

Mantle cell lymphomas expresses pan-B cell markers and usually coexpress CD5 and CD43 aberrantly, although a few cases may be CD5-negative.[26] The most characteristic feature is the nuclear expression of cyclin-D1, a cell cycle protein that can almost always be used to confirm the diagnosis (see Fig. 8C). Expression of cyclin-D1 is associated with a t(11;14) (q13;q32) translocation involving *CCND1* and *IGH* that brings the gene encoding cyclin-D1 under control of the immunoglobulin heavy chain gene promoter. Of note, cyclin-D1 is expressed by a variety of normal cells, including endothelial and proliferating epithelial cells, as well as nonlymphoid neoplasms and a small proportion of plasma cell myelomas.

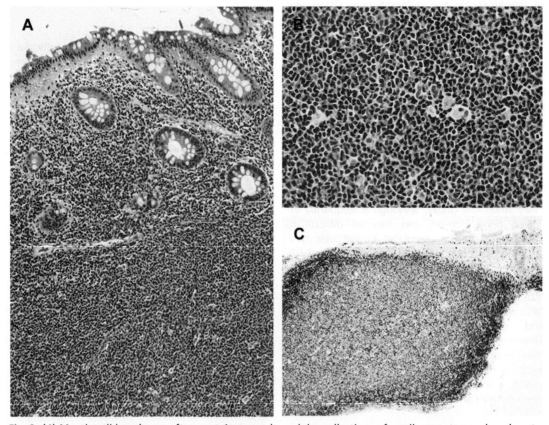

Fig. 8. (A) Mantle cell lymphoma often contains vaguely nodular collections of small, monotonous lymphocytes that may fill the submucosa and/or the mucosa (H&E, original magnification ×100). (B) At high magnification, the lymphoma cells can be seen to have homogeneous, dark chromatin, and angulated nuclear contours, with several nuclei having one or more flat edges. Scattered eosinophilic histiocytes are visible within the infiltrate (H&E, original magnification ×400). (C) A positive nuclear cyclin-D1 stain confirms the diagnosis (cyclin-D1 stain, original magnification ×100).

Key Features

- Classically presents as lymphomatous polyposis with numerous lymphomatous nodules/polyps throughout the GI tract

- Composed of small, mature-appearing lymphocytes with dark, angulated nuclei and interspersed epithelioid histiocytes

- Despite mature appearance, has an aggressive clinical course with relatively short overall survival

- Nuclear cyclin-D1 expression characteristic

Pitfalls

! Rarely, cases may be negative for CD5 (and, even more rarely, cyclin-D1).

! Appearance of lymphomatous polyposis is not specific for mantle cell lymphoma.

! Variants with larger cells and blastoid or pleomorphic appearance may be mistaken for DLBCL.

! Normal cells (such as endothelial and epithelial cells) also express cyclin-D1, as do a handful of other lymphoid neoplasms (such as a small subset of plasma cell myeloma).

Burkitt Lymphoma

Burkitt lymphoma (BL) classically produces a large and destructive mass centered on the distal ileum and/or cecum in young patients.[18,27] However, BL can involve any portion of the GI tract and has multiple forms. Endemic disease occurs in equatorial Africa and New Guinea, whereas sporadic tumors occur around the globe. An immunodeficiency-related form occurs in the setting of human immunodeficiency virus (HIV) infection. Most cases are associated with EBV infection. BL has a propensity for rapid-growth and striking proliferation; nearly 100% of cells show strong Ki-67 labeling. At low magnification, this is manifested in a starry-sky appearance, with sheets of monotonous, medium-sized lymphoma cells that have inconspicuous nucleoli, punctuated by tingible-body macrophages (the stars among the sky of lymphoma cells) that contain cellular debris (Fig. 9).

The cells of BL express CD20 and markers of germinal center origin (CD10 and BCL-6) but are negative for BCL-2. The diagnosis requires *MYC* rearrangements, which usually occur as the t(8;14)(q24;q32) translocation between *MYC* and *IGH* genes. Appropriate therapy is associated with survival rates of 80% to 90%. The term *atypical* BL has been used to describe highly proliferative lymphomas that lack the typical immunophenotype and/or monotonous cytologic features of BL, although this term is now out of favor; some such cases show *MYC* rearrangements in combination with rearrangements involving *BCL2* and/or *BCL6*.[28,29] These cases are termed double (or triple) hit lymphomas and tend to behave clinically

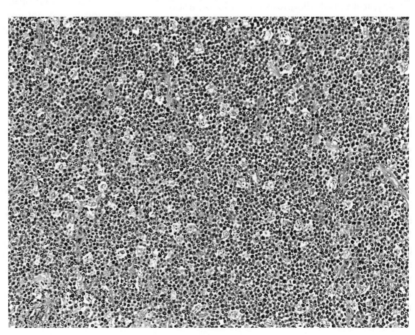

Fig. 9. BL characteristically has a starry-sky appearance created by the presence of numerous tingible-body macrophages scattered among the monotonous, medium-sized lymphoma cells. These macrophages contain phagocytosed nuclear debris and reflect the rapid cell turnover rate inherent to this type of lymphoma (H&E, original magnification ×200).

in a fashion intermediate between BL and DLBCL. The WHO's 2016 classification classifies these lymphomas as "high-grade B cell lymphoma with *MYC* and *BCL2* and/or *BCL6* rearrangements."[21] There are some calls to perform molecular studies for these rearrangements on all DLBCLs, whereas others do so only on cases that have a germinal center phenotype.[28,29]

Key Features

- Relatively rare, aggressive B-cell neoplasm of follicle center cell origin
- Typically has approximately 100% proliferative rate on Ki-67 stain
- Characteristic starry-sky appearance at low magnification
- Classically involves the right lower quadrant (ileum and right colon)
- Associated with rearrangements in *MYC* gene

Pitfalls

! May be confused with DLBCL

! Atypical Burkitt diagnosis out of favor; a subset of lymphomas formerly placed in this category are so-called double hit lymphomas

T-CELL LYMPHOMAS

Enteropathy-Associated T-Cell Lymphoma

Enteropathy-associated T-cell lymphoma (EATL) is an aggressive neoplasm that produces large and destructive masses, often in the jejunum (**Fig. 10**A).[1,30,31] Most cases arise in patients with celiac disease and, thus, EATL is closely associated with the HLA haplotypes DQ2 and DQ8. EATL may arise in patients with known celiac disease, sometimes in the setting of refractory sprue, although it may also occur as the sentinel event in patients with previously undiagnosed celiac disease.[18] Lymphomatous involvement of the mucosa results in ulcers, and most examples of ulcerative jejunitis reported in patients with refractory celiac disease likely represent EATL.

EATL consists of a diffuse and destructive infiltrate of intermediate-sized or large cells with pleomorphic nuclei that resemble DLBCL. Tumor cells are often accompanied by numerous eosinophils, and some cases have scattered eosinophilic abscesses (see **Fig. 10**B). Neoplastic T cells express CD3 but frequently lose expression of CD5. They are negative for CD4, although occasional tumors show some CD8 staining. Staining for cytotoxic granule-associated proteins like TIA-1 and granzyme B indicate a cytotoxic T-cell phenotype. CD56 is negative, and the cells express the alpha-beta subtype of the T-cell receptor. Infiltrates in small bowel biopsies from some patients with clinically refractory celiac disease show a similar antigen profile and clonal T-cell populations. High-grade tumors that contain pleomorphic cells may express CD30, resulting in diagnostic confusion with anaplastic large cell lymphoma.[1]

In the WHO's earlier classifications, a type II subtype of EATL was recognized, with a more monomorphic population of medium-sized lymphoma cells and a different antigen profile, including positivity for CD8 and CD56. This form of disease is now considered a completely separate entity as of the WHO's 2016 classification of lymphoid neoplasms, and is termed monomorphic epitheliotropic intestinal T cell lymphoma (MEITL).[21] Like EATL, this lymphoma is clinically aggressive but it is not associated with underlying celiac disease and seems to occur with increased frequency in patients of Asian and Hispanic descent. In addition to these differences, MEITL is more likely to express the gamma-delta subtype of T cell receptor.

EATL has a poor prognosis because of its inherently aggressive nature and occurrence in debilitated patients with nutritional compromise. Most cases present as ulcerated masses or with perforation, so they are first encountered in resection specimens. Median survival times are on the order of months.

Key Features

- T-cell lymphoma associated with celiac disease
- Clinically aggressive, leading to ulceration and perforation
- May follow a long history of (often refractory) celiac disease or may be the presenting event in patients with undiagnosed celiac disease
- Cytotoxic T-cell immunophenotype
- Very poor prognosis

Pitfalls

! Ulcerative jejunitis that is associated with celiac disease is probably synonymous with EATL.

! EATL can resemble DLBCL and other aggressive lymphomas.

! Some cases are CD30-positive, leading to potential confusion with anaplastic large cell lymphoma.

! Former category of type II EATL is considered a totally separate entity in the WHO's updated classification as of 2016.

Extranodal Natural Killer/T-Cell Lymphoma, Nasal Type

Although quite rare overall, extranodal natural killer (NK)/T-cell lymphoma, nasal type (ENKTL), has a propensity for involvement of the GI tract.[18,31–33] This lymphoma is a very aggressive lymphoma that can bear a resemblance to EATL and should be considered in the differential diagnosis when one is entertaining a diagnosis of a T-cell GI lymphoma. Tumors frequently ulcerate, owing to a tendency to infiltrate in a vaso-centric and vaso-destructive fashion (**Fig. 11**). This feature enhances the destructive nature of the lymphoma, leading to extensive tissue necrosis. ENKTLs are composed of variably sized cells that may have an anaplastic appearance. They express CD56 but are negative for CD4 and CD8. Surface expression of CD3 is also absent, although the CD3 epsilon antigen may be found in the cytoplasm. Like EATL, lesional cells have a cytotoxic phenotype, expressing TIA-1 and granzyme B. By definition, ENKTLs are related to EBV; in situ hybridization for EBV-encoded ribonucleic acid (EBER) should demonstrate its presence.

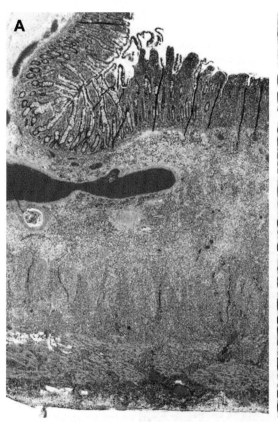

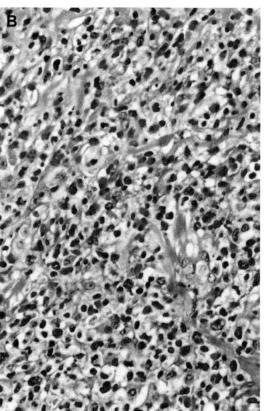

Fig. 10. (*A*) EATL is associated with underlying celiac disease (gluten-sensitive enteropathy) and leads to aggressive, transmural infiltrates of lymphoma cells as seen on the right side of this low-magnification photomicrograph. Note the blunt villi in the mucosa on the left side of the image, reflecting the underlying enteropathy (H&E, original magnification ×20). (*B*) At high magnification, numerous eosinophils can be seen in the infiltrate. This feature is common for EATL (H&E, original magnification ×400).

Key Features

- Rare T-cell lymphoma with cytotoxic T-cell phenotype
- Invariably associated with EBV infection
- Highly aggressive
- Angiocentric and angio-destructive infiltration pattern

Pitfalls

! It is easily mistaken for other T-cell lymphomas, including EATL and peripheral T-cell lymphoma, not otherwise specified.

! The moniker of nasal type refers to site of most common involvement, but it is not specific; the GI tract is the most common site of involvement outside the head and neck.

GENERAL APPROACH TO GASTROINTESTINAL LYMPHOMA DIAGNOSIS

Although it is impossible to outline a correct or best way to approach an atypical lymphoid infiltrate encountered on a biopsy of the GI tract, a pragmatic approach incorporating clinical, endoscopic, and histopathological findings is attainable. This approach begins, importantly, with correlating the endoscopic findings associated with the biopsy, as this information truly serves as the gross description of the process. If the endoscopic report (ideally with photographs) is not at hand, every effort should be made to obtain it, because it provides value to both parties in the diagnostic equation as well as to patients. For the pathologist, correlation of a suspicious lymphoid infiltrate with the finding of a mass lesion or ulcer can point toward a malignant diagnosis, whereas for the clinical physician, it provides a target for reexamination to either obtain more tissue for diagnosis or to follow the progress of therapy once a diagnosis is established. Although atypical lymphoid populations sampled in the setting of large and destructive masses or ulcers can be relatively easy to evaluate and diagnose, those that are patently atypical under the microscope but that come from endoscopically normal mucosa are often much more challenging. It is important to remember that this is true for both the pathologist and patients' clinical physicians because an unequivocal diagnosis of lymphoma in a biopsy taken from relatively normal-appearing mucosa (or mucosa with a nonspecific abnormality, such as erythema) can prove to be a management nightmare for an endoscopist who has absolutely no idea where to target follow-up biopsies.

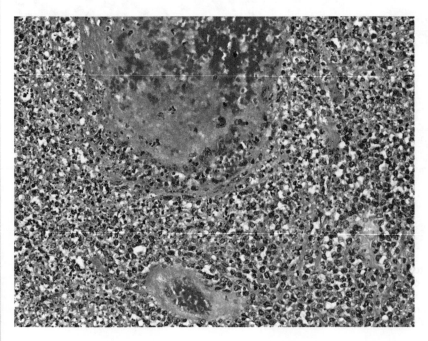

Fig. 11. The vaso-centric pattern of infiltration characteristic of extranodal NK/T-cell lymphoma is seen in this high-magnification photomicrograph. This tendency leads to enhanced tissue destruction due to a disruption of vascular flow (H&E, original magnification ×400).

If sufficient suspicion exists for a diagnosis of lymphoma once the clinical and histopathological information is brought together, the next step is typically the employment of immunohistochemistry to further explore the possibility. It can be tempting to take a comprehensive approach and to order a cadre of stains that cover several different types of lymphoma at the outset, but this approach can actually be counterproductive. First, a lymphoma panel of stains may actually give the pathologist too much information and lead to confusion, such as when BCL-2 stains normal primary follicles. In addition, this approach may lead to premature exhaustion of the tissue block when it contains tiny fragments of tissue. Thus, a tailored approach based on the morphology of the infiltrate and the pretest probability of different types of lymphoma (or benign, reactive conditions, such as follicular hyperplasia) is preferable.

A small panel of stains for CD3, CD20, and CD43 is a reasonable place to begin when working up a lymphoid infiltrate in the GI tract (or elsewhere). This combination of stains allows for an assessment of the immune-architecture of the process (such as B-cell follicles being surrounded by interfollicular T-cell zones) and provides information on the overall balance of T versus B cells in an infiltrate. Reactive, non-neoplastic lymphoid processes are often T cell–predominant, so a population that contains predominantly B cells, particularly with an unusual architecture or arrangement, is all the more suspicious for lymphoma. CD43 provides additional helpful information, because its expression pattern in a reactive condition should roughly parallel that of CD43 (unless the infiltrate contains many plasma cells, which also normally express CD43). Both MCL and chronic lymphocytic leukemia/small lymphocytic lymphoma (CLL/SLL) typically express CD43 aberrantly, so its presence on CD20-positive small B cells can point in the direction of one of these processes and prompt additional staining with CD5 and/or cyclin-D1. Also, a minority of MALT lymphomas

aberrantly expresses CD43, as discussed earlier, so confirmation of CD20 and CD43 coexpression can be extremely helpful in this situation, given the lack of another specific marker of neoplasia in this disease. Finally, expression of CD43 *without* CD3 or CD20 raises the possibility of a myeloid neoplasm (eg, myeloid sarcoma/GI involvement by acute myeloid leukemia). If suspicion remains and/or is augmented by the results of this first round of immunostaining, additional targeted studies can be ordered to search for the patterns described in earlier sections regarding specific lymphoma types. **Table 2** summarizes the key immunohistochemical differences among the small B cell lymphomas.

Whether or not to perform additional ancillary studies, such as cytogenetic, molecular diagnostic, or flow cytometric assays, in the diagnosis of GI lymphomas is a subject of debate. Because the tissue obtained for diagnosis by endoscopic biopsy is often scant, it is probably most prudent to save as much tissue as possible for the performance of immunohistochemistry rather than to attempt to send tissue for ancillary studies a priori. In addition, involvement of the tissue can be patchy, meaning that biopsy fragments sent for ancillary testing may not contain the lymphoid cells at all or may contain only necrotic cells in the case of an aggressive process, such as DLBCL, EATL, or ENKTL. Lymphomas consisting of large cells are also notoriously difficult to subject to flow cytometry, because such cells are inherently fragile and are often destroyed in the process of tissue disaggregation in preparation for flow cytometric analysis.

Specific and important molecular diagnostic studies, such as those of *MYC* gene rearrangements and specific translocations, including t(11;18) in MALT lymphoma and t(11;14) in MCL, can be a crucial part of diagnosis and treatment planning for certain diseases as discussed in prior sections. Using molecular diagnostic studies for immunoglobulin and/or T-cell receptor gene rearrangements in order to establish a diagnosis of lymphoma, however, can be fraught with risk

Table 2
Immunohistochemical markers for small B-cell lymphomas

Lymphoma	Marker						
	CD20	CD5	CD43	BCL-2	CD10	BCL-6	Cyclin-D1
Mantle cell	+	+	+	+ (diffuse)	−	−	+
Follicular	+	−	−	+ (follicles)	+	+	−
MALT	+	−	−/+	+ (diffuse)	−	−	−

because reactive, non-neoplastic lymphoid populations can frequently harbor small, clonal populations of T and/or B cells that, when subjected to amplification, can result in an overdiagnosis of lymphoma. Thus, it is probably most advantageous, again, to preserve as much tissue as possible for a good, H&E-stained section to assess morphology, followed by paraffin-based immunohistochemistry for specific subclassification that can be used to guide appropriate therapy.

SUMMARY

The GI tract is the most common extranodal site of involvement by lymphoma, with B cell tumors outnumbering T-cell tumors by a wide margin. DLBCL is the most common lymphoid neoplasm involving the GI tract, but a variety of other B- and T-cell neoplasms occur in the GI organs, often with characteristic associations and/or manifestations, such as the close association between *H pylori* gastritis and MALT lymphoma of the stomach, and the development of EATL in a background of celiac disease. Although the diagnosis of GI lymphomas can sometimes seem daunting to the general pathologist, a knowledge of the most commonly encountered entities, in combination with a reasoned and pragmatic approach to the diagnostic workup, makes it possible to approach most cases with confidence.

REFERENCES

1. Smith LB, Owens SR. Gastrointestinal lymphomas: entities and mimics. Arch Pathol Lab Med 2012; 136:865–70.
2. Owens SR. General approach to lymphomas of the gastrointestinal tract. In: Lamps LW, Bellizzi AM, Frankel WL, et al. Neoplastic gastrointestinal pathology: an illustrated guide. New York: Demos Medical; 2016. p. 75–85.
3. Owens SR, Smith LB. Molecular aspects of H. pylori-related MALT lymphoma. Patholog Res Int 2011; 2011:193149.
4. Cramer SF, Romansky S, Hulbert B, et al. The rectal tonsil: a reaction to Chlamydial infection? Am J Surg Pathol 2009;33:483–5.
5. Farris AB, Lauwers GY, Ferry JA, et al. The rectal tonsil: a reactive lymphoid proliferation that may mimic lymphoma. Am J Surg Pathol 2008;32:1075–9.
6. Kokima M, Itoh H, Motegi A, et al. Localized lymphoid hyperplasia of the rectum resembling polypoid mucosa-associated lymphoid tissue lymphoma: a report of three cases. Pathol Res Pract 2005;201:757–61.
7. O'Malley DP, Goldstein NS, Banks PM. The recognition and classification of lymphoproliferative disorders of the gut. Hum Pathol 2014;45:899–916.
8. Burke JS. Lymphoproliferative disorders of the gastrointestinal tract: a review and pragmatic guide to diagnosis. Arch Pathol Lab Med 2011;135: 1283–97.
9. Owens SR. Large cell lymphoma. In: Greenson JK, Lauwers GY, Montgomery EA, et al. Diagnostic pathology: gastrointestinal. 2nd edition. Philadelphia: Elsevier; 2016. p. 192–7.
10. Stein H, Warnke RA, Chan WC, et al. Diffuse large B-cell lymphoma, not otherwise specified. In: WHO classification of tumours of haematopoietic and lymphoid tissues. Lyon (France): IARC Press; 2008. p. 233–7.
11. Nakamura S, Jaffe ES, Swerdlow SH. EBV positive diffuse large B-cell lymphoma of the elderly. In: WHO classification of tumours of haematopoietic and lymphoid tissues. Lyon (France): IARC Press; 2008. p. 243–4.
12. Lamps LW, Owens SR. Neoplasms of the stomach. In: Lamps LW, Bellizzi AM, Frankel WL, et al. Neoplastic gastrointestinal pathology: an illustrated guide. New York: Demos Medical; 2016. p. 173–215.
13. Banks PM. Gastrointestinal lymphoproliferative disorders. Histopathology 2007;50:42–54.
14. Hwang HS, Park CS, Yoon DH, et al. High concordance of gene expression profiling-correlated immunohistochemistry algorithms in diffuse large B-cell lymphoma, not otherwise specified. Am J Surg Pathol 2014;38:1046–57.
15. Read JA, Koff JL, Nastoupil LJ, et al. Evaluating cell-of-origin subtype methods for predicting diffuse large B-cell lymphoma survival: a meta-analysis of gene expression profiling and immunohistochemistry algorithms. Clin Lymphoma Myeloma Leuk 2014;14:460–7.
16. Sehn LH, Gascoyne RD. Diffuse large B-cell lymphoma: optimizing outcome in the context of clinical and biologic heterogeneity. Blood 2015;125:22–32.
17. Owens SR. MALT lymphoma. In: Greenson JK, Lauwers GY, Montgomery EA, et al. Diagnostic pathology: gastrointestinal. 2nd edition. Philadelphia: Elsevier; 2016. p. 184–91.
18. Chen W, Owens SR, Frankel WL. Neoplasms of the small intestine. In: Lamps LW, Bellizzi AM, Frankel WL, et al. Neoplastic gastrointestinal pathology: an illustrated guide. New York: Demos Medical; 2016. p. 217–47.
19. Harris NL, Swerdlow SH, Jaffe ES, et al. Follicular lymphoma. In: WHO classification of tumours of haematopoietic and lymphoid tissues. Lyon (France): IARC Press; 2008. p. 243–4.
20. Foukas PG, de Leval L. Recent advances in intestinal lymphomas. Histopathology 2015;66: 112–36.

21. Swerdlow SH, Campo E, Pileri SA, et al. The 2016 revision of the World Health Organization classification of lymphoid neoplasms. Blood 2016;127: 2376–90.

22. Schmatz AI, Streubel B, Kretschmer-Chott E, et al. Primary follicular lymphoma of the duodenum is a distinct mucosal/submucosal variant of follicular lymphoma: a retrospective study of 63 cases. J Clin Oncol 2011;29:1445–51.

23. Damaj G, Verkarre V, Delmer A, et al. Primary follicular lymphoma of the gastrointestinal tract: a study of 25 cases and a literature review. Ann Oncol 2003;14:623–9.

24. Owens SR. Mantle cell lymphoma. In: Greenson JK,Lauwers GY, Montgomery EA, et al. Diagnostic pathology: gastrointestinal. 2nd edition. Philadelphia: Elsevier; 2016. p. 198–201.

25. Swanson BJ, Owens SR, Frankel WL. Neoplasms of the colon. In: Lamps LW, Bellizzi AM, Frankel WL, et al. Neoplastic gastrointestinal pathology: an illustrated guide. New York: Demos Medical; 2016. p. 265–314.

26. Hashimoto Y, Omura H, Tanaka T, et al. CD5-negative mantle cell lymphoma resembling extranodal marginal zone lymphoma of mucosa-associated lymphoid tissue: a case report. J Clin Exp Hematop 2012;53:185–91.

27. Leoncini L, Raphael M, Stein H, et al. Burkitt lymphoma. In: WHO classification of tumours of haematopoietic and lymphoid tissues. Lyon (France): IARC Press; 2008. p. 262–4.

28. Karube K, Campe E. MYC alteration in diffuse large B-cell lymphomas. Semin Hematol 2015;52:97–106.

29. Swerdlow SH. Diagnosis of "double hit" diffuse large B-cell lymphoma and B-cell lymphoma, unclassifiable, with features intermediate between DLBCL and Burkitt lymphoma: when and how, FISH versus IHC. Hematology Am Soc Hematol Educ Program 2014;2014:90–9.

30. Ferreri AJ, Zinzani PL, Govi S, et al. Enteropathy-associated T-cell lymphoma. Crit Rev Oncol Hematol 2011;79:84–90.

31. Isaacson PG, Chott A, Ott G, et al. Enteropathy-associated T-cell lymphoma. In: WHO Classification of tumours of haematopoietic and lymphoid tissues. Lyon (France): IARC Press; 2008. p. 289–91.

32. Chan JKC, Quintanilla-Martinez L, Ferry JA, et al. Extranodal NK/T-cell lymphoma, nasal type. In: WHO classification of tumours of haematopoietic and lymphoid tissues. Lyon (France): IARC Press; 2008. p. 285–8.

33. Swerdlow SH, Jaffe ES, Brousset P, et al. Cytotoxic T-cell and NK-cell lymphomas: current questions and controversies. Am J Surg Pathol 2014;38:e60–70.

UNITED STATES POSTAL SERVICE ® Statement of Ownership, Management, and Circulation (All Periodicals Publications Except Requester Publications)

1. Publication Title	2. Publication Number	3. Filing Date
SURGICAL PATHOLOGY CLINICS	025 – 478	9/18/2017

4. Issue Frequency	5. Number of Issues Published Annually	6. Annual Subscription Price
MAR, JUN, SEP, DEC	4	$206.00

7. Complete Mailing Address of Known Office of Publication (Not printer) (Street, city, county, state, and ZIP+4®)

ELSEVIER INC.
230 Park Avenue, Suite 800
New York, NY 10169

Contact Person
STEPHEN R. BUSHING

Telephone (Include area code)
215-239-3688

8. Complete Mailing Address of Headquarters or General Business Office of Publisher (Not printer)

ELSEVIER INC.
230 Park Avenue, Suite 800
New York, NY 10169

9. Full Names and Complete Mailing Addresses of Publisher, Editor, and Managing Editor (Do not leave blank)

Publisher (Name and complete mailing address)

ADRIANNE BRIGIDO, ELSEVIER INC.
1600 JOHN F KENNEDY BLVD. SUITE 1800
PHILADELPHIA, PA 19103-2899

Editor (Name and complete mailing address)

STACY EASTMAN, ELSEVIER INC.
1600 JOHN F KENNEDY BLVD. SUITE 1800
PHILADELPHIA, PA 19103-2899

Managing Editor (Name and complete mailing address)

PATRICK MANLEY, ELSEVIER INC.
1600 JOHN F KENNEDY BLVD. SUITE 1800
PHILADELPHIA, PA 19103-2899

10. Owner (Do not leave blank. If the publication is owned by a corporation, give the name and address of the corporation immediately followed by the names and addresses of all stockholders owning or holding 1 percent or more of the total amount of stock. If not owned by a corporation, give the names and addresses of the individual owners. If owned by a partnership or other unincorporated firm, give its name and address as well as those of each individual owner. If the publication is published by a nonprofit organization, give its name and address.)

Full Name	Complete Mailing Address
WHOLLY OWNED SUBSIDIARY OF REED/ELSEVIER, US HOLDINGS	1600 JOHN F KENNEDY BLVD. SUITE 1800 PHILADELPHIA, PA 19103-2899

11. Known Bondholders, Mortgagees, and Other Security Holders Owning or Holding 1 Percent or More of Total Amount of Bonds, Mortgages, or Other Securities. If none, check box → ☐ None

Full Name	Complete Mailing Address
N/A	

12. Tax Status (For completion by nonprofit organizations authorized to mail at nonprofit rates) (Check one)
The purpose, function, and nonprofit status of this organization and the exempt status for federal income tax purposes:
☒ Has Not Changed During Preceding 12 Months
☐ Has Changed During Preceding 12 Months (Publisher must submit explanation of change with this statement)

13. Publication Title	14. Issue Date for Circulation Data Below
SURGICAL PATHOLOGY CLINICS	JUNE 2017

15. Extent and Nature of Circulation			Average No. Copies Each Issue During Preceding 12 Months	No. Copies of Single Issue Published Nearest to Filing Date
a. Total Number of Copies (Net press run)			443	354
b. Paid Circulation (By Mail and Outside the Mail)	(1)	Mailed Outside-County Paid Subscriptions Stated on PS Form 3541 (Include paid distribution above nominal rate, advertiser's proof copies, and exchange copies)	284	248
	(2)	Mailed In-County Paid Subscriptions Stated on PS Form 3541 (Include paid distribution above nominal rate, advertiser's proof copies, and exchange copies)	0	0
	(3)	Paid Distribution Outside the Mails Including Sales Through Dealers and Carriers, Street Vendors, Counter Sales, and Other Paid Distribution Outside USPS®	65	56
	(4)	Paid Distribution by Other Classes of Mail Through the USPS (e.g., First-Class Mail®)	0	0
c. Total Paid Distribution (Sum of 15b (1), (2), (3), and (4))		▶	349	304
d. Free or Nominal Rate Distribution (By Mail and Outside the Mail)	(1)	Free or Nominal Rate Outside-County Copies included on PS Form 3541	38	50
	(2)	Free or Nominal Rate In-County Copies Included on PS Form 3541	0	0
	(3)	Free or Nominal Rate Copies Mailed at Other Classes Through the USPS (e.g., First-Class Mail)	0	0
	(4)	Free or Nominal Rate Distribution Outside the Mail (Carriers or other means)	0	0
e. Total Free or Nominal Rate Distribution (Sum of 15d (1), (2), (3) and (4))		▶	38	50
f. Total Distribution (Sum of 15c and 15e)		▶	387	354
g. Copies not Distributed (See Instructions to Publishers #4 (page #3))		▶	56	0
h. Total (Sum of 15f and g)		▶	443	354
i. Percent Paid (15c divided by 15f times 100)		▶	90.18%	85.88%

* If you are claiming electronic copies, go to line 16 on page 3. If you are not claiming electronic copies, skip to line 17 on page 3.

16. Electronic Copy Circulation	Average No. Copies Each Issue During Preceding 12 Months	No. Copies of Single Issue Published Nearest to Filing Date
a. Paid Electronic Copies ▶	0	0
b. Total Paid Print Copies (Line 15c) + Paid Electronic Copies (Line 16a) ▶	349	304
c. Total Print Distribution (Line 15f) + Paid Electronic Copies (Line 16a) ▶	387	354
d. Percent Paid (Both Print & Electronic Copies) (16b divided by 16c × 100) ▶	90.18%	85.88%

☒ I certify that 50% of all my distributed copies (electronic and print) are paid above a nominal price.

17. Publication of Statement of Ownership

☒ If the publication is a general publication, publication of this statement is required. Will be printed in the DECEMBER 2017 issue of this publication.

☐ Publication not required.

18. Signature and Title of Editor, Publisher, Business Manager, or Owner

STEPHEN R. BUSHING – INVENTORY DISTRIBUTION CONTROL MANAGER

Date 9/18/2017

I certify that all information furnished on this form is true and complete. I understand that anyone who furnishes false or misleading information on this form or who omits material or information requested on the form may be subject to criminal sanctions (including fines and imprisonment) and/or civil sanctions (including civil penalties).

PS Form 3526, July 2014 (Page 3 of 4)

PS Form 3526, July 2014 (Page 1 of 4 (see instructions page 4)) PSN: 7530-01-000-9931 PRIVACY NOTICE: See our privacy policy on www.usps.com

PRIVACY NOTICE: See our privacy policy on www.usps.com.

Printed and bound by CPI Group (UK) Ltd, Croydon, CR0 4YY

03/10/2024

01040383-0017